New Frontiers in Breast Imaging

New Frontiers in Breast Imaging

Edited by Cody Perez

hayle
medical

New York

Hayle Medical,
750 Third Avenue, 9th Floor,
New York, NY 10017, USA

Visit us on the World Wide Web at:
www.haylemedical.com

ISBN: 978-1-63241-583-7

Cataloging-in-Publication Data

New frontiers in breast imaging / edited by Cody Perez.
    p. cm.
Includes bibliographical references and index.
ISBN 978-1-63241-583-7
1. Breast--Imaging. 2. Breast--Radiography. 3. Breast--Diseases--Diagnosis.
4. Breast--Cancer--Diagnosis. I. Perez, Cody.
RC280.B8 N49 2019
616.994 49--dc23

Table of Contents

Preface

The examination of the form of the breast and the investigation of any underlying condition such as lesions and cancers is done through a medical diagnostic technique known as breast imaging. It comprises of a set of techniques such as mammography, xeromammography, galactography, ultrasound, magnetic resonance imaging (MRI) and scintimammography. For women in the age group of 50-74, mammography is recommended every two years. For women undergoing breast surgeries, such as breast reduction, breast enlargement and mastopexy, mammograms should be done less frequently. Digital breast tomosynthesis (DBT) provides higher degree of accuracy as compared to traditional mammography. Medical ultrasonography is used for both diagnosis and screening. This book is a valuable compilation of topics, ranging from the basic to the most complex advancements in the domain of breast imaging. The topics covered herein deal with the core techniques of breast imaging. With state-of-the-art inputs by acclaimed experts of this field, this book targets students and professionals.

This book is a comprehensive compilation of works of different researchers from varied parts of the world. It includes valuable experiences of the researchers with the sole objective of providing the readers (learners) with a proper knowledge of the concerned field. This book will be beneficial in evoking inspiration and enhancing the knowledge of the interested readers.

In the end, I would like to extend my heartiest thanks to the authors who worked with great determination on their chapters. I also appreciate the publisher's support in the course of the book. I would also like to deeply acknowledge my family who stood by me as a source of inspiration during the project.

Editor

Microwave Breast Imaging Techniques and Measurement Systems

Lulu Wang, Hu Peng and Jianhua Ma

Abstract

Electromagnetic waves at microwave frequencies allow penetration into many optically non-transparent mediums such as biological tissues. Over the past 30 years, researchers have extensively investigated microwave imaging (MI) approaches including imaging algorithms, measurement systems and applications in biomedical fields, such as breast tumor detection, brain stroke detection, heart imaging and bone imaging. Successful clinical trials of MI for breast imaging brought worldwide excitation, and this achievement further confirmed that the MI has potential to become a low-risk and cost-effective alternative to existing medical imaging tools such as X-ray mammography for early breast cancer detection. This chapter offers comprehensive descriptions of the most important MI approaches for early breast cancer detection, including reconstruction procedures and measurement systems as well as apparatus.

Keywords: microwave imaging, breast imaging, breast cancer detection, dielectric properties

1. Introduction

Medical imaging approaches, such as X-ray mammography, ultrasound and magnetic resonance imaging (MRI), play an important role in breast cancer detection [1]. X-ray mammography is the gold-standard method for breast cancer detection, but it has some limitations [2, 3], including harmful radiation, relatively high false-negative rates particularly with patients with dense breast tissue. Ultrasound presents good soft tissue contrast but fails in the presence of bone and air, and the image quality highly depends on operator [4]. MRI allows physicians to evaluate various parts of human body and determine the presence of certain diseases [5], but it is too expensive [6]. Therefore, it is important and necessary to develop a new imaging technique for early breast cancer detection.

In the late 1970s, Larsen et al. obtained the first microwave image of canine kidney [7]. Since then, MI has been intensively studied by many research groups [8–18], and the research objectives have been moved from imaging of organs to application-specific imaging for various tissues such as breast, joint tissues, blood and soft tissues. MI has been recommended as a safe, low-cost and low health risk alternative to existing medical imaging techniques including X-ray mammography and ultrasound. In the past many years, people paid too much attention to the MI algorithms. Several algorithms have been developed and validated numerically and in laboratory environments but they have not extensively validated in clinical environments. Recent clinical trial results demonstrated that more attention should be paid to the hardware implementation system, especially microwave sensors and sensor arrays, in clinical environments rather than laboratory environments.

This chapter presents the basic ideas of MI including currently available breast imaging methods which have been considered as important approaches for early breast cancer detection. The starting point for the development of MI methods is the formulation of the electromagnetic inverse scattering problem. Inverse scattering-based procedures address the data inversion in several different ways, depending on the target itself or on the imaging configuration and operation conditions. In this chapter, electrical properties of biological tissues, MI approaches and biomedical applications and several proof-of-concept apparatuses, including advantages, challenges and possible solutions, as well as future research directions are addressed.

2. Dielectric properties of biological tissues

The dielectric properties (DPs, relative permittivity ε_r and conductivity σ) of malignant tissues at the microwave spectrum change significantly compared to the normal tissue and the dielectric contrast can be detected and imaged by applying MI approaches [19]. The DPs of different types of biological tissues are very different due to water content difference, which are strongly nonlinear functions with frequency [20]. Choosing suitable operating frequencies for the MI system is a critical task, and the attenuation of RF signals increases with frequency due to increase in the conductivity, resulting in a lower penetration depth. Several computer models have been developed to investigate biological tissues. Debye and Cole-Cole models are the most commonly used models. The Debye model simulates the frequency dependence of DPs of tissues sufficiently [21]:

$$\varepsilon_r = \varepsilon_\infty + \frac{\varepsilon_s + \varepsilon_\infty}{1+j\omega\tau} - j\frac{\sigma}{\omega\varepsilon_0} \tag{1}$$

where ε_∞ means the permittivity value of the tissue, ε_s is the static permittivity of the tissue, and τ is characteristic relaxation time of the medium.

Cole-Cole model is defined as [22]:

$$\varepsilon^*(\omega) = \varepsilon_\infty + \frac{\varepsilon_s - \varepsilon_\infty}{1+(j\omega\tau)^{1-\alpha}} \tag{2}$$

where ε^* is the complex dielectric constant, ε_s and ε_∞ are static and infinite frequency dielectric constants, ω is the angular frequency and τ is a time constant. The exponent parameter α, which takes a value between 0 and 1, describes different spectral shapes. When $\alpha = 0$, the Cole-Cole model becomes to the Debye model.

Many research groups have investigated DPs of various biological tissues, including breast, heart, skin, liver, bone and lymph nodes [23–31]. Some factors that make effects on DPs of tissues include water content [20], change in the dielectric relaxation time [30], charging of the cell membrane [31], sodium content [31] and necrosis and inflammation causing breakdown of cell membrane [32].

3. Microwave imaging techniques

MI approaches can be classified as passive and active. Passive MI approaches use radiometric to measure temperature differences between normal and malignant tissues and identify the lesions based on the measurement differences. Active MI approaches span the high-MHz to low-GHz regime and appear to offer excellent opportunities to supplement the arsenal of screening tools to the radiologist, despite the fact that MI has yet to reach any demonstrated level of clinical feasibility [33]. This chapter focuses on active MI including tomography and radar-based techniques.

3.1. Microwave tomographic (MWT)

Microwave tomographic (MWT) provides quantitative information of DPs of the imaged object, which makes it possible to identify tissues and materials. One of the major limitations is heavy computation work. Based on the operating frequency of the measurement system, MMT can be grouped as single-frequency and multi-frequency approaches.

Larsen et al. [17] developed the first MWT system to produce a microwave canine kidney image at a frequency of 3.5GHz. The system consisted of one transmitting antenna and one receiving antenna, and antennas and the imaged object were immersed in coupling medium that made of water. During data collection, antennas moved to different positions. Such design was not convenient for practical implantation of MI theory, and long data acquisition time was required. To solve this problem, Hawley et al. [34] developed a new MWT system to measure blood content changes. This system consisted of a circular array of 64 waveguide antennas at an operating frequency of 2.45GHz, each waveguide antenna worked as transmitter and receiver, and mechanical movement was not required in the data collection.

A multi-frequency MWT system for breast cancer detection was developed by Meaney et al. (see **Figure 1**) [35]. The system was made of a cylindrical array of 16 monopole antennas that were placed around a breast phantom. The space between breast phantom and antennas was filled of matching medium that was made from glycerin and water mixture. This system was validated on various numerical breast models and phantoms, and simulation results showed that a small tumor (2 mm in diameter) can be imaged. A good agreement between simulation

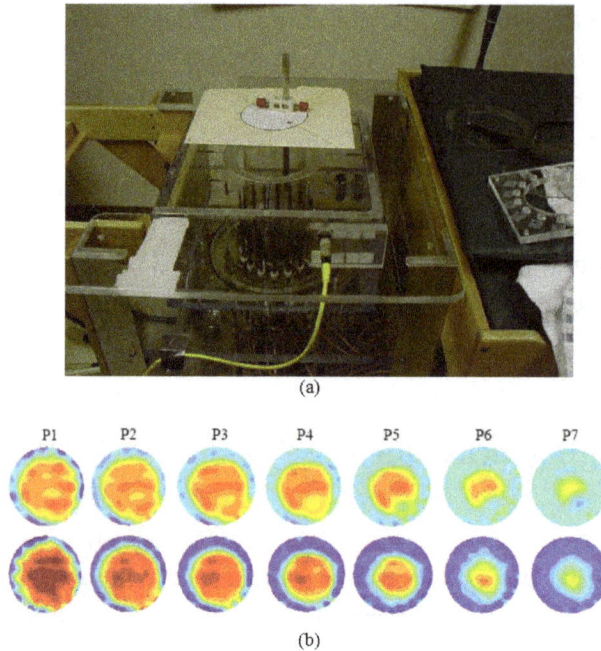

(a)

(b)

Figure 1. (a) Multi-frequency MWT system for breast cancer detection and (b) microwave (top row, permittivity, and bottom row, conductivity, at 1100 MHz) images in the same anatomically coronal view for the left breast of a woman with fatty to scattered radiographic density. P1–P7 indicates microwave tomograms spaced 1 cm apart beginning near the chest wall.

and experimental results was observed. The same research group also conducted a three-dimensional MWT system for clinical trial, and results showed that breast tumor as small as 1 cm in diameter could be detected [11]. Although clinical results did not achieve a good agreement with experimental results [35], their studies confirmed that it is possible to use MI for breast cancer detection.

3.2. Radar-based microwave imaging

Radar-based MI approaches can be classified into five groups: confocal microwave imaging (CMI), tissue sensing adaptive radar (TSAR), microwave imaging via space time (MIST), multi-static adaptive (MSA) MI, and holographic microwave imaging technique (HMI). This section presents various radar-based MI approaches for breast cancer detection.

A CMI system was developed by Hagness et al. [13, 14]. In their numerical studies, an array of 17 monopole transceivers was placed along the surface of breast model, and all antennas were equally spaced and spanning 8 cm. Results showed that a small tumor (2 mm in diameter) can be detected by using the 2D system [13], and a tumor with size of 6 mm in diameter can be detected by using the 3D system [14]. The CMI provides necessary imaging resolution and adequate penetration depth in the breast. It does not compensate for frequency-dependent propagation effects but has limited ability to discriminate against artefacts and noise. To overcome these challenges, they applied delay multiply-and-sum signal processing with CMI, where the scattered signals were time-shifted, multiplied in pair and the products were summed to form a synthetic focal point [15]. This method has an ability to produce higher resolution image and high interference rejection capability [16].

A TSAR prototype system as shown in **Figure 2(a)** was developed by Fear et al. [18]. During data acquisition, a patient was lying in prone position on the examination table with her breast extending through the breast hole and the antennas was scanned around the breast. In order to reduce the noise, the breast image was formed from the reflection signals without skin reflections. Clinical results (see **Figure 2(b)**) showed that the TSAR has an ability to detect and localize lesions with size greater than 4 mm in diameter. The major limitations of TSAR include the large reflections caused from the skin and expensive electronics for real-time imaging. To solve these problems, a Bayesian estimator was applied to enhance the reconstructed image [36].

A MIST beam-forming was developed by Bond et al. [16, 37–38]. A planar array of 16 horn antennas was placed close to the surface of the breast model, and a UWB signal was transmitted sequentially from each antenna. Numerical results demonstrated that a small tumor (2 mm in diameter) embedded in the heterogeneous breast tissue were successfully detected even with denser breast tissue. MIST offers significant improvement in performance over UWB MI approaches based on simpler focusing schemes. However, the system caused skin-breast artefacts in the image prior. The research team upgraded the imaging system (see **Figure 3(a)**) to overcome the challenges of detecting, localizing and resolving multiple or multifocal lesions [39]. The experimental results demonstrated that tumors with size of 4 mm in diameter could be imaged (see **Figure 3(b)**).

Recently, Smith et al. [40–43] proposed a near-field indirect HMI method, which involves recording the holographic intensity pattern and reconstructing the image by using Fourier transformation from the recorded intensity pattern. Compared to TSAR, indirect HMI has the ability to produce real-time image at a significantly low cost. However, more validation works are required on the theory and proof-of-concept for medical applications.

More recently, the authors proposed a far-field HMI method for imaging of biological objects [44–46]. Different from IHM, the 3D HMI uses physical displacement (scan of the distance)

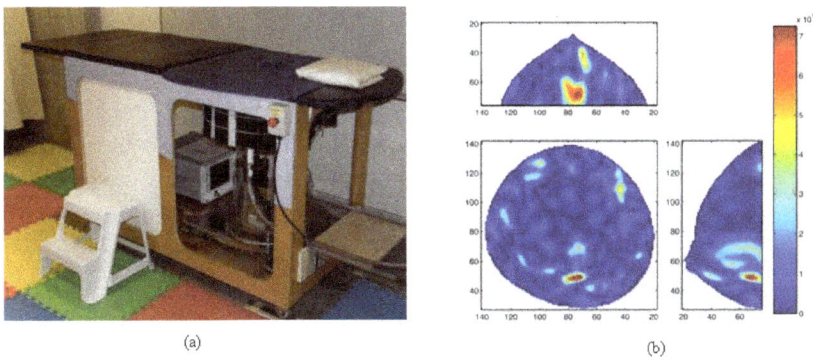

(a)

(b)

Figure 2. (a) TSAR prototype system and (b) TSAR images for patient.

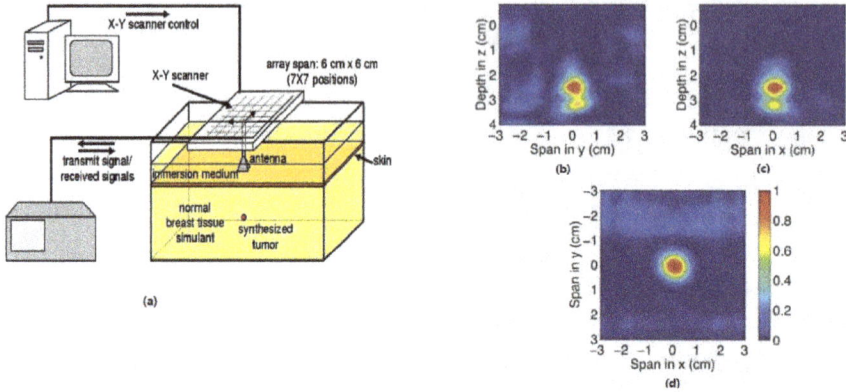

Figure 3. (a) MIST experimental system setup; reconstructed images with a 4-mm-diameter tumor; (b) yz-plane at x = 0.1 cm; (c) xz-plane at y = 0.1 cm and (d) xy-plane at z = 2.3 cm [39].

between the sensor array plane and the imaged object over a specified range (vertical) to obtain the depth information from sequenced 2D images. Both simulation and experimental results demonstrated that the HMI has several advantages in data collection, including that no matching medium was required and that the complex permittivity of the object was not required to calculate to generate an image that reduced the imaging reconstruction time.

3.3. Imaging systems

Most of existing active MI measurement systems involve hardware and software parts. The hardware system generally includes a microwave source generator, transmitting antenna(s) to send microwave signals toward the target object, receiving antennas(s) to measure the scattered electric field from the target object, a signal measurement controller to control antennas and antenna array plane, and a host computer that contains a matched software system to analyze the measured data using image processing algorithm to display the reconstructed image on a screen displaying unit. The transmitter and receiver can use the same sensor. The requirements for the hardware systems and the computational power are different due to the image algorithm differences. **Table 1** presents various developed MI systems.

3.3.1. Microwave sensor

To design an efficient and robust MI system, it is necessary to develop a sensor to match specific requirements including operating frequency, bandwidth, directivity, sensitivity, accuracy of the detection and many other factors such as compact size and low cost. Sensors should be designed specifically for lower frequencies to enhance electric field intensities inside biological tissues, due to more penetration inside the tissue when the frequency is relatively low; thus, more useful information of the object can be obtained. Various sensors have been developed for imaging of breast, including open-ended coaxial probe [47–57], tapered slot antenna (TSA) [59–63], bow-tie antenna [64–70], monopole antenna [71–78], dipole antenna [79, 80], waveguide antenna [81–84], patch antenna and Vivaldi antenna.

	Dartmouth College (USA)	Keele University (UK)	University of Bristol (UK)	University of Manitoba (Canada)	Auckland University of Technology (NZ)
Antenna	Circular array of 16 monopoles	Circular array of 24 ceramic-filled open-ended waveguides	Two spherical arrays consist of 31 and 60 ultra-wideband antennas	Circular array of doubled layers Vivaldi antennas	Spiral array of 16 open-ended waveguide antennas
Frequency	0.5–3 GHz	1.0–2.3 GHz	4–8 GHz	3–6 GHz	12 GHz
Test phantom	Real patients	Soft animal tissues	Real breasts	Various dielectric objects	Various dielectric objects
Immersion medium	0.9% saline ($\varepsilon_r = 76.6$, $\Sigma = 2.48$ S/m)	Metallic bath with coupling liquid	Matching ceramic	No matching medium, air only	No matching medium, air
Image	2D and 3D	2D	3D	2D	2D and 3D
Clinical trial	Yes	No	Yes	No	No

Table 1. Various MI measurement systems.

Open-ended coaxial probes were employed in MI systems to measure dielectric properties of biological tissues [47–56]. Advantages of using probes include that tissue manipulation or preparation is not required, dielectric-properties measurements can be integrated in a straightforward manner with surgical and pathology protocols, they are easy to use, they can respond at broadband frequencies and there is a capacity for noninvasive measurements. However, accuracy and reliability of the measurements depend on the aperture of probe as it is the only part of the system in direct contact with the imaged object.

A compact tapered slot antenna (TSA) was applied in an UWB MI system by Bialkowski et al. [58], and the benefits include high directivity, wide bandwidth, simple feed structure and relatively low in cost, which makes TSA become a popular choice for implementation of MI systems [59–63].

UWB bow-tie sensors were used by John et al. [70]. The system is made of an imaging cavity formed from 12 panels soldered together, and each panel is made of three UWB bow-tie sensors as shown in **Figure 4**. The coupling medium was filled in the cavity, and an image of a spherical object was reconstructed by using inverse scattering algorithm. Advantages of using bow-tie sensor include compact, wideband and easy-to-manufacture.

Researchers at Dartmouth College developed an MWT system that is made of a cylindrical array of 16 monopole antennas (see **Figure 1**), one antenna acting as transmitter and others acting as receivers, and sensors were placed in a coupling medium that is made of material close to fatty tissues. The system was validated on breast phantoms and real human subjects [35]. Advantages of using monopole antennas include easy to model, compact, can be placed at different geometries and can be impedance-matched across a wide bandwidth when immersed in a lossy medium.

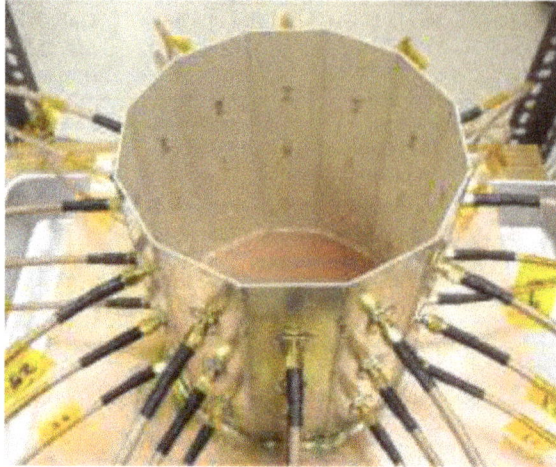

Figure 4. Imaging cavity demonstrated in John's publication [82].

Open-ended waveguide antennas were applied in the HMI system by the authors [46]. The HMI system was made of an array of 16 open-ended waveguide antennas, one acting as transmitter and other being receivers. During data collection, the transmitter continuously generated RF signals to the breast phantom and the scattered electric fields were measured by receivers. No matching medium was required in this measurement system.

3.3.2. Microwave sensor array

Investigators also studied the performance of producing high-resolution images at lower costs, including image algorithms, sensor design and sensor array geometry. People paid much attention to image algorithm and sensor design, but very little attentions have been paid to sensor arrays and their applications in the biomedical field. Most of the existing MI systems use circular- [18], planar- [38] and spherical [85]-shaped sensor array. The circular sensor array is more suitable for clinical settings. To generate a high-resolution image, a large number of sensors (from several to several hundreds) are required for the existing MI system. The image is improved with increasing the total number of sensors used in the system. However, limitations of increasing sensor numbers include the increased cost, size and complexity.

Recently, Klemm et al. [85] proposed a spherical array of 16 patch antennas for the clinical applicable CMI system. During data collection, the patient was lying in a prone position, which was felt to offer the best chance of the breast forming a gentle and uniformly curved shape. Experimental results showed that the image quality can be improved by improving the bandwidth of the array element.

More recently, the authors [46] proposed a spiral and random sensor array that contains 16 waveguide antennas for HMI system as shown in **Figure 5**. The experimental results showed that the breast phantom image can be improved by using spiral and random sensor arrays compared to the regular spaced sensor array. Color bar plots signal intensity on a linear scale.

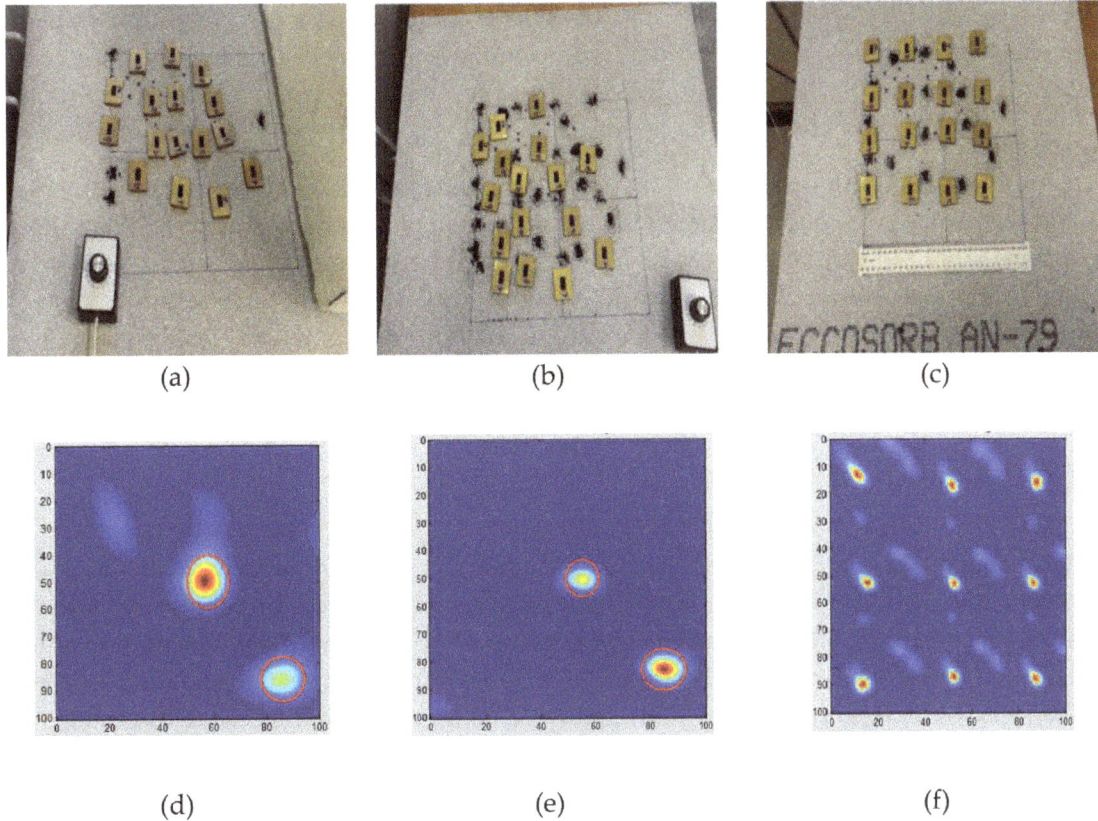

Figure 5. (a) Spiral array; (b) random array; (c) regularly spaced; reconstructed images of two inclusions using (d) spiral array; (e) random array and (f) regularly spaced array.

4. Challenges and future work

There are several major limitations for practical implementations of MI approaches. First, breast phantoms were made of simple materials, which cannot represent real human tissues accurately. Second, the electrical properties contrasts between the normal and the malignant tissues are much smaller than people thought, which caused more difficultly in imaging the structures. Choosing a suitable operating frequency range is also a challenging task. These challenges can be solved by developing a high dynamic system to capture the small difference in the scattered field or by developing a contrast agent to enhance the electrical properties of the malignant tissues. The spatial resolution is another major challenge. To enhance spatial resolution of an MI system, many researchers increased the number of microwave sensors for the implementation system. For example, the sensor number has been increased from 16 to 256 to increase the image quality [86]. However, the detection accuracy may be reduced due to the mutual coupling signals produced between sensors. Moreover, the system became very complex and the implementation costs increased significantly.

To address these problems, one single scanning antenna may be used instead of several antennas. Investigation of sensor arrays such as unequally spaced sensor arrays and applying compressive sensing approach [87, 88] may be another solution. Some recently proposed techniques such as multiple-input-multiple-output technique [89] may be able to reduce the complexity of the system. Finally, most of the existing experimental systems require the coupling medium between sensors and the imaged object, which increased the system cost significantly.

Many promising indicators suggested that MI systems in the future will be a successful clinical complement to conventional mammography. Investigations may improve the imaging algorithms and hardware implementation systems with particular focus on highly sensitive, compact and low-cost microwave sensors and sensor arrays to achieve high-quality images at relatively low cost. Significant contributions from existing MI commercial companies may be greatly helpful in developing the well-established MI modalities to clinical trials.

5. Conclusion

In conclusion, this chapter presented an exhaustive summary of MI approaches with particular focus on implementations of microwave breast imaging theory, including image algorithms, experimental setups, microwave sensors and sensor arrays. Several MI implementation apparatuses were reviewed in detail. MI systems have direct impacts on spatial resolution, operating frequencies, detection accuracy and quality of imaging. Several advantages of existing MI approaches, open challenges, possible solutions and future research directions were also discussed. Successful clinical trials of MI for breast imaging made the worldwide excitation, and this achievement confirmed that MI has potential to become a low-risk alternative to existing medical imaging tools such as X-ray mammography for breast cancer detection. However, MI-based techniques are still far from maturity due to the fact that many challenges have to be addressed before MI can be implemented in clinical environments.

Acknowledgements

This work was supported in part by the National Natural Science Foundation of China (NSFC) under Grant 61701159, in part by the Natural Science Foundation of Anhui Province under Grant 101413246, in part by the Foundation for Oversea Master Project from the Ministry of Education, China, under Grant 2160311028, and in part by the start-up funding from the Hefei University of Technology under Grant 407037164.

Author details

Lulu Wang[1]*, Hu Peng[1] and Jianhua Ma[2]

*Address all correspondence to: luluwang2015@hfut.edu.cn

1 School of Instrument Science and Opto-electronics Engineering, Hefei University of Technology, Hefei, China

2 School of Biomedical Technology, Southern Medical University, Guangzhou, China

References

[1] Fass L. Imaging and cancer: A review. Molecular Oncology. 2008;**2**(2):115-152

[2] Kerlikowske K, Gard CC, Sprague BL, Tice JA, Miglioretti DL. One vs. two breast density measures to predict 5- and 10-year breast cancer risk. Cancer Epidemiology, Biomarkers and Prevention: A Publication of the American Association for Cancer Research, Cosponsored by the American Society of Preventive Oncology. 2005; **24**(6):889

[3] O'Halloran M, Conceicao RC, Byrne D, Glavin M, Jones E. FDTD modeling of the breast: A review. Progress in Electromagnetics Research B. 2009;**18**:1-24

[4] Chan V, Perlas A. Basics of Ultrasound Imaging. New York: Springer; 2011

[5] Jacobs MA, Ibrahim TS, Ouwerkerk R. MR imaging: Brief overview and emerging applications. Radiographics. 2007;**274**:1213-1229

[6] Baltzer PA, Benndorf M, Dietzel M, Gajda M, Runnebaum IB, Kaiser WA. False-positive findings at contrast-enhanced breast mri: A bi-rads descriptor study. Breast Diseases: A Year Book Quarterly. 2011;**22**(1):44-45

[7] Wang Z, Lim EG, Tang Y, Leach M. Medical applications of microwave imaging. IEEE Press, New York, 1985.

[8] Fallahpour M, Case JT, Ghasr M, Zoughi R. Piecewise and Wiener filter-based SAR techniques for monostatic microwave imaging of layered structures. IEEE Transactions on Antennas and Propagation. 2014;**62**(1):1-13

[9] De Zaeytijd J, Franchois A, Eyraud C, Geffrin JM. Fullwave three-dimensional microwave imaging with a regularized Gauss–Newton method—Theory and experiment. IEEE Transactions on Antennas and Propagation. 2007;**55**(11):3279-3292

[10] Chandra R, Zhou H, Balasingham I, Narayanan RM. On the opportunities and challenges in microwave medical sensing and imaging. IEEE Transactions on Biomedical Engineering. 2015;**62**(7):1667-1682

[11] Meaney PM, Goodwin D, Golnabi A, Zhou T, Pallone M, Geimer S, Burke G, Paulsen K. Clinical microwave tomographic imaging of the calcaneus: A first-in-human case study of two subjects. IEEE Transactions on Biomedical Engineering. 2012;**59**(12): 3304-3313

[12] Semenov SY, Corfield DR. Microwave tomography for brain imaging: Feasibility assessment for stroke detection. International Journal of Antennas and Propagation. 2008;2548301-2548308

[13] Shea JD, Hagness SC, Van Veen BD. Hardware acceleration of FDTD computations for 3-D microwave breast tomography. IEEE Antennas and Propagation Society International Symposium. 2009. pp. 1-4

[14] Mashal A, Sitharaman B, Li X, Avti PK. Toward carbon-nanotube-based theranostic agents for microwave detection and treatment of breast cancer: Enhanced dielectric and heating response of tissue-mimicking materials. IEEE Transactions on Biomedical Engineering. 2010;**57**(8):1831

[15] Van Veen BD, Hagness SC, Bond EJ, Li X. Space-time microwave imaging for cancer detection. US Patent. 2009;US 7570063 B2

[16] Koutsoupidou M, Karanasiou IS, Kakoyiannis CG, Groumpas E, Conessa C, Joachimowicz N. Evaluation of a tumor detection microwave system with a realistic breast phantom. Microwave and Optical Technology Letters. 2017;**59**(1):6-10

[17] Mohammed AM, Abbosh S, Mustafa D, Ireland D. Microwave system for head imaging. IEEE Transactions on Instrumentation and Measurement. 2014;**63**(1):117-123

[18] Fear EC, Bourqui J, Curtis C, Mew D. Microwave breast imaging with a monostatic radar-based system: A study of application to patients. IEEE Transactions on Microwave Theory and Techniques. 2013;**61**(5):2119-2128

[19] Schulz S, Pusch S, Pohl E, Dielkus S, Herbst-Irmer R, Meller A. Investigation of tumor using an antenna scanning system. IEEE Microwave Symposium. 2014;**171**:1401-1406

[20] Lazebnik M, Watkins CB, Hagness SC, Booske JH. The dielectric properties of normal and malignant breast tissue at microwave frequencies: Analysis, conclusions, and implications from the Wisconsin/Calgary study. IEEE Antennas and Propagation Society International Symposium. 2007. pp. 2172-2175

[21] Lazebnik M, Okoniewski M, Booske JH, Hagness SC. Highly accurate Debye models for normal and malignant breast tissue dielectric properties at microwave frequencies. IEEE Microwave and Wireless Components Letters. 2007;**17**(12):822-824

[22] Said T, Varadan VV. Variation of Cole-Cole model parameters with the complex permittivity of biological tissues. In: 2009. MTT'09. IEEE MTT-S International Microwave Symposium Digest; IEEE; 2009. pp. 1445-1448

[23] Kim T, Oh J, Kim B, Lee J, Jeon S, Pack J. A study of dielectric properties of fatty, malignant and fibro-glandular tissues in female human breast. Asia-Pacific Symposium on Electromagnetic Compatibility and International Zurich Symposium on Electromagnetic Compatibility. 2008;216-219

[24] Garrett JD, Fear EC. Average dielectric property analysis of complex breast tissue with microwave transmission measurements. Sensors. 2015;**15**(15):1199-1216

[25] Fu F, Xin SX, Chen W. Temperature- and frequency-dependent dielectric properties of biological tissues within the temperature and frequency ranges typically used for magnetic resonance imaging-guided focused ultrasound surgery. International Journal of Hyperthermia. 2014;**30**(1):56

[26] O'Rourke AP, Lazebnik M, Bertram JM, Converse MC, Hagness SC, Webster JC. Dielectric properties of human normal, malignant and cirrhotic liver tissue: In vivo and

ex vivo measurements from 0.5 to 20 Ghz using a precision open-ended coaxial probe. Physics in Medicine and Biology. 2007;**52**(15):4707-4719

[27] Zhang L, Liu P, Shi X, You F, Dong X. A comparative study of a calibration method for measuring the dielectric properties of biological tissues on electrically small open-ended coaxial probe. IEEE International Conference on Biomedical Engineering and Biotechnology. 2012. pp. 658-661

[28] Zhang L, Shi X, You F, Liu P, Dong X. Improved circuit model of open-ended coaxial probe for measurement of the biological tissue dielectric properties between megahertz and gigahertz. Physiological Measurement. 2013;**34**(10):N83

[29] Yamamoto T, Koshiji K, Fukuda A. Development of test fixture for measurement of dielectric properties and its verification using animal tissues. Physiological Measurement. 2013;**34**(9):1179

[30] Lazebnik M, Mccartney L, Popovic D, Watkins CB, Lindstrom MJ, Harter J. A large-scale study of the ultrawideband microwave dielectric properties of normal, benign and malignant breast tissues obtained from cancer surgeries. Physics in Medicine and Biology. 2007;**52**(20):6093-6115

[31] Abeyrathne CD, Halgamuge MN, Farrell PM, Skafidas E. An ab-initio computational method to determine dielectric properties of biological materials. Scientific Reports. 2013;**3**(5):1796

[32] Rossmanna C, Haemmerich D. Review of temperature dependence of thermal properties, dielectric properties, and perfusion of biological tissues at hyperthermic and ablation temperatures. Critical Reviews in Biomedical Engineering. 2014;**42**(6):467-469

[33] Ibrahim WMA, Algabroun HM. The Family Tree of Breast Microwave Imaging Techniques. In: 4th Kuala Lumpur International Conference on Biomedical Engineering; Springer: Berlin Heidelberg; 2008

[34] Nikawa Y. Microwave diagnosis using MRI and image of capillary blood vessel. IEEE Asia Pacific Microwave Conference. 2009. pp. 595-598

[35] Meaney PM, Fanning MW, Raynolds T, Fox CJ, Fang Q, Kogel CA. Initial clinical experience with microwave breast imaging in women with normal mammography. Academic Radiology. 2007;**14**(2):207-218

[36] O'Halloran M, Byrne D, Elahi MA, Conceição RC, Jones E, Glavin M. Confocal Microwave Imaging. An Introduction to Microwave Imaging for Breast Cancer Detection, Part of the series Biological and Medical Physics, Biomedical Engineering. Springer International Publishing, AG Switzerland. 2016. pp. 47-73.

[37] Salvador SM, Fear EC, Okoniewski M, Matyas JR. Exploring joint tissues with microwave imaging. IEEE Transactions on Microwave Theory and Techniques. 2010;**58**(8):2307-2313

[38] Ricci E, Maggio F, Rossi T, Cianca E, Ruggieri M. UWB radar imaging based on space-time beamforming for stroke detection. IFMBE Proceedings. 2015;**45**:946-949

[39] Li X, Davis S K, Hagness S C, Van D W, Van Veen B D. Microwave imaging via space-time beam forming: Experimental investigation of tumor detection in multilayer breast phantoms. IEEE Transactions on Microwave Theory & Techniques, 2004, **52**(8):1856-1865.

[40] Smith D, Livingstone B, Elsdon M, Zheng H. The development of indirect microwave holography for measurement and imaging applications. 2015 IEEE Microwave Symposium. 2015;**722**:1-4

[41] Smith D, Yurduseven O, Livingstone B. The use of indirect holographic techniques for microwave imaging. IEEE Microwave Techniques. 2013;**10**:16-21

[42] Yurduseven O, Smith D, Livingstone B, Schejbal V, You Z. Investigations of resolution limits for indirect microwave holographic imaging. International Journal of RF and Microwave Computer-Aided Engineering. 2013;**23**(4):410-416

[43] Smith D, Yurduseven O, Livingstone B, Schejbal V. Microwave imaging using indirect holographic techniques. IEEE Antennas and Propagation Magazine. 2014;**56**(1):104-117

[44] Wang L, Al-Jumaily AM, Simpkin R. Imaging of 3-D dielectric objects using far-field holographic microwave imaging technique. Progress in Electromagnetics Research B. 2014;**61**:135-147

[45] Wang L, Al-Jumaily AM, Simpkin R. Three-dimensional far-field holographic microwave imaging: An experimental investigation of dielectric object. Progress in Electromagnetics Research B. 2014;**61**(1):169-184

[46] Wang L, Al-Jumaily AM, Simpkin R. Investigation of antenna array configurations using far-field holographic microwave imaging technique. Progress in Electromagnetics Research M. 2015;**42**:1-11

[47] Bobowski JS, Johnson T. Permittivity measurements of biological samples by an open-ended coaxial line. Progress in Electromagnetics Research B. 2012;**40**(40):159-183

[48] Reinecke T, Hagemeier L, Ahrens S, Klintschar M. Permittivity measurements for the quantification of edema in human brain tissue Open-ended coaxial and coplanar probes for fast tissue scanning. IEEE Sensors conference. 2014, Nov, 681-683

[49] Sato Y, Hirata A, Fujiwara O. In-vivo measurement of complex relative permittivity for human skin tissues using open-ended coaxial probe. IEEE Transactions on Electronics Information and Systems. 2011;**131**(131):2040-2045

[50] Huang R, Zhang D. Analysis of open-ended coaxial probes by using a two-dimensional finite-difference frequency-domain method. IEEE Transactions on Instrumentation and Measurement. 2008;**57**(5):931-939

[51] Michiyama T, Nikawa Y, Kuwano S. Measurement of complex permittivity for soft material using easy sticking open ended coaxial probe. Transactions of the Institute of Electronics Information and Communication Engineers C. 2010;**93**:167-174

[52] Jung JH, Cho JH, Kim SY. Accuracy enhancement of wideband complex permittivity measured by an open-ended coaxial probe. Measurement Science and Technology. 2016;**27**(1):015011

[53] Habibi M, Klemer DP, Raicu V. Two dimensional dielectric spectroscopy: Implementation and validation of a scanning open-ended coaxial probe. Review of Scientific Instruments. 2010;**81**(7):255-258

[54] Brusson M, Rossignol J, Binczak S, Laurent G. Determination of burn depth in the ablation of atrial fibrillation using an open-ended coaxial probe. Sensors & Actuators B Chemical. 2015, **209**: 1097-1101.

[55] Misra DK, Mckelvey JA. A quasistatic method for the characterization of stratified dielectric materials using an open-ended coaxial probe. Microwave & Optical Technology Letters. 2010;**7**(7):650-653

[56] Misra DK. Evaluation of the complex permittivity of layered dielectric materials with the use of an open-ended coaxial line. Microwave and Optical Technology Letters. 2015;**11**(11):183-187

[57] Meaney P M, Gregory A P, Epstein N R, Paulsen K D. Microwave open-ended coaxial dielectric probe: interpretation of the sensing volume re-visited. BMC Medical Physics. 2014, **14**(1):1-11.

[58] Tiang SS, Ain MF, Abdullah MZ. Compact and wideband wide-slot antenna for microwave imaging system. IEEE RF and Microwave Conference. 2011. pp. 63-66

[59] Gopikrishna M, Krishna DD, Aanandan CK, Mohanan P. Compact linear tapered slot antenna for UWB applications. Electronics Letters. 2008;**44**(20):1174-1175

[60] Costa JR, Medeiros CR, Fernandes CA. Performance of a crossed exponentially tapered slot antenna for UWB systems. IEEE Transactions on Antennas and Propagation. 2009;**57**(5):1345-1352

[61] Azim R, Islam MT, Misran N. Compact tapered-shape slot antenna for UWB applications. IEEE Antennas and Wireless Propagation Letters. 2011;**10**(3):1190-1193

[62] Wu J, Zhao Z, Liu J, Nie ZP, Liu QH. A compact linear tapered slot antenna with integrated Balun for UWB applications. Progress in Electromagnetics Research C. 2012;**29**:163-176

[63] Lu WJ, Zhang ZY, Liu R, Zhu HB. Design concept of a narrow-wideband antenna for spectrum sensing applications. IEEE China-Japan Joint Microwave Conference. 2011. pp. 1-4

[64] Mehdipour A, Mohammadpour-Aghdam K, Faraji-Dana R, Sebak AR. Modified slot bow-tie antenna for UWB applications. Microwave and Optical Technology Letters. 2008;**50**(2):429-432

[65] Hirata A. Double-sided printed bow-tie antenna with notch filter for UWB applications. Journal of Electromagnetic Waves and Applications. 2012;**23**(2):247-253

[66] Sayidmarie KH, Fadhel YA. A planar self-complementary bow-tie antenna for UWB applications. Progress in Electromagnetics Research C. 2013;**35**:253-267

[67] Kumar R, Surushe G. Design of microstrip-fed printed uwb diversity antenna with tee crossed shaped structure. Engineering Science and Technology, an International Journal. 2016;**19**(2):946-955

[68] Jalilvand M, Li X, Kowalewski J, Zwick T. Broadband miniaturised bow-tie antenna for 3D microwave tomography. Electronics Letters. 2014; 50(4):244-246

[69] Ünal Ø, Türetken B, Canbay C, Ünal Ø, Türetken B. Spherical conformal bow-tie antenna for ultra-wide band microwave imaging of breast cancer tumor. Applied Computational Electromagnetics Society Journal. 2014;29(2):124-133

[70] John S, Mark H, Paul C, Mahta M. A preclinical system prototype for focused microwave thermal therapy of the breast. IEEE Transactions on Biomedical Engineering. 2012;59(9):2431-2438

[71] Ojaroudi M, Kohneshahri G, Noory J. Small modified monopole antenna for UWB application. IET Microwaves Antennas and Propagation. 2009;3(5):863-869

[72] Ni W, Nakajima N. Small printed inverted-l monopole antenna for worldwide interoperability for microwave access wideband operation. IET Microwaves Antennas and Propagation. 2010;4(1):1714-1719

[73] Halili K, Ojaroudi M, Ojaroudi N. Ultrawideband monopole antenna for use in a circular cylindrical microwave imaging system. Microwave and Optical Technology Letters. 2012;54(9):2202-2205

[74] Golezani JJ, Abbak M, Akduman I. Modified directional wide band printed monopole antenna for use in radar and microwave imaging applications. Progress in Electromagnetics Research Letters. 2012;33:119-129

[75] Latif S, Flores-Tapia D, Pistorius S, Shafai L. A planar ultrawideband elliptical monopole antenna with reflector for breast microwave imaging. Microwave and Optical Technology Letters. 2014;56(4):808-813

[76] Ojaroudi N, Ojaroudi M, Ebazadeh Y. UWB/omni-directional microstrip monopole antenna for microwave imaging applications. Progress in Electromagnetics Research C. 2014;47:139-146

[77] Ojaroudi N, Ojaroudi M, Ghadimi N. UWB omnidirectional square monopole antenna for use in circular cylindrical microwave imaging systems. Wireless Personal Communications. 2015;11(3):1350-1353

[78] Ojaroudi M, Civi OA. Bandwidth enhancement of small square monopole antenna using self-complementary structure for microwave imaging system applications. Applied Computational Electromagnetics Society Journal. 2015;30(12):1360-1365

[79] Saenz E, Guven K, Ozbay E, Ederra I, Gonzalo P. Decoupling of multifrequency dipole antenna arrays for microwave imaging applications. International Journal of Antennas and Propagation. 2010;4:252-260

[80] Ahdi Rezaeieh S, Bialkowski K, Zamani A, Abbosh A. Loop-dipole composite antenna for wideband microwave-based medical diagnostic systems with verification on pulmonary edema detection. IEEE Antennas and Wireless Propagation Letters. 2015;15:1

[81] Ali M, Tailor A. Broadband coplanar waveguide-fed slot antenna for wireless local area networks and microwave imaging applications. Microwave and Optical Technology Letters. 2007;**49**(4):846-852

[82] Saleh W, Qaddoumi N. Potential of near-field microwave imaging in breast cancer detection utilizing tapered rectangular waveguide probes. Computers and Electrical Engineering. 2009;**35**(4):587-593

[83] Diener L. Microwave near-field imaging with open-ended waveguide—Comparison with other techniques of nondestructive testing. Research in Nondestructive Evaluation. 2009;**7**(2-3):137-152

[84] Brovko AV, Murphy EK, Yakovlev VV. Waveguide microwave imaging: Neural network reconstruction of functional 2-D permittivity profiles. IEEE Transactions on Microwave Theory and Techniques. 2009;**57**(2):406-414

[85] Klemm M, Craddock IJ, Leendertz JA, Preece A. Radar-Based breast cancer detection using a hemispherical antenna array-experimental results. IEEE Transactions on Antennas and Propagation. 2009;**57**(6):1692-1704

[86] Kurrant D, Bourqui J, Curtis C, Fear E. Evaluation of 3d acquisition surfaces for radar-based microwave breast imaging. IEEE Transactions on Antennas and Propagation. 2015;**63**(11):1-1

[87] Craven D, O'Halloran M, Mcginley B, Conceicao RC, Kilmartin L, Jones E. Compressive sampling for time critical microwave imaging applications. Healthcare Technology Letters. 2014;**1**(1):6-12

[88] Bevacqua MT, Scapaticci R. A compressive sensing approach for 3D breast cancer microwave imaging with magnetic nanoparticles as contrast agent. IEEE Transactions on Medical Imaging. 2016;**35**(2):665-673

[89] Qi Y. Application of sparse array and MIMO in near-range microwave imaging. Proceedings of SPIE - The International Society for Optical Engineering. 2011;**8179**(4): 81790X-81790X-12

2

Detection and Diagnosis of Breast Diseases

Mohammed Ali Alnafea

Abstract

Cancer is a disease that starts in a localized organ or tissue and then grows out of control. Breast cancer is an important health problem as in the Western world; it is the second most frequent cause of cancer death in women (after lung cancer). The incidence rate, however, rises dramatically over the age of 50 years. This is may be due to several risk factors, such as family history, genetics, early menstruation, late menopause, and other factors, that have not yet been identified. The problems of breast diseases have prompted global governments to put constant efforts to increase patient's recovery level against this disease. Early and accurate detection with mass screening programs helps improves a woman's chances for successful treatment. It also minimizes pain, suffering, and anxiety that surround patients and their families. The current and the most cost-effective technique used for screening and diagnosis of breast cancer is X-ray mammography. It is the state-of-the-art for earlier detection to improve both prognosis and survival rate. This is may be due to its good availability, high sensitivity, and relatively low cost/patient. The goal of this chapter is to introduce the problems caused by breast cancer. Starting with an overview of the requirement for breast tumor imaging and the diagnostic techniques used for breast cancer assessment are briefly described, highlighting the advantages and disadvantages of each technique. In addition, the problems associated with a relatively new functional breast imaging technique namely scintimammography were introduced and discussed. The intention that the chapter provide the reader with sufficient background on the available diagnostic techniques of breast tumor imaging approach, as well as an overview of the literature.

Keywords: breast cancer detection, molecular imaging, scintimammography

1. Introduction

Most women experience breast changes in their life. This is due to normal growth and changes in hormone levels. However, lumps, bumps, breast pain, nipple discharges, or skin irritation are examples of breast problems that have similar symptoms. The vast majority of lesions and abnormalities occurs in the breast are not cancer but are far more frequent than malignant ones [1–7]. Benign breast constitutes a heterogeneous group of lesions including various abnormalities, inflammatory lesions, epithelial and stromal proliferations, and neoplasms [3–5]. However, cancer is a disease that starts in a localized organ or tissue and then grows out of control. Breast cancer is an important health problem as it is the most common malignancy in women in Western countries. It is the second most frequent cause of cancer death in women (after lung cancer) [8, 9]. The incidence rate, however, rises dramatically over the age of 50 years. This is may be due to several risk factors such as family history, genetics, early menstruation, late menopause medication, and other factors that have not yet been identified. The above problems have prompted global governments to put constant efforts to increase patient's recovery level against this disease. Early and accurate detection with mass screening programs helps improves a woman's chances for successful treatment. It also minimizes pain, suffering, and anxiety that surround patients and their families. The goal of this chapter is to introduce the problems caused by breast cancer, starting with the requirements for breast imaging, an overview of the methods for diagnosing breast abnormalities with the focus on molecular imaging of the breast.

2. Requirements for breast imaging

The goal of breast evaluation is to classify findings as normal physiologic variations, clearly benign, or possibly malignant. The size, shape, and appearance of the female breast are not constant but undergo a number of changes during the lifetime of women. For instance, changes occur with pregnancy, breast feeding, and during the menstrual cycle. In addition, the age of the subject not only influences the shape but also parenchymal density of the breast. That is why young women tend to have dense breasts (more fibro-glandular tissue), creating a rounded appearance. On the other hand, postmenopausal women have breasts containing a large amount of fat. This makes the X-ray mammogram far more effective in older women as the fat content is more radio-translucent (appears darker) compared to glandular tissue (appears under-exposed) in younger women [10]. The above discussion suggests that both the shape and parenchymal density of the breast impose particular constraints on the choice of imaging modality. The imaging technique should be powerful for initial detection and subsequent follow-up of the diseases.

At present, no single technique was used for all cases of breast cancer detection without showing certain clinical or technical limitations. This implies necessity to address the specific needs that can help for breast tumors imaging to overcome these limitations. For instance, breast compression often needed as it holds the breast still and enhances the spatial resolution. It also evens out the breast thickness and reduces scatter in X-ray or γ-ray imaging [11], thus increasing image sharpness. Moreover, it spreads out the tissue so that the overlying breast tissue will not obscure small abnormalities. Since the breast is an external organ and extends to the chest wall, it requires appropriate views to be obtained. For instance, in X-ray mammography, a lateral (from the side) view of the breast allows separation of the chest wall from lesions deep within the breast. On the other hand, in single photon γ-ray emission imaging, one needs to separate the breast from the heart by employing an appropriate prone (face down) position. However, it has been claimed that with prone imaging view, there is a possibility of missing a small low-intensity medial lesion because of attenuation. This implies that another image is needed but in the lateral view. In addition, shielding the camera from the background cardiac flux is very useful in tumor detection in terms of contrast and resolution.

3. Interpreting imaging test

The usefulness of diagnostic imaging tests, which is their ability to detect a patient or subject with disease or exclude a patient or subject without disease. In other words, the idea in using any diagnostic test is to be able to correctly diagnose the disease and easily interpret the results. The latter is achieved by calculating the probability that a patient has a disease. The diagnostic test performance is usually measured by calculating four important statistical parameters or terms. These are the test's sensitivity, specificity, positive predictive value (PPV), and negative predictive value (NPV) [12, 13]. **Table 1** illustrates these parameters and their relationship. In breast tumor γ-ray imaging, these parameters are dependent on clinical history, biological factors such as size, site, or location, the type of the lesion, and patient's age. The test parameters may also depend on the physical and the practical aspects as well as on the imaging technology parameters. Sensitivity and specificity are properties of a test that tell us how good the diagnostic test is at predicting the disease and whether it is to be used or not [12]. Sensitivity is the proportion of people with the disease who have a positive test for the disease [12]. Specificity is the proportion of people without the disease who test negative [12]. A high sensitivity test means that the test has a low rate of false-negatives and high specificity means that the test has a low rate of false-positives. In brief, the text here and **Table 1** simply provide a practical application, hence of what these concepts mean in clinical practice and how they can be used in practical settings to aid the diagnostic process.

In clinical practice, the decision to send patients for breast biopsies is arbitrary, i.e., there is no fixed test threshold. Instead, the decision is usually based on the needs of patients and clinicians for the different clinical situations. As a result, for any given image of a breast lesion, there is a kind of trade-off between the sensitivity and specificity, i.e., sensitivity can only

Test outcome	Condition as determined by "gold" standard		
	True	False	
Positive	True positive	False positive	⇒Positive predictive value
Negative	False negative	True negative	⇒Negative predictive value
	⇓ Sensitivity	⇓ Specificity	

Table 1. The main diagnostic test parameters [12, 13] demonstrating the practical application and the relationship of these four terms.

increase by decreasing the specificity of a test. For instance, if the decision is to only select patients with extremely abnormal images to have breast biopsy, then the test will become extremely specific but not very sensitive. In this case, many patients falsely diagnosed as not having breast diseases or breast cancer. On the other hand, if the decision is to send patients with borderline abnormal images to have biopsy, the test will then become more sensitive but less specific. As a result, many patients who do not have breast cancer sent for an unnecessary biopsy, i.e., the diagnostic tests are useless. This sensitivity specificity trade-off of the diagnostic test is accurately illustrated by the analysis of the receiver operating characteristic (ROC) curve at each test threshold or cut-point. This curve is a plot of the true positive rate against the false positive rate for the different possible thresholds of the diagnostic test. The area under the ROC curve is a measure of test accuracy, i.e., how well the test separates or classifies the patient population into those with the abnormality and those without. An area of 1 represents excellent performance test and an area of 0.5 represents a fail test.

To know the probability that the imaging test is giving the correct diagnosis, the positive and negative predictive values are needed. The PPV of a test is the probability of a patient having the disease following a positive test result [13]. The NPV is the probability of a person not having the disease following a negative test result [13]. These test performance measures are influenced by the probability of disease at any point in time of the total abnormality in the population tested [13]. The predictive values also vary as a function of disease prevalence and patient subpopulation. Thus, a combined measure of diagnostic performance, the likelihood ratio, is a clinically useful diagnostic test performance measure. Negative likelihood ratios measure the ability of the test to accurately rule out disease, and positive likelihood ratios measure the ability of the test to accurately detect disease. In summary, both sensitivity and specificity terms of a diagnostic test suffer from limitations in clinical practice, as they cannot estimate the probability of breast cancer in an individual patient. However, PPV and NPV help to overcome this problem, but they both vary according to disease prevalence and populations.

4. Diagnosis of breast disease

Breast lesion investigations may include self or clinical breast examination, X-ray mammography, and biopsy. In addition, a variety of other efficient complementary imaging modalities provide additional information to achieve a definite breast diagnosis. The following subsections give an overview of the main diagnostic techniques used for breast tumor imaging.

4.1. X-ray mammography and screening

Mammography is a low energy (25–32 keV) X-ray examination of the soft tissues of the breast. It uses the variation in density between normal mammary features and abnormal tissue structures (lesion) to produce the image. The X-ray images are either captured on a film or directly stored on a digital computer. The former is one of the widely used current techniques based on screen-film technology. X-ray mammography considered the gold standard in breast imaging as it is fast, available, and has a lower cost than other breast imaging techniques. It has two main applications: as a screening method in asymptomatic patients and as a diagnostic method in symptomatic populations. The former application is extremely important and its introduction in the past three decades has significantly reduced the mortality rate of breast cancer in many countries [14, 15]. This is because the screening services accurately detect micro-calcifications and nonpalpable soft tissue masses, which have been beyond other imaging methods, due to the high spatial resolution (~50–100 µm). Normally, screening is achieved by exposing the breast to X-rays after gently compressed between two plates and then taking two views for each breast. A craniocaudal (imaging from above to below) and lateral views are generally taken. A lead grid is used to reduce scattering photons that reach the film. Diagnostic mammography evaluates the entire breast as well as characteristics of the mass. It is used for assessing the size of the lesion, for pre-surgical localization of suspicious areas of breast, and in the guidance of needle biopsies. The reported sensitivity (the fraction of patients actually having the disease and correctly diagnosed as positive) in lesion detection varied between 69 and 90% [16] depending on the breast density. The specificity (the fraction of patients without the disease, correctly diagnosed as negative) is the major drawback of conventional mammography. A variation in specificity between 87 and 97% and a low positive predictive value as low as 15% has also been reported [17]. This 'less than perfect' performance may be due to several confounding factors, e.g., poor mammographic technique, observer error, the lesions are nonpalpable or at a cellular level, and/or the lesions are obscured by the normal breast tissues. The presence of scars or tissue distortion may hide true small tumors on the mammogram. Nevertheless, conventional mammography remains a valuable and cost-effective technique for breast tumor diagnosis. Over the last three decades, considerable efforts are carried out to improve the current screen-film mammographic technique. These improvements include image quality, acquisition techniques, and interpretation protocol in order to reduce some of the mammographic limitations [18].

The use of digital imaging in general radiography has increased rapidly in recent years. This has extended to mammographic imaging. "Digital mammography" (DM) is a possible current direction in breast imaging compared to film-based conventional mammography. This is due to the presence of X-ray detector, which is considered the heart of DM. A number of technologies and several types of integrated digital detector system are in use nowadays. DM has the potential to improve contrast resolution compared with film-screen imaging. This is because DM detectors like other detectors characterized by sensitivity, spatial resolution properties, quantum detection efficiency, noise, and linearity of response.

This has improved diagnostic capability and relatively outweighs the potential reduction in limiting spatial resolution. DM technique offers many inherent advantages over the conventional screen film-based technology [19, 20]. For instance, processing with digital systems increase dynamic range (two to four times the dynamic range of typical film-screen), improved quantum efficiency, signal-to-noise-signal, and storage and display mechanisms.

Moreover, DM detector provides features for automatic control of exposure factors of the image acquisition. This represents the spatial pattern of X-ray transmitted by the breast tissue accurately. The use of computer-assisted image interpretation claimed to be helpful for the physician. This may enhance different features such as computer-aided diagnosis, which may further improve the visibility of lesions and improve mammographic sensitivity [21]. Therefore, repeated exposures (which are sometimes, needed when using conventional mammography) are not required and this may reduce the radiation dose. The advantage of digital imaging systems compared with film-screen imaging is the ability to manipulate and possibly enhance the displayed image. The breast dose levels required by current digital imaging systems are, in general, similar to those of a modern mammographic film-screen combination. However, developments in detector design and optimization of beam quality may eventually result in a reduction in radiation dose. With the use of DM, a number of image processing operations can be introduced to correct for spatial nonuniformities in detector responses. In addition, it is also possible to improve the effective spatial resolution of the detector. It also overcomes a number of limitations inherent in the screen-film image receptor used in conventional mammography. Consequently, this improved the diagnostic image quality as well as reduced the doses to the breast tissues.

Furthermore, it does not need either cassettes or dark rooms or processors, and thus allegedly saves space and time in archiving and retrieving DM images. However, DM requires large disk space for saving image data. Despite several advantages, DM does not yet reach the level of detail to replace screen film mammography. However, with continuous technical improvements of the digital system, this may be expected to change in the near future. Both conventional and DM systems suffer from substantial technical and clinical limitations. For instance, these systems are unreliable in imaging patients with dense parenchyma tissue especially in the younger female population due to more glandular tissue. Mammographic findings are nonspecific (cannot always differentiate benign from malignant disease) and often underestimate the size of the detected lesion. X-ray-based imaging is also not useful for breast diagnosis following surgery or radiotherapy, as the patient's breasts in these cases have architectural distortion.

Moreover, both the tube spectrum and the peak potential (KVp) are important parameters affecting the image quality in film-screen and digital mammography. Automatic selection of proper target/filter combination in modern mammography systems may be affected by improper KVp. In conventional devices, the user depends on central laboratory calibration and has no easy way to calibrate the instrument during use. It is worth mentioning that X-ray mammography is not always useful for nonpalpable tumors. Another group of women with a known family history of breast cancer was recommended not to repeat X-ray mammography. In other words, those close carrying a mutation in BRCA1 (human gene called breast cancer 1, early onset) or BRCA2 (breast cancer 2) genes. Those groups are at high genetic risk of cancer. Some even have opted for preventative bilateral mastectomy. It is preferred not to repeat scan in this group due to X-ray dose and thus, a more sensitive diagnostic test would be advisable. Once the diagnostic tests particularly X-ray mammography indicates or suspects breast cancer, breast biopsies are then performed. Breast biopsy is an invasive procedure used to remove tissue or cells from the breast for microscopic examination. This technique generally performed under local anesthesia. Several types of biopsy are available depending on location, type, and size of lesion. Fine needle aspiration biopsy is performed by inserting a very thin needle to the lesion for taking a small sample of cells, fluid, or tissue. Core needle biopsy is used with a large needle to remove a small cylindrical shape of tissue. Surgical biopsy involves removing part (incisional biopsy) or entire (excisional biopsy) lesion tissue.

In addition, a special wire localization technique may be used during surgery for deeply seated lesion. This technique usually performed under X-ray or ultrasound guidance. There are special instruments and techniques that help to guide the needle biopsy. These include stereotactic biopsy with a 3D mammographic technique to find the exact location of breast lesion and vacuum-assisted biopsy using a tube to gently suck the breast lesion and a knife to remove tissue. This technique is much less traumatic than open biopsy. Moreover, a sentinel node (the first lymph node to receive drainage from a breast cancer cell) biopsy may often be used to determine whether cancer cells have spread to other tissue. In summary, invasive breast biopsies play an important role for evaluating breast cancer particularly nonpalpable lesions. These surgical procedures are important for staging (see **Table 2**) and are considered the "gold standard" [17] to determine the presence or absence of breast cancer. However, invasive breast biopsy procedures are expensive, time consuming, and are often associated with emotional stress. It

Stage	Tumor size	Lymph node involvement	Metastasis
0	Carcinoma *in situ*	N0	M0
I	≤2 cm	N0	M0
IIA	No evidence of tumor	N1	M0
	≤2 cm	N1	M0
	2–5 cm	N0	M0
IIB	2–5 cm	N1	M0
	5 cm<	N0	M0
IIIA	No evidence of tumor	N2	M0
	≤2 cm	N2	M0
	2–5 cm	N2	M0
	5 cm<	N1	M0
	5 cm<	N2	M0
IIIB	Of any size	N0	M0
	Of any size	N1	M0
	Of any size	N2	M0
IIIC	Of any size	N3	M0
IV	Of any size	Any N	M1

Note: Beyond stage IIIB, the tumor is usually extended to either the skin or the chest wall and thus can be of any size. The N0 = no regional lymph node, N1 = metastasis in movable ipsilateral axillary lymph node(s), N2 = metastasis in ipsilateral axillary lymph node(s) fixed or matted, and N3 = metastasis in ipsilateral infraclavicular lymph node(s) or clinically apparent.

Table 2. The staging of breast cancer, adapted from Ref. [22].

also causes scar and tissue distortion that complicate the future mammography. As a result, additional imaging tests are being used to reduce the trauma, cost, avoid, or minimize unnecessary invasive breast biopsies, and more importantly to further improve breast cancer diagnosis.

4.2. Complementary diagnostic techniques

From the previous discussion, it is clear that there are some clinical situations where there are significant limitations to use mammography in isolation. In such cases, there is a great need to use sensitive tests to achieve a high confidence and accurate diagnostic decision. The use of breast biopsies is necessary if breast cancer is indicated or suspected in such cases. Of the performed breast biopsies, ≈60–80% [17] are negative of breast cancer or have benign lesions. In these cases, breast biopsies are considered unnecessary. This has led many breast cancer experts to propose complementary imaging modalities to provide additional diagnostic information and reduce unnecessary breast biopsies. Over the last two decades, complementary diagnostic techniques such as ultrasonography (US), magnetic resonance imaging (MRI), and radionuclide breast imaging techniques have emerged as potential investigations for the detection and diagnosis of breast cancer. The radionuclide breast imaging technique, unlike X-ray mammography, is not affected by breast density. This has prompted a number of investigators to evaluate the feasibility of radionuclide breast imaging techniques in a screening context particularly for women with dense breast.

4.2.1. Ultrasonography

US uses high frequency acoustic waves that reflect at boundaries with different acoustic properties. It is a noninvasive technique, easily available, and relatively cheap. Breast US provides unique information in assessing both palpable and nonpalpable breast abnormalities. For instance, it clearly differentiates between solid masses and cystic lesions. It is considered to be useful in cancer staging, measuring tumor sizes, easy accessing lesions located in peripheries, and reducing the number of unnecessary biopsies. It allows accurate needle placement during biopsy and is very useful for aspiration of cysts. The members of the European group for breast cancer screening recommended using US as a complementary method to X-ray mammography. In addition, the use of high frequency transducers has improved spatial resolution and thus claimed to be useful in axillary node evaluation. However, breast US technique is time consuming and operator/observer dependent. It has also a number of other limitations that may be due to the overlapping in sonographic characteristics. For instance, it cannot detect calcifications (micro calcifications or macro calcifications) in ductal carcinoma in situ (DCIS). It could also miss solid lesions especially in a fatty breast and if detected cannot determine whether a solid mass is benign or malignant. For these reasons, US is not used in some institutions as a screening technique for asymptomatic breast cancer as it is difficult to ensure that the entire breast has been scanned.

4.2.2. Magnetic resonance imaging

Magnetic resonance imaging (MRI) images is created by the recording of signals generated after radio-frequency excitation of nuclear particles exposed to strong magnetic field. Breast

MRI is a nonionizing tomographic functional technique that may be used when the diagnosis is uncertain with mammography [23]. The technique is valuable for specific clinical indications such as patients with (1) axillary adenopathy (enlargement or inflammation of lymph gland), (2) possible tumor recurrence after surgery or radiotherapy, (3) lesions overlying implants, or (4) those requiring staging of multi-focal carcinoma (two or more discrete lesions in one breast) [24]. Breast MRI with dedicated breast coil has excellent soft tissue resolution that enhances the ability to both identify the location and in some cases determines the full extent of the lesion. The use of intravenous contrast agent, gadolinium, which accumulates in tissues with a dense blood vessel network, also increases the sensitivity of breast MRI [16]. However, the reported specificity (ability to determine if lesion is benign or malignant) is 56–72% [24]. This technique has a limited application in patients with implanted metal devices or other metallic materials inside the body. In addition, several clinical limitations have been reported in the literature suggested not to use MRI in pre-menopausal women. For example, changes that do occur in the T_1 value of the breast tissue during the menstrual cycle [24] mean that patients should be scanned between the 6th and 16th day of the cycle. In summary, researchers have concluded that breast MRI is very sensitive, but not very specific and thus, cannot be used alone to rule out cancer. MRI is limited by lack of availability and inconsistent quality, and the technique is too expensive for routine use in breast cancer screening in the general patient population.

4.2.3. Radionuclide breast imaging techniques

The need to improve breast cancer detection and to reduce unnecessary invasive breast biopsies has stimulated researchers to investigate functional imaging modalities. These techniques produce a range of different imaging approaches such as positron emission tomography (PET), single photon emission computed tomography (SPECT), planar imaging, and dedicated imaging instrumentation with and without breast compression. These imaging techniques of the breast potentially offer additional information in breast cancer diagnosis. This is because these imaging methods rely on the physiological and biochemical characteristics of a lesion. Thus, it is considered as the best hope to differentiate between benign/normal and malignant diseases. These functional techniques are also used to assess and monitor the effect of cancer prevention drugs. The current radionuclide imaging techniques used for breast tumor imaging are briefly discussed.

4.2.3.1. Positron emission mammography

In PET, a small amount of positron emitter radiotracer, ^{18}F fluorodeoxyglucose (FDG), is administered intravenously to the patient [25]. It is then distributed in the body, and as it decays, the radionuclide emits a positron in any random direction. If the positron while travelling interacts with an electron within the body, the two particles then annihilate and produce two γ-rays of 511 keV each. Either a whole body scanner or a breast-specific positron emission mammography (PEM) camera [26] is used to detect the two γ-rays in coincidence (two events that are detected within ≈12 ns). PEM is increasingly used in North America not only in cancer diagnosis but also in staging, planning, and monitoring anticancer therapy. This information can be helpful in eliminating unnecessary axillary dissection [27], biopsies, and in determining the appropriate treatment. The diagnosis of viable tumor tissue following chemotherapy is another application of PET [28, 29]. Imaging with ^{18}F-FDG has shown considerable promise in breast cancer imaging, but the exact role is still in evolution. Wahl [30] recommended that it is best applied to solve difficult clinical cases in specific patients rather than routinely. There are at least four reasons that limit the wide use of PEM for routine cancer diagnosis. The first one is the high cost (over £2 million) of PET coincidence imaging equipment, i.e., cyclotron, scanner, and radiochemistry facility [25]. The second one is the difficulty of producing and labeling the short half-life PET radionuclides [21]. The third reason is the lack of medical centers with the required experience to develop more advanced methodology appropriate for breast oncology. In particular, more data is still needed concerning the metabolism of different PET radiopharmaceuticals in breast tumors. The final reason is the lack of oncologists with a high knowledge of PET methodology [30].

4.2.3.2. Scintimammography

Scintimammography (SM) is a promising noninvasive functional imaging technique. It has been proposed to complement X-ray mammography and to improve patient selection for biopsy. This single photon imaging of the breast involves injecting the patient in the arm vein with a small amount (555–740 MBq [31]) of radiopharmaceutical. The most commonly used radiopharmaceutical for SM is ^{99m}Tc labeled sestamibi. After injection, the radiopharmaceutical distributes in the breast tissue as well as in other body organs. It accumulates more in the target object (breast lesion) with uptake ratio nearly 9:1 tumor-to-background-ratio (TBR) [32]. A standard full-size clinical gamma camera is then used to scan the patient and thus measure the 3D distribution of the radioactivity. SM imaging using full size clinical γ-camera includes a range of different imaging approaches such as planar (2D) imaging or SPECT technique. The latter technique gives a 3D image but is not widely used because it is difficult to accurately localize the lesion [33]. In contrast, planar SM is the technique that is more widely used in clinical practice because it provides better lesion localization particularly the prone images with lateral views [33]. In this case, the gamma camera is usually equipped with a low energy high resolution (LEHR) parallel-hole collimator and two views (prone and supine) are taken, to the diagnosed breast. Since the energy imaged is 140 keV representing the photopeak, 20% energy window (symmetric ±10%) is often used and thus, centered over the photopeak. The main clinical applications of planar SM imaging are summarized here and the details are found in literatures [33–39]. In brief, SM with a general purpose γ-camera introduced to evaluate patients with dense breast tissue and prior to breast biopsy [34]. The technique is considered valuable for many clinical applications such as evaluating the axillary lymph nodes, investigating patients with micro calcifications [35], assessing multi-focal and multi-centric breast cancer diseases [36]. It is also useful for imaging patients following surgery, chemotherapy, hormonal replacement therapy, and radiotherapy as well as for patients with breast implants [33]. The technique may also assist in the differentiation of benign and malignant breast abnormalities by measuring the radiotracer uptake in the lesion as compared with surrounding breast tissue. Studies such as Refs. [37, 38] suggested that SM may be used as a second-line diagnostic test in cases where the sensitivity of mammography is decreased or there is a doubt about the presence of a lesion.

In summary, SM using conventional γ-camera is considered as a useful complementary imaging modality to aid the diagnosis and the detection of breast cancer [39]. It may also help to assess patients recommended for biopsy and this may reduce the number of unnecessary or benign breast biopsies. However, the major drawback of the current standard clinical gamma camera SM imaging systems is the use of mechanical collimator. This causes the camera imaging system to utilize a very small fraction, ~0.01%, of the total number of the emitted photons. This limits the statistics and hence the quality and diagnostic value of the observed images. The collimator sensitivity and resolution are a trade-off and the camera is also limited by its intrinsic spatial resolution. As a result, these factors make it difficult to practically image cases of smaller, nonpalpable lesions (<1 cm) that may be deep seated or those close to the chest wall. These have stimulated the development of newly dedicated (breast specific) instrumentations that used for breast tumor imaging applications.

4.2.3.3. Dedicated breast cameras

Recent years have seen considerable interest by scientists in developing new compact medical imaging detectors. These instruments proposed for different clinical applications with the aim to improve image quality by building cameras of suitable size and shape for the part of the body under investigation. Among these designed detectors is the small-dedicated gamma camera for functional breast tumor imaging. The justification for this development is that a standard full size clinical gamma camera designed for whole body imaging and thus, is not been optimized for breast tumor imaging. In other words, there are a number of shortcomings with such general purpose gamma camera such as the limiting sensitivity. On average (50% [40]) for lesions <1 cm such as DCIS particularly, the medially located tumors. In addition, several studies [41–52] have pointed out that due to the large FoV of the camera and the bulky collimators, it is difficult to position the camera close to the breast, and thus, imaging breast tissue adjacent to the chest wall may not be possible. This may, ultimately, decrease the spatial resolution of the camera imaging system and thus affect the diagnostic value of the test in detecting such a small lesion size. To overcome some of the limitations offered by conventional gamma camera on breast imaging, Gupta et al. [41] reported the first preliminary clinical data that performed with breast-specific detectors and then compare it with the data obtained from standard full-size camera. A limited number of patients were investigated in this study but interestingly reported a higher sensitivity for the dedicated camera. Following this and due to the large research activities, new generation of detectors have been designed and developed for breast tumor imaging. For instance, the position-sensitive photo-multiplier tubes (PSPMT), semiconductor arrays, and scintillation crystals are coupled to an array of solid-state photodetectors. **Table 3** summarizes the features and the physical parameters of some of the currently under investigation and the commercially available dedicated breast camera. In general, these small FoV detectors have led to the improvement of the overall spatial resolution of such imaging system.

The commercially available dedicated breast camera has two detectors and is designed and optimized to image only the breasts. It possesses a high intrinsic spatial resolution and the camera is also equipped with ultra-high resolution parallel-hole collimator and thus, optimized

Cameras and study (reference)	Crystal sizes (mm³)	FoV sizes (cm²)	Intrinsic resolution (mm)	Spatial resolution (mm)	Energy resolution (%)
CsI(TI) [47]	2 × 2 × 3	10 × 10	2	9	n/a
CsI(Si) [49]	3 ×3 × 6	21 × 21	3	6.5	n/a
NaI(TI) [50]	3 ×3 × 6	15 × 20	3	6.3	10%
LumaGEM NaI(TI) [42, 50]	2 ×2 × 6	12.8 × 12.8	2.2	3.4	10%
LumaGEM 32000S/12K² (CZT) [51]	2.5 ×2.5 × 5	16 × 20	1.58	2.5	6%
LumaGEM (CsI) 5600 crystal [52]	3 × 3× 6	10 × 10	1.7	n/a	n/a

All cameras are based on PSPMT(s) principle. The CZT detector array absorbs the γ-rays directly and converts their energy into electrical signal without the conversion to visible light as in the case with a scintillation detector. The spatial resolution is measured with general purpose collimator at 10 cm distance except the LumaGEM cameras that based on ultra-high resolution collimators.

Note: n/a, not available.

Table 3. Physical characteristics and specifications of dedicated gamma cameras proposed for scintimammography.

for high-resolution SM. The main advantage of such cameras is the ability to separate the breast from the chest wall by positioning the camera close to the breast. Thus, the camera can be used in areas with limited space (e.g., medial view can be possible), where the use of a full-sized camera is impractical or impossible. The use of moderate breast compression capabilities may improve both the signal-to-noise ratio (SNR) and the spatial resolution [42] and thus increase the sensitivity for detecting smaller lesions. The proposed clinical indications for such dedicated cameras are similar to the full size clinical gamma camera SM. There are some recent clinical studies associated with using these dedicated gamma cameras. For instance, a clinical preliminary study by Brem et al. [43, 44] using dedicated breast camera demonstrated a slight improvement in resolution and tumor sensitivity particularly for lesions ≤1 cm. Rhodes et al. reported [45] on SM, performed on 40 women with small mammographic abnormalities (<2 cm) scheduled to undergo biopsy. The SM examination identified (33/36) malignant lesions confirmed at biopsy. The authors concluded that this preliminary study suggested an important role for the dedicated SM camera in women with dense breasts.

In another study, Brem et al. [46] evaluated 94 women (median age 55 years) who presented with normal mammographic and physical examination results but all subjects were considered at high risk of developing breast cancer. Of these women, 35 had a history of previous breast carcinoma or atypical ductal hyperplasia. The authors concluded that with this camera, they could depict small (8–9 mm) nonpalpable lesions in women at a high risk of breast cancer. In summary, while these studies using breast-specific cameras are promising, all are considered preliminary in nature because they are based on very few cases. Additional studies with a larger sample size are needed to accurately assess and reach scientific conclusions concerning these proposed cameras. They also need to be cost competitive with the general purpose gamma cameras in order to be widely used in breast tumor imaging applications. In addition, the smallest lesion sizes that can be detected with these cameras claimed to be 3–3.3 mm [47] compared to 4–5 mm [48] with conventional camera. However, the evidence published to date did not demonstrate a statistically significant difference in lesion detection. The spatial resolution of these proposed cameras may further improve by increasing the pixel size but there are practical limitations in the development of cameras with small pixel sizes, including cost and detector design. More importantly, due to the use of collimator, these dedicated cameras suffer from low detection efficiency.

4.3. Summary of the role of different imaging modalities

In many centers, the current evaluation and primary diagnosis of breast are based on combination of physical examination, mammography, and breast biopsy. Mammography represents a significant contribution and remains the gold standard for breast tumor imaging. This is because mammography is relatively simple, cost-effective, and relatively, highly sensitive. However, in many clinical cases, mammography may be nonspecific and lesions may not be detected. This is because the breast lesion can be indistinguishable from normal breast tissue or obscured by the dense parenchyma. Mammography is also not reliable following radiation therapy, surgery, and hormonal replacement therapy. Consequently, breast biopsies are used for many cases as a second-line diagnostic test to evaluate a suspicious lesion. Unfortunately, many breast biopsies are performed on normal patients, which results in high cost and patient's stress. Thus, other noninvasive imaging techniques are needed and can be used as complementary functional methods to minimize unnecessary breast biopsies.

MRI and US are adjunctive imaging techniques to mammography. Breast US is relatively inexpensive and is currently the commonest complementary method. This technique is also useful particularly when there is a cyst in the breast, but has lower accuracy in solid lesions. Breast MRI with contrast is a sensitive and relatively specific technique for some certain indications but are too expensive to be used routinely. Both MRI and US are useful tools in breast diagnosis, in particular for solving problems in selected applications. For the aforementioned reasons, the use of complementary imaging techniques, to aid in the diagnosis, is necessary. Thus, additional imaging methods are needed for investigation, detection, and diagnosis of breast cancer. Functional breast γ-ray imaging techniques have aided breast cancer diagnosis.

Among the currently used techniques are planar SM with ^{99m}Tc labeled sestamibi and PET with ^{18}F-FDG. Both radionuclide techniques have been emerged as potential investigation for the detection and diagnosis of breast cancer. Consequently, it is increasingly used particularly for imaging patients with dense breasts. Having discussed commercial imaging methodologies, various weaknesses in each approach has led to the need for new complimentary imaging methods. Of these approaches, SM is one of the most promising approach. The current research in this area is focusing on dedicated collimator-based cameras. These dedicated cameras also suffer from low detection efficiency. In addition, this is an unattractive option for many health providers, due to limited clinical applications of such an imaging system. This provides the motivation for investigating the application of collimator-less method in breast tumor imaging. A gamma camera, employing a low energy high resolution (LEHR) parallel-hole collimator is used, to generate an image of the resulting radionuclide distribution. The LEHR collimator geometrically selects γ-photons from a predetermined direction and as a result, a very small fraction of the total emitted photons reaches the detector. Thus, this limits the detection efficiency and spatial resolution of the observed image–collimator are trade-off.

Factors like these have generated massive research aimed to improve the accuracy and efficiency of the current SM imaging systems and reduce the overall costs of breast surgical biopsies procedures but without the need for the new dedicated camera instrumentation development. This is one of the primary motivations to carry out research using a simple coded aperture (CA) mask, instead of a collimator, coupled to a standard clinical gamma camera for breast tumor imaging without the need for a new dedicated camera instrumentation development. This is particularly attractive at general hospital level, where the cost of running an additional dedicated imaging system may be prohibitive. In addition, the smallest lesion sizes that can be detected with dedicated cameras claimed to be 4–5 mm compared to 8–10 mm with conventional camera. The spatial resolution of these proposed cameras may further improve by increasing the pixel size, but there are practical limitations in the development of cameras with small pixel sizes, including cost and detector design. CA imaging as originally developed for astronomical applications is well suited for detecting faint pseudo-point like objects in a nonzero background. Thus, it appears to be well matched to the imaging objectives in SM. While related prior work has also considered, this approach is characterized by gross simplifications in terms of clinical reality [53, 54].

Acknowledgements

This work funded by the National Plan for Science, Technology and Innovation (MAARIFAH), King Abdulaziz City for Science and Technology, Kingdom of Saudi Arabia, Award Number (MED_2516).

Author details

Mohammed Ali Alnafea

Address all correspondence to: alnafea@ksu.edu.sa

Department of Radiological Sciences, College of Applied Medical Sciences, King Saud University, Riyadh, Saudi Arabia

References

[1] Caleffi M, Filho DD, Borghetti K, et al. Cryoablation of benign breast tumors: Evolution of technique and technology. Breast. 2004;**13**:397-407

[2] Kelsey JL, Gammon MD. Epidemiology of breast cancer. Epidemiologic Reviews. 1990; **12**:228-240

[3] Fitzgibbons PL, Henson DE, Hutter RV. Benign breast changes and the risk for subsequent breast cancer: An update of the 1985 consensus statement. Cancer Committee of the College of American Pathologists. Archives of Pathology & Laboratory Medicine. 1998;**122**:1053-1055

[4] Sarnelli R, Squartini F. Fibrocystic condition and "at risk" lesions in asymptomatic breasts: A morphologic study of postmenopausal women. Clinical and Experimental Obstetrics & Gynecology. 1991;**18**:271-279

[5] Akobeng AK. Understanding diagnostic test 1: Sensitivity, specificity and predictive value. Acta Paediatrica. 2006;**96**:338-341

[6] Cook MG, Rohan TE. The patho-epidemiology of benign proliferative epithelial disorders of the female breast. The Journal of Pathology. 1985;**146**:1-15

[7] La Vecchia C, Parazzini F, Franceschi S, et al. Risk factors for benign breast disease and their relation with breast cancer risk. Pooled information from epidemiologic studies. Tumori. 1985;**71**:167-178

[8] Harris JR, Lippman ME, Verone U, Willett W. Breast cancer. New England Journal of Medicine. 1992;**327**:319-328

[9] The American Cancer Society. Cancer Facts and Figures 2006. http://www.cancer.org. Retrieved on September. 2006

[10] Stefanoyiannis AP, Costaridou L, Skiadopoulos S, Panayiotakis G. A digital equalisation technique improving visualisation of dense mammary gland and breast periphery in mammography. European Journal of Radiology. 2003;**45**:139-149

[11] Pani R, Scopinaro F, Pellegrini R, Soluri A, Weinberg IN, De Vincentis G. The role of Compton background and breast compression on cancer detection in scintimammography. Anticancer Research. 1997;**17**(3B):645-1649

[12] Altman DG, Bland JM. Diagnostic test 1: Sensitivity and specificity. British Medical Journal. 1994;**308**:1552

[13] Altman DG, Bland JM. Diagnostic test 2: Predictive value. British Medical Journal. 1994; **309**:102

[14] Skaane P, Hofvind S, Skjennald A. Randomized trial of screen-film versus full-field digital mammography with soft-copy reading in population-based screening program: Follow-up and final results of Oslo II study. Radiology. 2007;**244**(3):708-717

[15] Duffy SW, Tabr L, Chen HH, Holmqvist M, Yen MF, Abdsalah S, Epstein B, Frodis E, Ljungberg E, Hedborg-Melander C, Sundbom A, Tholin M, Wiege M, Kerlund A, Wu HM, Tung TS, Chiu YH, Chiu CP, Huang CC, Smith RA, Rosn M, Stenbeck M, Holmberg L. The impact of organized mammography service screening on breast carcinoma mortality in seven Swedish counties. Cancer. 2002;**95**:458-496

[16] Kacl GM, Liu PF, Debatin JF, Garzoli E, Caduff RF, Krestin GP. Detection of breast cancer with conventional mammography and contrast-enhanced MR imaging. European Radiology. 1998;**8**(2):194-200

[17] Kopans DB. The positive predictive value of mammography. American Journal of Roentgen. 1992;**158**:521-526

[18] Hendee WR. History and status of X-ray mammography. Health Physics. 1995;**69**(5): 636-648

[19] Sankararaman S, Karellas A, Vedanthan S. Physical characteristics of a full field digital mammography system. Nuclear Instruments and Methods in Physics Research A. 2004;**533**(14):560-570

[20] James JJ. The current status of digital mammography (review). Clinical Radiology. 2004;**59**:1-10

[21] Adler DD, Wahl RL. New methods for imaging the breast: Techniques, findings, and potential. American Journal of Roentgenology. 1995;**164**:19-30

[22] Singletary SE, Allred C, Ashley P, Bassett LW, Berry D, Bland KI, Borgen PI, Clark G, Edge SB, Hayes DF, Hughes LL, Hutter RVP, Morrow M, Page DL, Recht A, Theriault RL, Thor A, Weaver DL, Wie HS, Greene FL. Revision of the American joint Committee on cancer staging system for breast cancer. Journal of Clinical Oncology. 2002;**20**:3628-3636

[23] Weinreb JC, Newstead G. MR imaging of the breast. Radiology. 1995;**196**:593610

[24] Rankin SC. MRI of the breast. British Journal of Radiology. 2000;**73**(872):806-818

[25] Sharp PF, Gemmell HG, Smith FW. Practical Nuclear Medicine. USA: Oxford University Press; 1998. ISBN: 0-19-26284-0. 1-12

[26] Wahl RL. Current status of PET in breast cancer imaging, staging, and therapy. Seminars in Roentgenology. 2001;**36**(3):250-260

[27] Adler LP, Crowe JP, Alkaisi NK, Sunshine JL. Evaluation of breast masses and axillary lymph nodes with [F-18] 2-deoxy-2-fluoro-D-glucose PET. Radiology. 1993;**187**(3):743-752

[28] Strauss LG, Conti PS. The application of PET in clinical oncology. Journal of Nuclear Medicine. 1991;**32**(4):632-648

[29] Strauss LG. PET in clinical oncology: Current role for diagnosis and therapy monitoring in oncology. The Oncologist. 1997;**2**:381-388

[30] Price P. Is there a future for PET in oncology? European Journal of Nuclear Medicine. 1997;**24**(6):587-589

[31] Bombardieri E, Aktolun C, Baum RP, Bishof-Delaloye A, Buscombe J, Chatal JF, Maffioli L, Moncayo R, Mortelmans L, Reske SN. Breast scintigraphy: Procedure guidelines for tumour imaging. European Journal of Nuclear Medicine and Molecular Imaging. 2003;**30**(12):B107-B114

[32] Maublant J, Zheng Z, Rapp M, Ollier M, Michelot J, Veyre A. In vitro uptake of Technetium-99m-Teboroxime in carcinoma cells: Comparison with Technetium-99m-Sestamibi and Thallium-201. Journal of Nuclear Medicine. 1993;**24**(34):1949-1952

[33] Schillaci O, Buscombe JR. Breast scintigraphy today: Indications and limitations. European Journal of Nuclear Medicine and Molecular Imaging. 2004;**31**:S35-S45

[34] Wiesenberger AG, Barbosa F, Green TD, Hoefer R, Keppel C, Kross B, Majewski S, Popor V, Wojcik R, Wymer DC. A combined scintimammography/stereotactic core biopsy X-ray. Nuclear Science Symposium Conference Record. 2000;**3**

[35] Fondrinier E, Muratet JP, Anglade E, Fauvet R, Breger V, Lorimier G, and Jallet P. Clinical experience with 99mTc-MIBI scintimammography in patients with breast microcalcifications. Breast. 2004;**13**(4):316-320

[36] Schillaci O, Scopinaro F, Spanu A, Donnetti M, Danieli R, Di Luzio E, Madeddu G, David V. Detection of axillary lymph node metastases in breast cancer with ^{99m}Tc tetrofosmin scintigraphy. International Journal of Oncology. 2002;**20**(3):483-487

[37] Imbriaco M, Del Vecchio S, Riccardi A, Pace L, Di Salle F, Di Gennaro F, Salvatore M, Sodano A. Scintimammography with ^{99m}Tc-MIBI versus dynamic MRI for non-invasive characterization of breast masses. European Journal of Nuclear Medicine and Molecular Imaging. 2001;**28**:1

[38] Buscome JR, Cwikla JB, Holloway B, Hilson AJW. Prediction of the use fullness of combined mammography and scintimammography in suspected primary breast cancer using ROC curves. Journal of Nuclear Medicine. 2001;**42**:3-8

[39] Fahey FH, Grow KL, Webber RL, Harkness BA, Harkness BA, Bayram E, and Hemler PF. Emission tuned-aperture computed tomography: A novel approach to scintimammography. Journal of Nuclear Medicine. 2001;**42**(7):1121-1127

[40] Scopinaro F, Ierardi M, Porfiri LM, Tiberio NS, De Vincentis G, Mezi S, Cannas P, Gigliotti T, Marzetti L. ^{99m}Tc-MIBI prone scintimammography in patients with high and intermediate risk mammography. Anticancer Research. 1997;**17**:1635-1638

[41] Gupta P, Waxman A, Nguyen K, Phillips E, Yadagar J, Silberman A, Memsic L. Correlation of ^{99m}Tc-sestamibi uptake with histopathologic characteristics in patients with benign breast diseases. [Abstract]. Journal of Nuclear Medicine. 1996;**37**(5):1122-1122

[42] Coover LR, Caravaglia G, Kunh P. Scintimammography with dedicated breast camera detects and localizes occult carcinoma. Journal of Nuclear Medicine. 2004;**45**(4):553-558

[43] Brem RF, Schoonjans JM, Kieper DA, Majewski S, Goodman S, Civelek C. High-resolution scintimammography: A pilot study. Journal of Nuclear Medicine. 2002;**43**:909-915

[44] Brem RF, Kieper DA, Rapelysea JA, Majewski S. Evaluation of a high resolution, breast-specific, small-field-of-view gamma camera for the detection of breast cancer. Nuclear Instruments and Methods in Physics Research Section A. 2003;**497**(1):39-45

[45] Rhodes DJ, O'Connor MK, Phillips SW, Smith RL, Collins DA. Molecular breast imaging: A new technique using ^{99m}Tc-scintimammography to detect small tumours of the breast. Mayo Clinic Proceedings. 2005;**80**:24-30

[46] Brem RF, Rapelyea JA, Zisman G, Mohtashemi K, Raub J, Teal CB, Majewski S, Welch BL. Occult breast cancer: Scintimammography with high-resolution breast-specific gamma camera in women at high risk for breast cancer. Radiology. 2005;**237**(1):274-280

[47] Scopinaro F, Pani R, De Vincentis G, Soluri A, Pellegrini R, Porfiri LM. High resolution scintimammography improves the accuracy of technetium-99m methoxyisobutylisonitrile scintimammography: Use of a new dedicated gamma camera. European Journal of Nuclear Medicine and Molecular Imaging. 1999;**40**:1279-1288

[48] Taillefer R. The Role of ^{99m}Tc-sestamibi and other conventional radiopharmaceuticals in breast cancer diagnosis. Seminars in Nuclear Medicine. 1999;**XXIX**(1):16-40

[49] Hartsough N, Pi B, Gormley J, Conwell R, Ashburn W. Performance characteristic of a compact, quantized gamma camera. [Abstract]. Journal of Nuclear Medicine. 1999;**40**:227

[50] Itti E, Patt BE, Diggles LE, MacDonald L, Iwanczyk JS, Mishkin FS and Khalkhali I. Improved scintimammography using a high-resolution camera mounted on an upright mammography gantry. Nuclear Instruments and Methods in Physics Research. 2003;**497**(1):1-8

[51] Gamma Medica. LumaGEM. http://www.gammamedica.com/products/luma.html. Retrieved on July 2006

[52] Gamma Medica. LumaGEM. http://www.gammamedica.com/articles/DiScan.pdf. Retrieved on July 2006

[53] Alnafea MA, Wells K, Spyrou NM, Saripan MI, Guy M and Hinton P. Preliminary results from a Monte Carlo study of breast tumour imaging with low energy high-resolution collimator and a modified uniformly-redundant array-coded aperture. Nuclear Instrument and Method A. 2006;**563**:146-149

[54] Alnafea MA, Wells K, Spyrou NM, and Guy M. Preliminary Monte Carlo study of coded aperture imaging with a CZT gamma camera system for scintimammography. Nuclear Instrument and Method A. 2007;**573**:122-125

3

Diagnostic System in Electrical Impedance Mammography

Alexander Karpov, Andrey Kolobanov and
Marina Korotkova

Abstract

Electrical impedance mammography (EIM) belongs to nonlocal techniques of image creation. It is based on a number of data collection methods, including the cross-sectional approach, the back-projection method with the weight function applied horizontally and vertically, and the static image method. The analysis of data acquired by applying the above methods enabled to work out the EIM diagnostic system. It involves the following diagnostic categories: structural percentile limits and the mammary gland structure, age-related percentile limits and age-related electric conductivity, outlying values statistics and early diagnostics of breast cancer, D-statistics and distortion of the mammographic scheme in the presence of breast cancer, diagnostic table, and the assessment of the electrical impedance image.

Keywords: electroimpedance mammography, breast cancer, high-risk group

1. Introduction

Modern academic research and clinical practice avail of various tomography systems of electrical impedance diagnostics [1–7]. Electrical impedance mammography (EIM) represents one of the most rapidly developing imaging modalities designed for breast cancer detection [8–22].

EIM belongs to noninvasive techniques of image creation. It measures electromagnetic phenomena and assesses their changes via external scanning.

Since electric current distribution is not limited by two-dimensional plane, the data obtained reflect the change of electric conductivity in three-dimensional space, thus providing for the layer-by-layer image of the object. Based on the reconstruction of internal distribution from a set of external points, EIM refers to tomography techniques of image construction.

There exist two types of techniques creating tomographic images: local and nonlocal. The local technique implies the passage of one direct ray through the body causing the creation of one pixel in the image. The pixel value depends solely on the substance that the ray meets on its way. X-ray, magnetic resonance, and positron emission all belong to local or hard-field tomography techniques.

The nonlocal technique is characterized by all points on the object affecting the measurement result. This is the so-called cross measurement. The pixel value depends both on the object structure and the structure of the surrounding tissues. Electrical impedance, ultrasound reflection, and optical tomography belong to the category of nonlocal or soft-field tomography techniques.

Thus, EIM is a noninvasive technique featuring nonlocal properties of tomographic image creation.

2. Diagnostics system in electrical impedance mammography

Modern electrical impedance mammography systems, both commercial and experimental, differ in the following characteristics: alternating current parameters, electrode number and arrangement configuration, method of data collection, and algorithm of image reconstruction. Electrical impedance mammograph, MEIKv5.6, developed and manufactured by "PKF "Sim-technika," Russia was used for the creation of electrical impedance images [22].

The mammograph has the following significant characteristics:

- Noninvasive technology of image creation

- 3D-tomography system

- Form of "soft-field" tomography

- "Nonlocal" method of tomographic image creation

- 50 kHz frequency and 0.5 mA amplitude alternating current

- Planar positioning of electrodes

- 256 electrode panel

- Cross-sectional approach to data collection. The cross-sectional approach is a variation of the complementary method, when all electrodes are involved in measurement pairwise.

- Back-projection method as an algorithm of image reconstruction

- Static image

- Quantitative diagnostic information

The analysis of data obtained via the MEIKv5.6 electrical impedance mammograph allowed to pick out the following diagnostic categories:

- Structural percentile limits and mammary gland structure

- Age-related percentile limits and age-related electric conductivity

- Outlier statistics and early detection of breast cancer

- D-statistics and distorted mammographic scheme in the presence of breast cancer

- Diagnostic table and EIM image evaluation

2.1. Structural percentile limits and mammary gland structure

The analysis in hand is based on data acquired from 1632 electromammographic examinations of normal women of various age groups. It is essential that the test groups contained about the same number of women: 380 women aged 20–30, 428 women aged 31–40, 449 women aged 41–50, and 375 women aged 51–60. The analysis of the electrical impedance mammograms was carried out "blindly", i.e., without taking the women's age into account.

The fluctuations of the electrical impedance index values made from 0.01 standard units, the lower range value, to 0.68 standard units, the upper range value. To define the structure of electric conductivity index distribution, we extracted eight property ranges with the 0.09 step and calculated the number of observations in each range (**Table 1**).

Figure 1 shows data distribution by the electric conductivity index. The conductivity index mean value constituted 0.29, median, and 0.26, mode.

A bell-shaped curve, similar mean, median, and mode values allow us to declare the quantitative variable (electric conductivity index in this case) distribution as normal. Mean value and

Electric conductivity index	Number of observations
0.05–0.14	0
0.15–0.24	67
0.25–0.34	279
0.35–0.44	471
0.45–0.54	435
055–0.64	299
0.65–0.74	75
0.75–0.84	6
Total	1632

Table 1. Distribution of mean electric conductivity index frequencies.

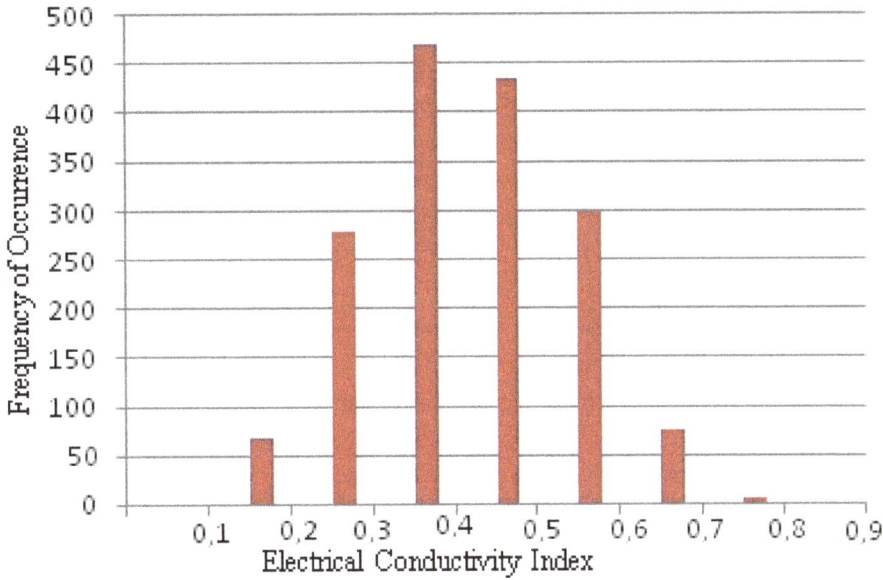

Figure 1. Histogram of mean electric conductivity index frequency distribution.

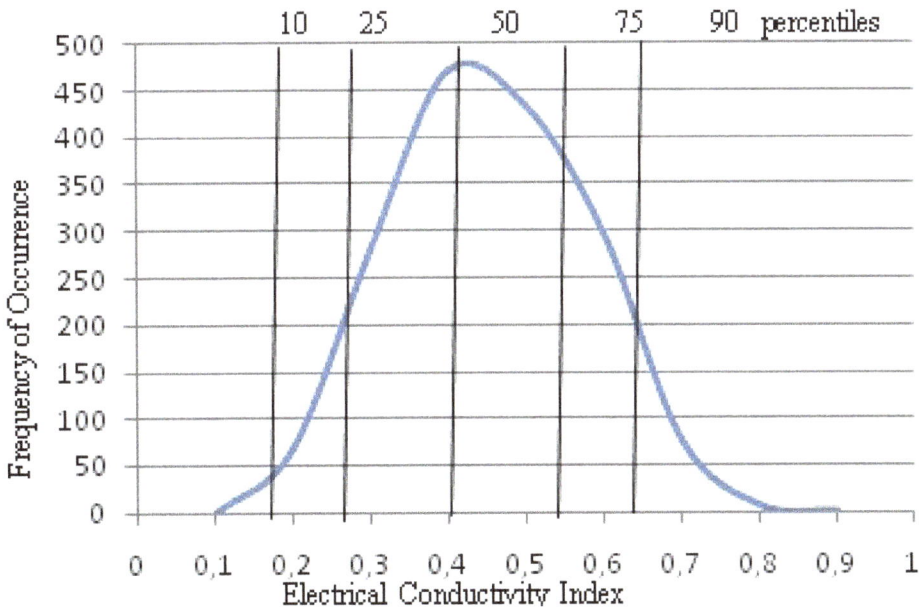

Figure 2. Frequency polygon and percentile ranges.

standard deviation are generally used for normal distribution characterization. We see the implementation of the 10th, 25th, 50th, 75th, and 90th percentile as most rational since it does not require the knowledge of the variable distribution form (**Figure 2**).

In accordance with the proposed assessments, the values within the first range (below the 10th percentile) should be considered as distinctly low, within the second range (10th–25th percentile) as low, the third and fourth ranges (25th–75th percentile) as mean, within the fifth range (75th–90th percentile) as high, and the sixth range (above the 90th percentile) as distinctly high.

The mammary gland structure allows to distinguish a few kinds of tissues performing various functions (epithelial, connective, nerve, blood, and lymph). The age involution of the mammary gland consists in the reduction of ductal epithelium proliferation, in the substitution of the secretory epithelium by a connective tissue with different correlations of tissue elements. The electric conductivity index (IC) obtained from the electrical impedance scanning is a quantitative variable, which characterizes the mammary gland structure. A low index is typical of a gland containing a big number of cell elements and thereafter high ion concentration. This causes us to regard the mammary gland structure with the conductivity index percentile limit <10 percentile as representing the ductal type. This is confirmed by the fact that the proportion of the test-group women aged 20–30 with the ductal type of the mammary gland structure and indices fitting in the first channel (<10 percentile) exceeded 70%. A high electric conductivity index is typical of a gland containing big number of fat lobules and a lot of connective tissue and therefore low ion concentration. Thus, the mammary gland structure with the conductivity index percentile limit >90 percentile should be estimated as representing the amorphous type. This is confirmed by the fact that the proportion of women aged 51–60 with the involutive type of the mammary gland structure and indices fitting in the sixth channel (>90 percentile) also exceeded 70%. The mammary gland structure with the conductivity index percentile limit between the 25th and 75th percentile should be estimated as representing the mixed type. This is proved by the fact that this percentile channel included data of women of all age-groups. Different combinations of structures determining tissue electric conductivity produce a wide range of conductivity index values.

Table 2 presents a summary table of the mammary gland structure assessment from the perspective of EIM execution.

Thus, the mammary gland structure can be assessed from the perspective of electrical impedance mammography with a view to the electric conductivity index. As is well-known, the mammary gland structure conditions its density, which is why the distinguished ranges of electric conductivity correspond to different types of breast density. The so-called dense breasts, which correlate with the ductal structural type, are characterized by low values of

Structural type	Electric conductivity	Percentile limits
Amorphous	Above 0.66	>90‰
Mixed with the predominance of the amorphous component	0.57–0.65	75–90‰
Mixed	0.30–0.56	25–75‰
Mixed with the predominance of the ductal component	0.22–0.29	10–25‰
Ductal	Below 0.22	<10‰

Table 2. Types of mammary gland structure from the perspective of electrical impedance mammography.

electric conductivity index. High index values are typical of the amorphous structure when the mammary gland chiefly consists of the adipose and connective tissues. The peculiarity of this approach to the mammary gland structure assessment is a quantitative expression of the mamma's anatomic and histological composition. The results of the mammary gland density assessment from the perspective of electrical impedance mammography with a view to the electric conductivity index are presented in **Table 3**. The assessment is done in line with the American College of Radiology (ACR) terms [23].

2.2. Age-related percentile limits and age-related electric conductivity

The analysis in hand is based on data acquired from over 2000 electromammographic examinations of normal women aged 20–80. The analysis of the electrical impedance mammograms was carried out using the percentile limits approach, the women's age taken into account. It should be noted that modern medical, biological, and clinical research has been increasingly employing the percentile approach as a method of concise description of distributions. This approach does not require the knowledge of distribution form, i.e., it is nonparametric. The use of percentile curves is routine for many diagnostic modalities, e.g., they are widely used for the assessment of fetal development in ultrasound diagnostics. 5, 50, and 95 percentile limits for the electric conductivity index were calculated in each age group, which allowed to draw percentile curves (**Figure 3**) and make a table summarizing percentile limits of normal age-related electric conductivity of the mammary glands (**Table 4**).

Percentile limits of age-related electric conductivity can be used for the formation of breast cancer risk groups. The conductivity index values below the 5th percentile must be regarded as distinctly low, whereas the values exceeding the 95th percentile as distinctly high.

The risk group for breast cancer should thus include patients exhibiting abnormally low age-related electric conductivity values, i.e., below the 5th percentile, which witnesses for extremely high density of the glandular tissue ductal component. High density of the ductal

	EIM classification	Electric conductivity	ACR classification
Type Ia	Amorphous	above 0.66	Predominantly fat, parenchyma below 25%
Type Ib	Mixed with the predominance of the amorphous component	0.57–0.65	
Type II	Mixed	0.30–0.56	Fat with some fibroglandular tissue, parenchyma between 25 and 50%
Type III	Mixed with the predominance of the ductal component, high density of the ductal component	0.22–0.29	Heterogeneously dense, parenchyma 50–75%
Type IV	Ductal, extremely high density of the ductal component	below 0.22	Extremely dense, parenchyma 75–100%

Table 3. Mammary gland structure and density types from the perspective of EIM execution in accordance with the ACR classification.

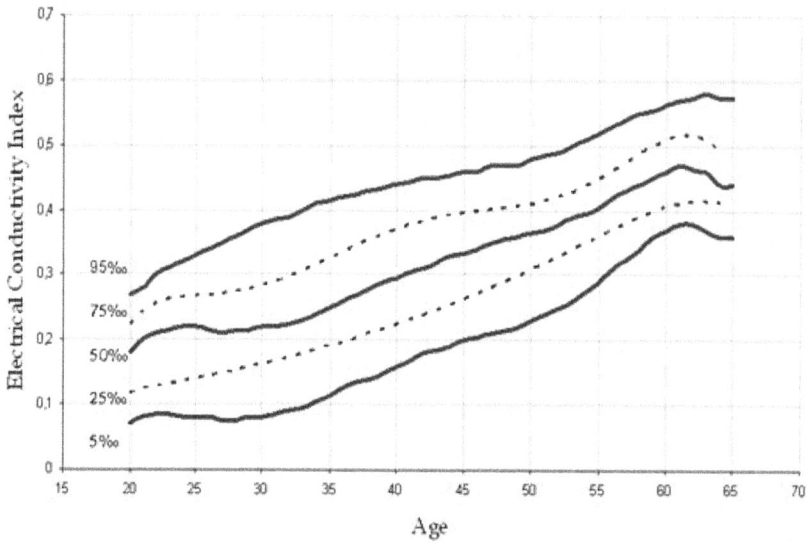

Figure 3. Percentile curves of age-related electric conductivity of the mammary gland.

Age range, years	5 percentile	50 percentile	95 percentile
20–29	0.18	0.28	0.44
30–39	0.16	0.40	0.53
40–49	0.22	0.51	0.63
50–59	0.32	0.58	0.72
60–69	0.43	0.57	0.78
over 70	0.50	0.57	0.64

Table 4. Age-related percentile limits of the mean electric conductivity index.

component carries potential threat since it is often conjoined by the insufficient trophic function of the connective tissue, which is known to be provided by the main substance thereof. Dyscrasia may result in dystrophic processes, including those in the basal membrane.

Abnormally high values of age-related electric conductivity, i.e., exceeding the 95th percentile, correlate with menstrual disorders, the latter standing for hormonal changes.

2.3. Outlier statistics and early detection of breast cancer

Unlike other tomographic modalities which only avail of visual evaluation feature, electrical impedance scanning also provides quantitative information. These unique data are used for diagnostic purposes. A detailed description thereof demands a short reference to outlier statistics.

Provided that all value variations come from a single general population, they are expected to differentiate by virtue of random causes only and stay within the range of M ± 2 standard deviation. However, we sometimes come across values, which differ dramatically from the rest of the totality. Such values are often referred to as outliers. In this case, checking the values for the presence of outliers is highly desirable. If such a difference is a result of an error or its cause is unknown, the outlier value should be excluded from the assessment. Elimination of values that are "too remote" from the center of a sample is called sample *censoring*.

There are two basic types of methods implemented for outlier elimination [24]:

(a) Elimination method with the general standard deviation given.

(b) Elimination method with the general standard square deviation not given.

In the first case, X and standard deviation are calculated with a view to the results obtained from the sample aggregate; in the second case, the sample is stripped of the suspicious results before the calculations are made. Normalized deviate, which serves a nondimensional characteristic of the variable deviation from the arithmetical mean, is one of the criteria used to determine the outliers (1).

$$t = x - M/\sigma \qquad (1)$$

where "t" is the outlier detection criterion, "x" is an outlier, "M" is the mean value for a variant group, and "σ" is a standard deviation. "ttable" stands for standard values of the outlier detection criterion, the values are shown in the table. The values of ttable= 2, P = 0.95 are often used for large selections.

The "three sigma" rule applied for the assessment of the measurement results distributed in accordance with the normal law is one of the simplest outlier detection methods. This rule implies the following: if $Xoutlier - X > 3S_x$, where S_x–is an assessment of the standard deviation measurement, the result is hardly probable and may be considered as a miss. The X and S_x values are calculated without regard to the extreme values of $Xoutlier$.

In this paragraph, we will comment on the results of an electrochemical test of the MEIK v5.6 electrical impedance mammograph. The figure below shows a prototype installation filled with water. The mammograph was used to acquire an electrical impedance scan of the physiological saline solution (**Figure 4A**). The mean electric conductivity index (IC) made 1.85,

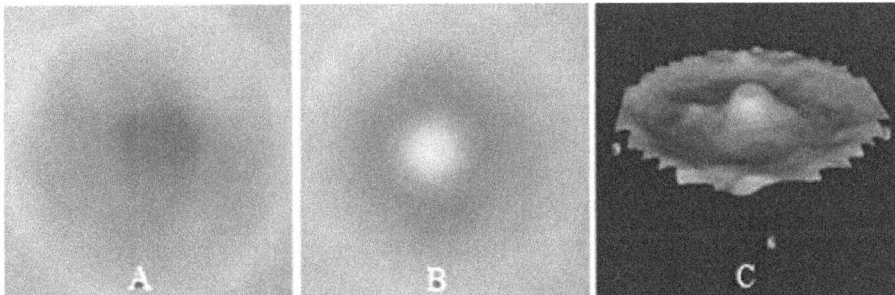

Figure 4. Electroimpedance scans (11 mm deep) of water: A–homogeneous, B–with a metal coin in the middle, C–a 3D image.

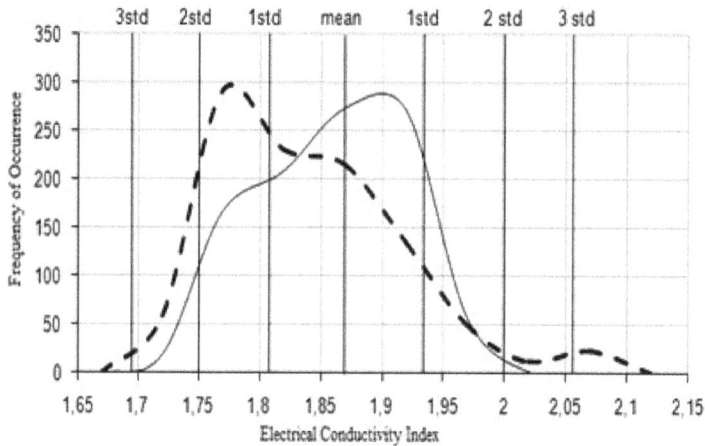

Figure 5. Histograms of electric conductivity distribution of water (continuous curve) and of water with a coin (dotted curve).

whereas the standard deviation amounted to 0.075 and three standard deviations to 0.22. Then, a metal coin was put into the water, 1 cm deeper than the mammograph panel with electrodes (**Figure 4B**). When overlapped, the conductivity distribution histograms (**Figure 5**) allow to see that the IC of the coin (dotted curve) is higher than the IC of water (continuous curve) by a value exceeding three standard deviations. This is typical of outliers; however, in this particular case, it speaks for the presence of an object whose IC value is significantly different from that of the medium, neither does the object belong to the general observation population.

The above mentioned fully applies to medical and biological measurements. **Figure 6** shows an electrical impedance mammogram of a patient suffering from breast cancer, the quantitative parameters being: IC = 0.56, standard deviation–0.12. At 3 o'clock next to the areola, we can see an indistinctly contoured focus with the IC of 0.94. Thus, the IC in the area of interest exceeds the IC of the mammogram by a value going over 3 standard deviations. On the right, we present X-ray and ultrasound images of the same case.

The given example proves that the electric properties of malignant tumors differ significantly from those of the surrounding tissue. It is a well-known fact that cancer cells exhibit an increased electrical activity. Some of the characteristic features of cancer cells that affect their electrical activity are:

1. Cancer cells have cell membranes that exhibit different electrochemical properties and a different distribution of electrical charges than normal tissues [25].

2. A change in mineral content of the cell, particularly an increase in the intracellular concentration of positively charged sodium ions and an increase in the negative charges on the cell coat (glycocalyx) are two of the major factors causing cancer cells to have lower membrane potential than normal cells [25].

3. Cancer cells exhibit both lower electrical membrane potentials and lower electrical impedance than normal cells [26, 27].

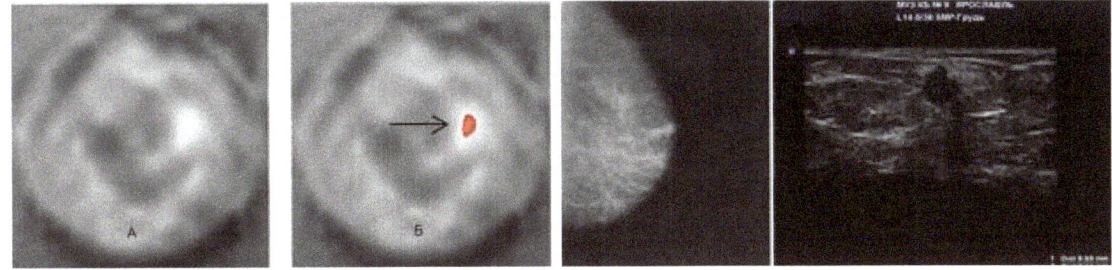

Figure 6. On 3 o'clock next to the areola, a focus is visualized (A), highlighted–arrow (B), less than 10 mm in size. X-ray: A lesion of less than 1 cm in size with a radiant contour in the upper-outer segment. US: a lesion of an irregular shape, with nonhomogeneous structure, 9 × 9 mm without vascularization.

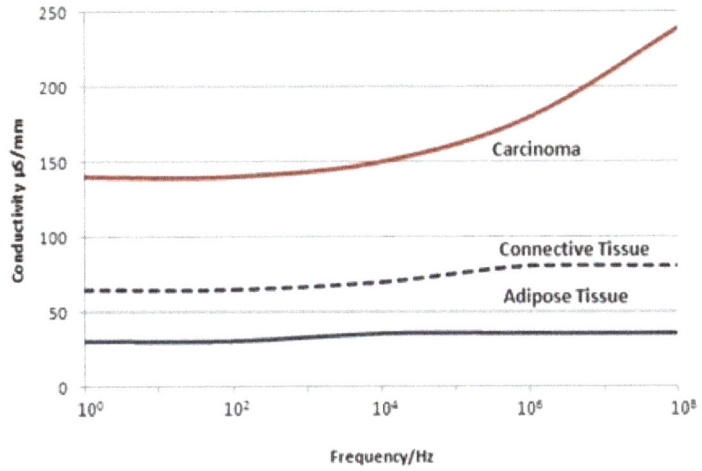

Figure 7. Influence of the current frequency on the electric conductivity of the mammary gland tissues.

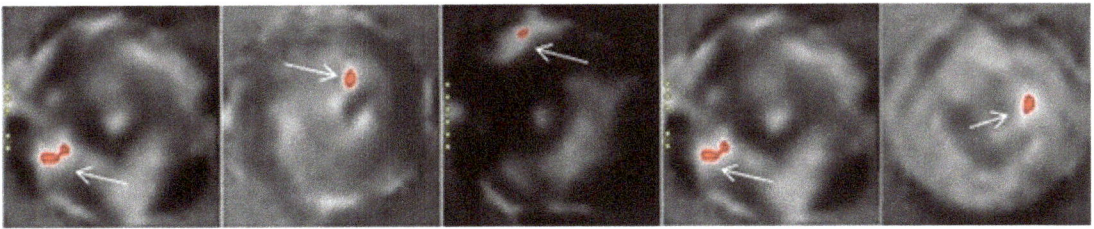

Figure 8. High electrical conductivity area (>3 std) outside the lactiferous sinus zone, which is highlighted (arrow).

From **Figure 7**, it becomes clear that the mammary gland carcinoma has three times higher electric conductivity than the surrounding tissues [28].

This knowledge can be applied to early detection of breast cancer. To perform this task one is to search for areas with abnormal values of IC>3 std, which is typical of an oncologic process with tumors not exceeding 1 cm. To make the search easier, the mammograph highlights abnormal conductivity areas with red (arrow) (**Figure 8**).

2.4. D-statistics and distorted mammographic scheme in the presence of breast cancer

As the disease connected by the breakup of the epithelium basal membrane progresses, various phenomena can occur in the tumor and the surrounding tissues. These processes are always accompanied by alterations of electrical properties of the tumor mass. Increased vascularization leads to electrical conductivity increase due to ionic conduction. Replacement of dead tumor cells by collagen fibers leads to electrical conductivity decrease. While purulent inflammation areas emerge, permittivity decreases as a result of the cell membranes death. Lymphocytic infiltration causes the tumor and the surrounding tissues impedance to increase, because of a significant local concentration of cell membranes. Thus, tumor growth is regularly accompanied by the alteration of the electrical properties both of the tumor and the surrounding tissues.

As noted previously, the electrical impedance approach enables to conduct a quantitative analysis of the image involving the assessment of the following parameters: mean electric conductivity index, histogram of electric conductivity distribution, comparison of the electric conductivity distribution histogram with the referent values.

To refer the patient to the norm or pathology category, the divergence in the distribution form criterion, also known as the λ-criterion or the Kolmogorov-Smirnov criterion [29], is used in Eq. (2).

$$\lambda = \left| \sum N1(xij)/n1 - \sum N2(xij)/n2 \right| \max \sqrt{n1 n2/n1 + n2} \tag{2}$$

where $N1$ stands for observation quantities within the ranges, $n1$–within the sample aggregate, A_1; and $N2$ and $n2$–the same for A_2.

Dx statistics, to be more exact, a subaggregate when calculating the Kolmogorov-Smirnov criterion Eq. (3).

$$D(xij) = \left| \sum N1(xij)/n1 - \sum N2(xij)/n2 \right| \max \tag{3}$$

where $N1$ stands for observation quantities within the ranges, $n1$–within the sample aggregate, A_1; $N2$ and $n2$–the same for A_2.

This nonparametric criterion enables to determine the statistical significance of divergences in the distribution of any characteristic of norm or pathology including the distribution of electric conductivity on electrical impedance tomograms.

The Dx statistics allows to define the area of one of the distributions, which is not shared by the other (**Figure 9**). The Dx value reflects the proportion of observations or data, which distinguishes experiment (patient) from control (norm). This value is essential for substantiation of diagnosis as well as for assessing the parameter information capacity.

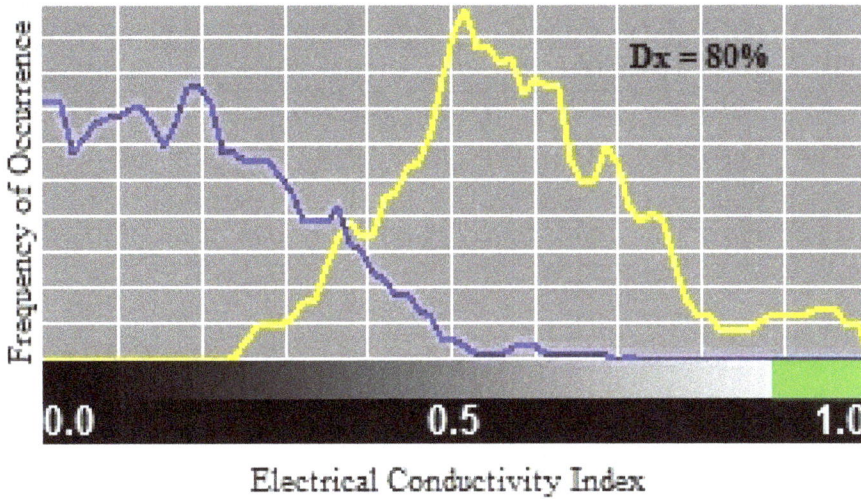

Figure 9. Assessment of distribution divergence by their area.

High information capacity of the divergences revealed enables to refer the patient to this or that category (e.g., norm or cancer) with great probability. To determine the informative value of distribution divergence Kulback's information measure is applied Eq. (4).

$$J = 10 \lg P1/P2 * 0.5(P1 - P2) \qquad (4)$$

where J = information value of the range, $P1$–probability of patients' suffering from disease A1 getting into the range, $P2$–the same for disease A2.

It shows how informative the Dx statistics applied is, how this parameter contributes to diagnosing the disease, e.g., cancer. The assessment of distribution divergence (Dx) produced results standing in direct relationship with the information capacity, according to Kulback (Table 5). This relationship must be recognized as fairly regular and consistent [29].

In the presence of cancer, the histogram of the affected gland is shifted. Table 6 sums up data on comparative electric conductivity obtained from patients suffering breast cancer, benign changes of the mammary gland as well as from normal women with different types of mammary gland structure.

In the course of oncologic process development, general and local electric conductivity naturally tends to change. The distortion of the mammographic scheme can be observed as early

Distribution divergence	Information capacity	Reliability
below 20%	Very low	No
20–30%	Relatively low	Yes
30–50%	Good	Yes
50–65%	High	Yes

Table 5. Distribution divergence and information capacity.

	Number of patients	Comparative electric conductivity (affected–normal gland)					
		<20%	20–30%	30–40%	40–50%	50–60%	>60%
Cancer	310	101 (33%)	67 (22%)	44 (14%)	37 (12%)	26 (8%)	35 (11%)
Healthy	161	157 (98%)	4 (2%)	0	0	0	0
Healthy acinar-ductal type	20	18 (90%)	1 (5%)	1 (5%)	0	0	0
Healthy amorphous type	32	28 (88%)	2 (6%)	2 (6%)	0	0	0
Benign	68	59 (87%)	7 (10%)	2 (3%)	0	0	0

Table 6. Comparative electric conductivity of the mammary glands, data acquired from patients suffering from breast cancer, benign lesions, and normal women.

Diagnostic criteria	Electrical impedance mammography points
Shape	
• Round, oval	1
• Lobular, irregular	2
Contour	
• No	0
• Sharp	1
• Hyperimpedance, indistinct	2
Surrounding tissues	
• *Preserved*	0
• Structure alteration/displacement	1
• Thickening/extrusion/retraction	2
Internal electrical structure	
• Hyperimpedance ($IC_{roi} < IC_{av} - 2std$)	0
• Isoimpedance$IC_{roi} = IC_{av} \pm 2std$)	1
• Hypoimpedance ($IC_{roi} > IC_{av} + 2std$)	2
• Animpedance ($IC_{roi} > IC_{av} + 3std$)	3
Comparative electrical conductivity	
• Divergence between the histograms <20%	0
• Divergence between the histograms 20–30%	1
• Divergence between the histograms 30–40%	2
• Divergence between the histograms >40%	3

Table 7. Diagnostic criteria for differentiation of volumetric lesions in electroimpedance mammography.

as at onset of the disease that is why this criterion was added to the EIM breast cancer diagnostic scale (**Table 7**). Below (**Figure 10**), we provide examples of the distorted mammographic scheme from three patients with breast cancer.

2.5. Diagnostic table and EIM image assessment

A volumetric lesion is an extensional involvement detected on several scan planes. Image analysis implies the assessment of the lesion shape, contour, internal electric structure, and changes in the surrounding tissues.

A diagnostic table was made to regularize the description of volumetric lesions. **Table 7** presents assessment parameters each being given a certain set of points.

Using the numerical score for the assessment of volumetric lesions in electrical impedance mammography allows to compare this information to BI-RADS ACR categories (**Table 8**).

The EIM point scale enables to standardize the description of volumetric lesions when carrying out electrical impedance mammography examination as well as use the algorithm of patients' supervision worked out by the specialists of the American College of Radiology.

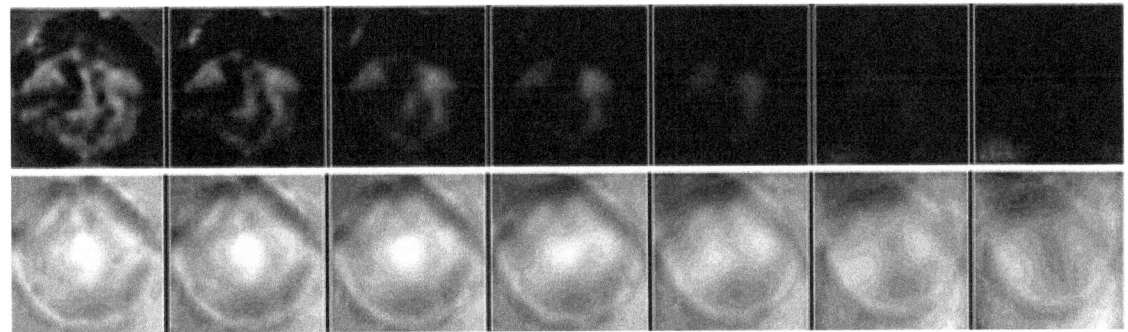

Figure 10. Electroimpedance mammographic scheme distortion (the top images show the affected gland, the bottom line contains images of the normal breast).

EIM	ACR
Common scale	*BI-RADS categories*
No score	BI-RADS 0 poor image
0–1	BI-RADS 1 lesion is not defined
2–3	BI-RADS 2 benign tumors–routine mammography
4	BI-RADS 3 probably benign findings
5–7	BI-RADS 4 suspicious abnormality–biopsy
>8	BI-RADS 5 highly suggestive of malignancy–treatment/biopsy

Table 8. EIM scale and ACR BI-RADS.

3. Conclusion

EIM diagnostic system is a clear and logical system involving determination of the mammary gland structure and density, allowing for cancer diagnostics for various types of breast as well as formation of breast cancer risk groups.

Author details

Alexander Karpov*, Andrey Kolobanov and Marina Korotkova

*Address all correspondence to: karpovay@medyar.ru

Clinical Hospital, Yaroslavl, Russia

References

[1] Barber DC, Brown BH. Applied potential tomography. Journal of Physics E-Scientific Instruments. 1984;**17**(9):723-733

[2] Brown BH, Seagar AD. The Sheffield data collection system. Clinical Physics and Physiological Measurement. 1987;**8**(Suppl A):91-97

[3] Electrical impedance tomography. Edited by D.S.Holder, IOP. 2005

[4] Karpov A, Korotkova M, et al. Electrical impedance potential mammography for visualization of objects (Electrochemical tests). Journal of Physics: Conference Series. 2010;**224**:012032

[5] Akhtari-Zavare M, Latiff L. Electrical impedance tomography as a primary screening technique for breast cancer detection. Asian Pacific Journal of Cancer Prevention. 2015;**16**(14):5595-5597

[6] Shetiye P, Ghatol A, et al. Detection of breast cancer using electrical impedance and RBF neural network. International Journal of Information and Electronics Engineering. 2015;**5**(5):P356-360

[7] Prasad NS, Houserkova D, Campbell J. Breast imaging using 3D electrical impedance tomography. Biomedical Papers of the Medical Faculty of the University of Palacky, Olomouc Czechoslovakia. 2008;**152**(1):151-154

[8] Cherepenin V, Karpov A, Korjenevsky A, Kornienko V, Mazaletskaya A, Mazurov D, Meister D. A 3D electrical impedance tomography (EIT) system for breast cancer detection. Physiological Measurement. 2001;**22**:9-18

[9] Cherepenin V, Karpov A, Korjenevsky A, Kornienko V, Kultiasov Y., Ochapkin M,Trochanova O, Meister J. Three-dimensional EIT imaging of breast tissues: System design and clinical testing. Medical Imaging. 2002;**V21**N6:662-667

[10] Karpov A, Korjenevsky A, Mazurov D, Mazaletskaya A. 3D electrical impedance scanning of breast cancer. World Congress on Medical Physics and Biomedical Engineering, Chicago; 2000; p. 62

[11] Halter RJ, Hartov A, Paulsen KD. A broadband high-frequency electrical impedance tomography system for breast imaging. IEEE Transactions on Biomedical Engineering. 2008;**55**(2 Pt 1):650-659

[12] Jossinet J. A hardware design for imaging the electrical impedance of the breast. Clinical Physics and Physiological Measurement. 1988;**9**Suppl A:25-28

[13] Kerner TE, Paulsen KD, Hartov A, Soho SK, Poplack SP. Electrical impedance spectroscopy of the breast: Clinical imaging results in 26 subjects. IEEE Transactions on Medical Imaging. 2002;**21**(6):77-80, 95-100

[14] Kim, BS, Boverman, G, Newell, JC, Saulnier, GJ, Isaacson, D. The complete electrode model for EIT in a mammography geometry. Physiological Measurement. 2007;**28**(7):S57-S69

[15] Raneta O., Ondruš D., Bella V. Utilisation of electrical impedance tomography in breast cancer diagnosis. Klinická Onkologie. 2012;**25**(1):36-41

[16] Karpov A, Korotkova M. Diagnostic criteria for mass lesions differentiating in electrical impedance mammography. Journal of Physics: Conference Series. 2013;**434**:012053

[17] Chakraborti K, Selvamurthy W. Clinical application of electrical impedance tomography in the present health scenario of India. Journal of Physics: Conference Series. 2010;**224**:012069

[18] Zain N., Kanaga K. A review on breast electrical impedance tomography clinical accuracy. ARPN Journal of Engineering and Applied Sciences. v2015;**10**(15):P6230-6234

[19] Pak D, Rozkova N, et al. The electroimpedance computer tomography in screening of diseases of the breast. Medical Visualization. 2012;**2**:P35-42

[20] Zain N, Chelliah K. Breast imaging using electrical impedance tomography: Correlation of quantitative assessment with visual interpretation. Asian Pacific Journal of Cancer Prevention. 2014;**15**(3):1327-1331

[21] Korotkova M, Karpov A, et al. Electrical impedance imaging characteristics of nodular and edematous-infiltrative forms of breast cancer. Breast Cancer Symposium. San Antonio. 2011:6-10

[22] Korotkova M, Karpov A. Standards for Electrical Impedance Mammography In book "Imaging of the Breast. Technical Aspects and Clinical Implication". Edited by Tabar L, Croatia, 2014

[23] Breast Imaging Reporting and Data System (BI-RADS). 4th ed. Reston: American College of Radiology; 2003

[24] Zaydel A. Error of Measurement of Physical Quantities. 1985

[25] Cure JC. On the electrical characteristics of cancer. Paper presented at the Second International Congress of Electrochemical Treatment of Cancer. 1995; Florida

[26] Cone CD. Variation of the transmembrane potential level as a basic mechanism of mito-
      sis control. Oncology. 1970;**24**:438-470

[27] Blad B, Baldetorp B. Impedance spectra of tumour tissue in comparison with normal tis-
      sue: A possible clinical application for electrical impedance tomography. Physiological
      Measurement. 1996;**17**Suppl 4A:A105-A115

[28] Jossinet J. The impedivity of freshly excised human breast tissue. Physiological Measure-
      ment. 1998;**19**:61-75

[29] Gubler E. Quantitative methods for analysis and identification of pathology. Leningrad.
      1978

4

Breast Ultrasound Tomography

Nebojsa Duric and Peter Littrup

Abstract

Both mammography and standard ultrasound (US) rely upon subjective criteria within the breast imaging reporting and data system (BI-RADS) to provide more uniform interpretation outcomes, as well as differentiation and risk stratification of associated abnormalities. In addition, the technical performance and professional interpretation of both tests suffer from machine and operator dependence. We have been developing a new technique for breast imaging that is based on ultrasound tomography which quantifies tissue characteristics while also producing 3-D images of breast anatomy. Results are presented from clinical studies that utilize this method. In the first phase of the study, ultrasound tomography (UST) images were compared to multi-modal imaging to determine the appearance of lesions and breast parenchyma. In the second phase, correlative comparisons with MR breast imaging were used to establish basic operational capabilities of the UST system. The third phase of the study focused on lesion characterization. Region of interest (ROI) analysis was used to characterize masses. Our study demonstrated a high degree of correlation of breast tissue structures relative to fat subtracted contrast-enhanced MRI and the ability to scan ~90% of the volume of the breast at a resolution of 0.7 mm in the coronal plane.

Keywords: breast, ultrasound, 3-D imaging, tomography, cancer

1. Introduction

Breast cancer is the most common cancer among women, accounting for one-third of cancers diagnosed. Statistically, ~230,000 new cases of invasive breast cancer and ~63,000 in situ breast carcinomas are diagnosed in the US annually; breast cancer is the third leading cause of cancer death among women, causing ~40,000 deaths in the US every year [1]. According to SEER statistics, approximately 61% of women are found to have localized breast cancers at the time of diagnosis; about 31% are found to be regional disease; another 5% are diagnosed with distant metastases while about 3% are unstaged [2]. The 5-year survival rate for women with localized cancer is 98%; for those with regional disease, it drops to 84%; for those diagnosed with distant stage, the survival rate drops dramatically to 23%; while for unstaged cancers the 5-year survival rate is about 58%. **Figure 1** illustrates the dependence of survival on cancer stage.

There are many reasons why cancers are not detected early but some of the major factors relate to limited participation in breast screening and the performance of screening mammography.

1.1. Limited participation in screening

National cancer screening statistics indicate that only 51% of eligible women undergo annual mammograms [4]. That rate is even lower for African American women and/or those of lower socioeconomic groups. Access, fear of radiation and discomfort are some of the factors that contribute to the low participation rate. Greater participation would lead to detection of breast cancer at an earlier stage leading to longer survival. Increased participation and improved breast cancer detection would have the greatest effect on the statistic of nearly 1 in 3 women who are diagnosed each year with later stage (regional or greater) breast cancer, totaling approximately 60,000 women per year in the USA. The net effect would be an increase in survival time and a corresponding decrease in mortality rates. This is also suggested in a recent meta-analysis, whereby increased participation and sensitivity lead to additional invasive cancer detection and greater mortality reduction [4].

1.2. Limited performance of mammography

For women with dense breast tissue, who are at the highest risk for developing breast cancer [5–8], the performance of mammography is at its worst [9]. Consequently, many cancers are

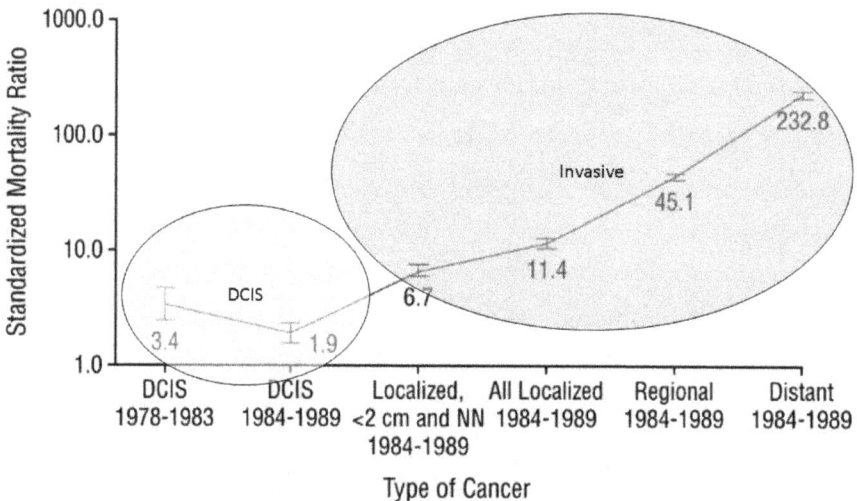

Figure 1. The dependence of mortality rates on cancer type and stage. From Kerlikowske et al. [3].

missed at their earliest stages when they are the most treatable. Improved cancer detection for women with denser breasts would decrease the proportion of breast cancers diagnosed at later stages, which would significantly lower the mortality rate.

1.3. The breast screening challenge

X-ray mammography detects about 5 cancers per 1000 screens [10]. However, its positive predictive value (PPV) is low and its sensitivity is greatly reduced in women with dense breast tissue [10]. Although digital breast tomosynthesis (DBT) may improve upon some of the limitations of standard mammography, it is unlikely to create a paradigm shift in performance [11] while generating even higher levels of ionizing radiation [12]. MRI can significantly improve on these limitations by virtue of its volumetric, radiation-free imaging capability. Studies have shown that MRI can have a positive impact in the breast management continuum ranging from risk assessment to diagnosis and treatment monitoring [12, 13]. However, MRI can have a high false positive rate, requires contrast injection and the exams can be both long and costly [14]. Furthermore, MR has long been prohibitively expensive for routine use and there is a need for a low-cost equivalent alternative. Yet, for high-risk women, MRI is now viewed as the gold standard for breast cancer detection and screening [15–23]. Positron emission tomography is also limited by cost and radiation concerns.

Recent studies have demonstrated the effectiveness of hand held ultrasound imaging in detecting breast cancer, particularly for women with dense breasts (**Table 1**). These studies have shown that up to 4.5 extra cancers were detected per 1000 screens [24–34]. A striking aspect of the added detections is that they are predominantly node negative invasive cancers which would have potentially progressed to a later stage before possible mammographic detection. Moreover, there is little risk of over detection of ductal carcinoma in situ (DCIS). The sensitivity of mammography is greater for DCIS than it is for invasive cancer, with DCIS making up approximately 25% of mammographic screen-detected breast cancers [35].

We have examined the data from these studies to extract the statistics of cancer detection by imaging mode (**Table 1**). The results are summarized in **Figure 2**. It is striking to note that ultrasound (US) almost doubles the cancer detection rate in dense breasts. However, despite these successful study outcomes, handheld ultrasound is unlikely to be adopted for screening because it is operator dependent, and its imaging aperture is small, which hinders whole breast imaging. Furthermore, ultrasound's increased sensitivity to invasive cancer is offset by lowered sensitivity to DCIS by virtue of mammography's greater ability to detect microcalcifications. Although such a trade-off may be justified by the fact that mortality from invasive cancers is much higher than that from DCIS, a combined screening [mammography plus automated breast ultrasound (ABUS)] would provide a comprehensive screen. It has therefore been proposed that ABUS be used for screening, supplemental to mammography.

Author (Year)	Center	Type	Exams	US only cancers	Yield per 1000
Brem et al. (2014)	Multi	ABUS	15,318	30	1.96
Berg et al. (2012)	Multi	HHUS	7473	32	4.28
Hooley et al. (2012)	Single	HHUS	935	3	3.21
Kelly et al. (2010)	Multi	AWBU	6425	23	3.58
Corsetti et al. (2008)	Multi	HHUS	9157	37	4.04
Crystal et al. (2003)	Single	HHUS	1517	7	4.61
Leconte et al. (2003)	Single	HHUS	4236	16	3.78
Kolb et al. (2002)	Single	HHUS	13,547	37	2.73
Kaplan (2001)	Single	HHUS	1862	6	3.22
Buchberger et al. (2000)	Single	HHUS	8103	32	3.95
Gordon et al. (1995)	Single	HHUS	12,706	44	3.46

Table 1. Summary of studies used in the analysis.

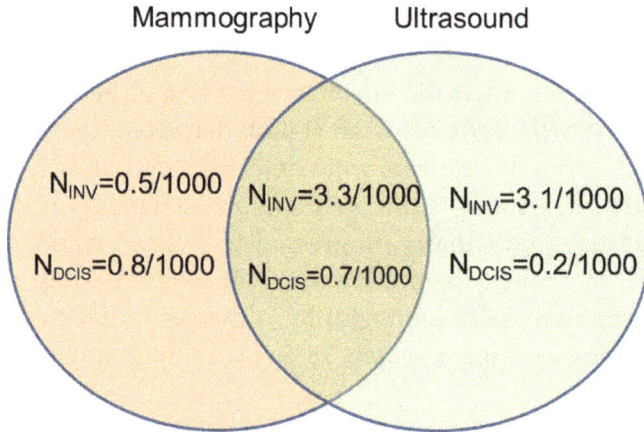

Figure 2. Venn diagram summarizing comparative cancer detection rates for screening mammography and ultrasound.

To that end, automated breast ultrasound (ABUS) has been introduced as a way of overcoming these issues, mainly by reducing operator dependence and increasing the field of view. For example, the GE Invenia ABUS ultrasound system for breast cancer screening, originally developed by U-Systems., recently received screening approval, adjunctive to mammography, from the FDA, because it demonstrated an ability to detect cancers missed by mammography in dense breasts. The SomoInsight screening study [24], indeed showed that ABUS plus mammography outperformed mammography alone, leading to the first FDA approval for ultrasound screening for breast cancer.

The fundamental quandary of breast screening today is the knowledge that (i) mammography misses cancers in dense breasts, (ii) that Automated Breast ultrasound (ABUS) detects cancers that mammography misses and yet (iii) screening continues largely with mammography only. This paradox is amplified even further by the proliferation of state breast density notification laws in the USA which mandate that this information be available to women undergoing breast cancer screening. The primary reason this paradox exists today is that ABUS screening increases call back rates (up to a factor of two in case of the SomoInsight study [23]). The improvement in classification performance, measured by the area under the ROC curve, is modest because the increase in sensitivity is partially offset by an increase in false positives thus slowing its adoption. Technically, with its basic B-mode capability, ABUS has the same issue with false positives as hand held ultrasound. It is therefore unlikely that ABUS will be widely adopted for screening in the foreseeable future without more tissue-specific imaging capability. Improved lesion characterization would help lower the barriers to adoption of screening ultrasound.

1.4. Potential role of UST

Ultrasound tomography (UST) is an emerging technique that has the potential for tissue-specific imaging and characterization, by virtue of its transmission imaging capability [36–61]. Improved specificity would lower call back rates and lower the barriers to adoption. An adjunctive use of UST would have the potential to improve specificity relative to current ABUS and provide a comprehensive screen that would uncover invasive cancers otherwise missed by mammography. Detection of such early stage invasive cancers would provide women with curative treatment, the opportunity for which might be otherwise lost.

Conventional reflection ultrasound exploits differences in acoustic impedance between tissue types to provide anatomical images of breast tumors [62, 63]. However, reflection is just one aspect of a multi-faceted set of acoustic signatures associated with the biomechanical properties of tissue. UST is a technique that moves beyond B-mode imaging by virtue of its transmission capabilities. The latter provides additional characterization by measuring tissue parameters such as sound speed and attenuation (ATT) [64–68]. These parameters can be used to characterize lesions in a quantitative manner, a capability not available in current whole breast ultrasound systems. By merging reflection images with images of the bio-acoustic parameters of sound speed and attenuation, UST offers the possibility of exploiting differences in anatomical and physical properties of tissue to accurately differentiate cancer from normal tissue or benign disease. UST parameters are also quantitative, which allows new consideration of second and third-order statistical image analyses, or radiomics. Ultrasound has previously not been suitable for the burgeoning applications of radiomics due to its lack of true quantitative parameters such as sound speed (m/s) and attenuation (dB/cm/MHz). Initial assessments of UST performance was carried out, as described below.

In an initial attempt to assess the potential of UST in breast imaging, studies were carried out at the Karmanos Cancer Institute, Detroit, MI, USA. Informed consent was obtained from all patients, prospectively recruited in an IRB-approved protocol following HIPAA guidelines. Patients were scanned at the Alexander J Walt Comprehensive Breast Center. Standard multi-modality imaging was available for all patients. The Walt Breast Center houses SoftVue, a UST system manufactured by Delphinus Medical Technologies, Inc (Novi, MI). SoftVue embodies a number of attributes that differentiate it from conventional imaging modalities:

- *Water-based pulse coupling*: SoftVue utilizes a water filled imaging chamber that is kept at body temperature. Its primary purpose is to couple the sound energy between the transducer and the breast tissue.

- *Closed geometry probe*: A circular ring transducer surrounds the breast while both are immersed in water. There is no compression of the breast since the transducer is offset from the breast with water acting as the pulse coupling agent. The closed transducer geometry allows collection of signals that pass through the entire width of the breast, a requirement for transmission imaging and the reconstruction of sound speed and attenuation images. These parameters provide quantitative information in absolute units that are tied to externals standards (km/s and dB/cm, respectively).

- *Operator independence*: Unlike mammography and other ABUS systems, multiple positionings are not required for larger breasts. Once the patient is positioned on the table, the operator simply presses the button and the exam is performed automatically without further intervention from the operator.

- *Scan time*: SoftVue scan time is 1–2 min per breast (depending on breast size). This scan duration minimizes intra-slice and inter-slice motion artifacts.

- *Image reconstruction time.* In this study, reconstruction time for a bilateral breast exam was ~30 min for the average patient and current hardware/software processing ability.

SoftVue was used to scan the recruited patients for this study. Coronal image series were produced by tomographic algorithms for reflection, sound speed and attenuation. All images were reviewed by a board-certified radiologist who has more than 20 years of experience in breast imaging and US-technology development. Symptomatic study participants were scanned with a SoftVue UST system. Pathological correlation was based on biopsy results and standard imaging (e.g. US definitive cyst).

Tomographic algorithms were used to generate images stacks of reflectivity, sound speed and attenuation for each patient. Lesions were identified based on correlation with standard imaging so that the tumor sound speed (SS) and attenuation (ATT) could be assessed. An example each type of image is shown in **Figure 3**.

In the first phase of the study, correlative comparisons with multi-modal imaging were carried out to assess lesion properties relative to mammography, US and MR. In the second

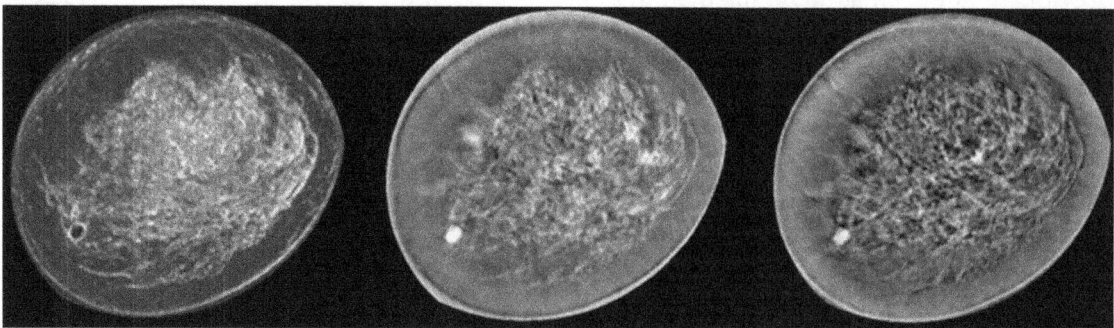

Figure 3. From left to right, reflection, sound speed and attenuation image slices depicting breast parenchyma and a fibroadenoma at 7 o'clock.

phase, MR breast imaging was used to establish basic operational capabilities of the UST system including the identification and characterization of parenchymal patterns, determination of the spatial resolution of UST and an estimate the breast volume that can imaged with UST. The third phase of the study focused on lesion characterization. Region of interest (ROI) analyses were performed on all identified lesions using all three UST image types. Combinations of the ROI generated quantitative values were used to characterize all masses, particularly in relation to relative differences with surrounding peritumoral regions.

2. Multi-modal comparisons

Since the patients were recruited at KCI on the basis of having a suspicious finding, standard imaging such as mammography, US and sometimes MRI were available, as well as the radiology and pathology reports. These images and the associated reports were used to retroactively locate the lesions in the UST image stacks for visual comparison. **Figures 4–7** show examples of UST images in relation to the other modalities. When MRI was available, the images were projected into the coronal plane for easier comparison with the UST whose native format is coronal.

Figure 4 shows a 9mm IDC at 3 o'clock. CC and MLO mammographic views of the affected breast are shown on the left with the lesion identified by arrows. The UST views corresponding

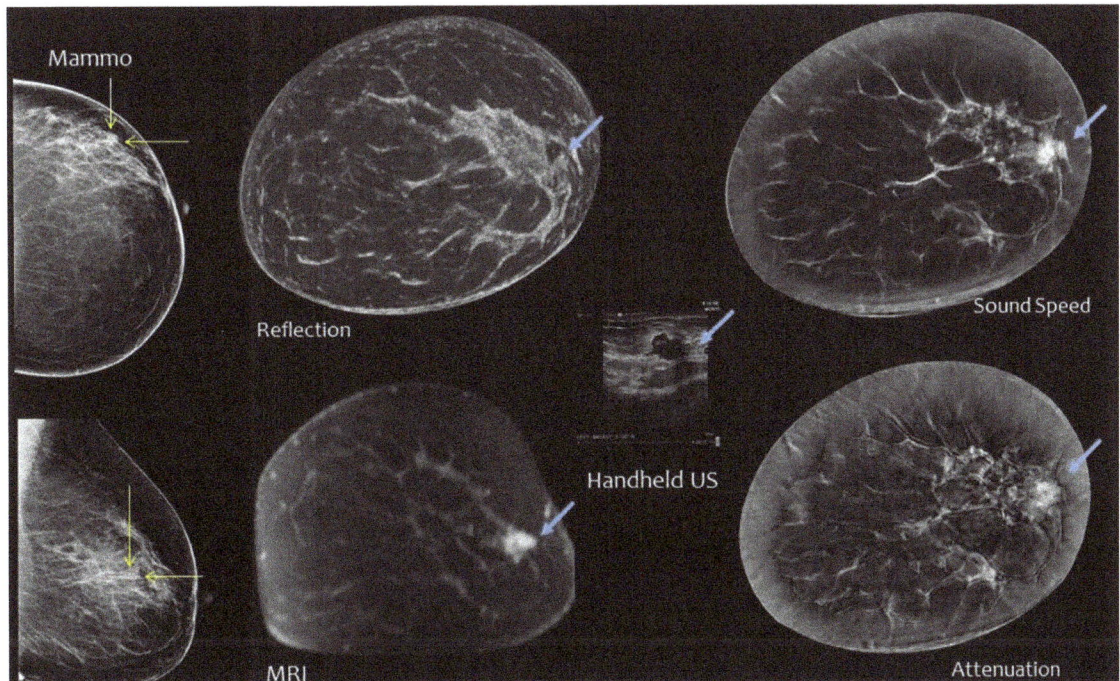

Figure 4. A 9 mm IDC at 3 o'clock. CC and MLO mammographic views of the affected breast are shown on the left with the lesion identified by arrows. The coronal UST views are shown in the form of reflection, sound speed and attenuation images. The corresponding ultrasound and MR images are also shown.

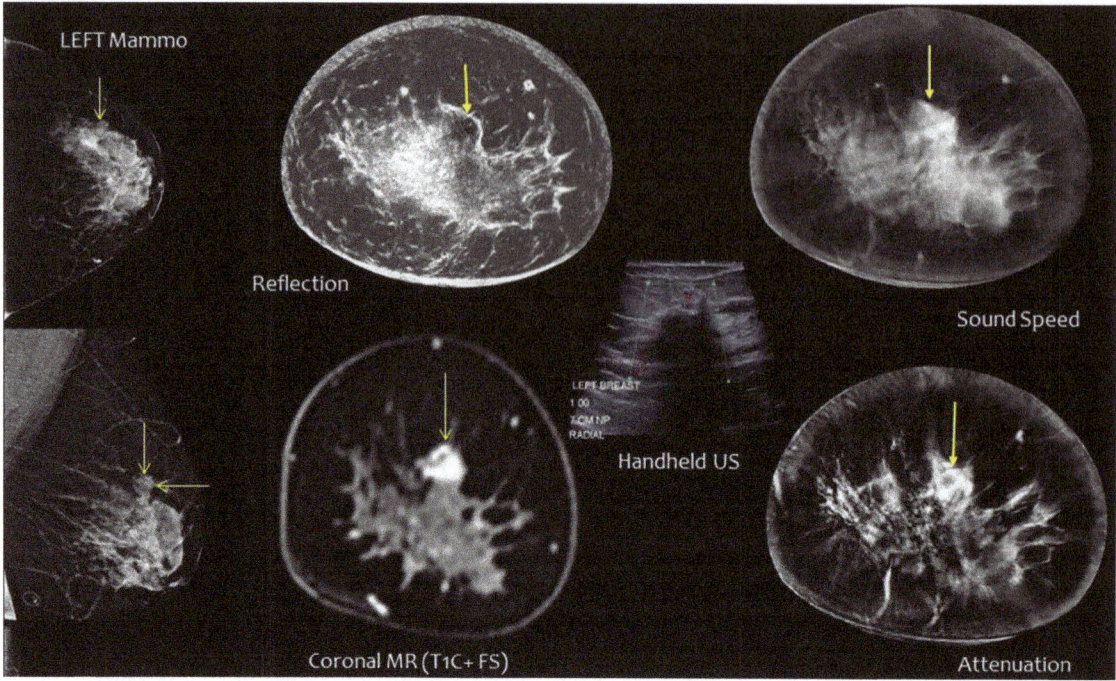

Figure 5. Multimodality images compared to UST reflection, sound speed and attenuation. An IDC is shown at 12 o'clock.

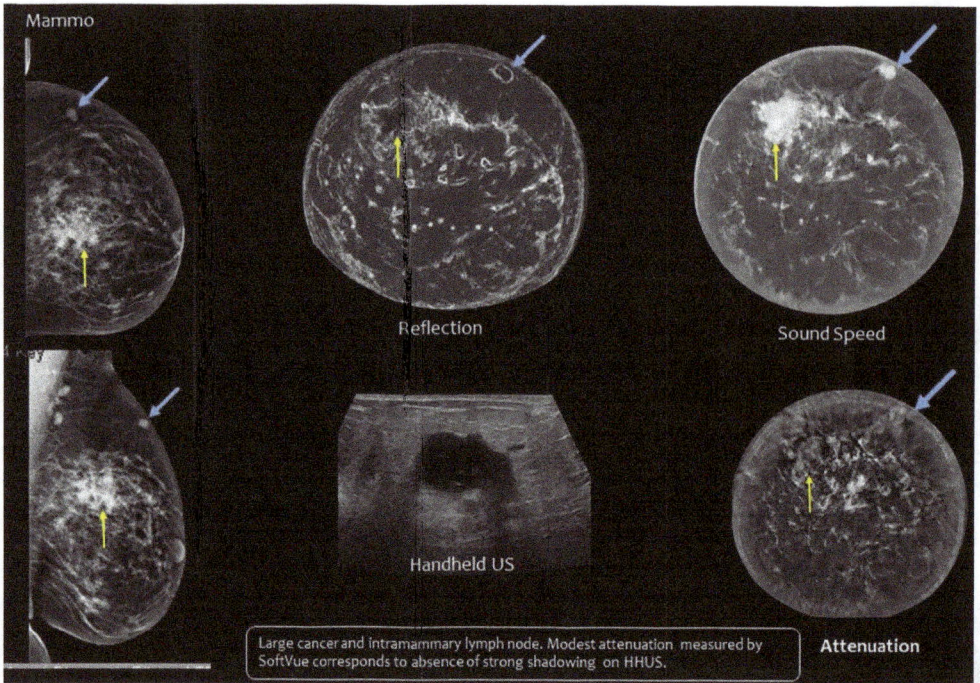

Figure 6. Multimodality images vs UST reflection, sound speed and attenuation showing an IDC and intramammary lymph node.

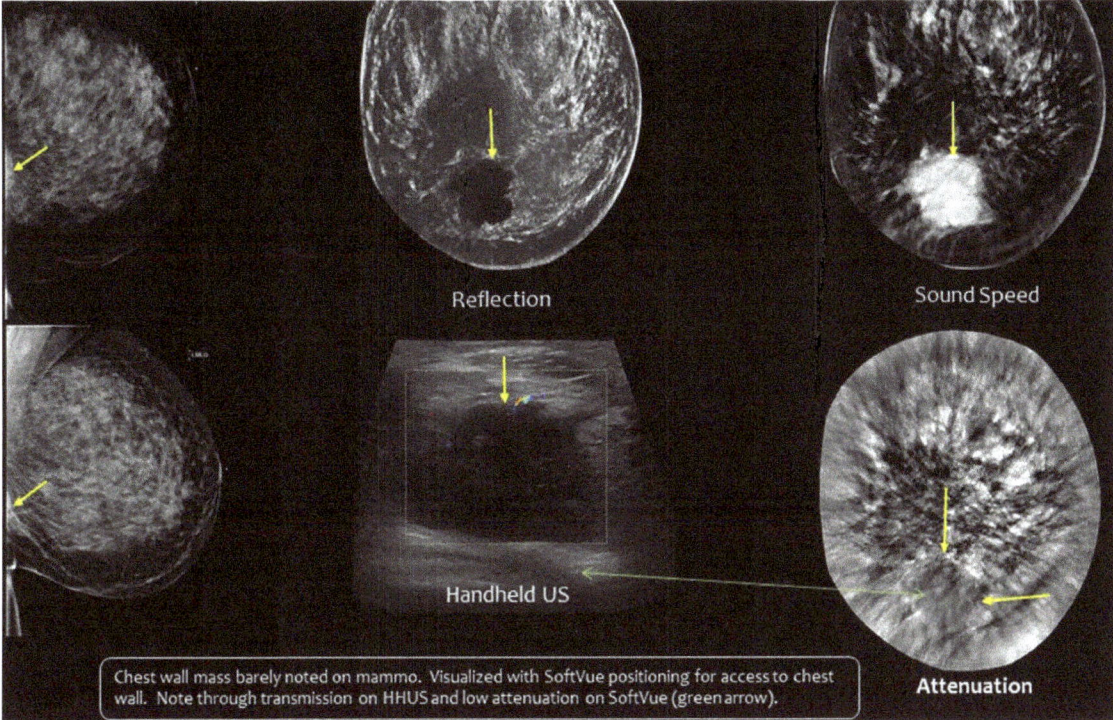

Reflection   Sound Speed

Handheld US

Chest wall mass barely noted on mammo. Visualized with SoftVue positioning for access to chest wall. Note through transmission on HHUS and low attenuation on SoftVue (green arrow).

Attenuation

Figure 7. Illustrating the chest wall access achievable by UST relative to mammography.

to the coronal planes that contain the lesions are across the top with reflection, sound speed and attenuation images laid out from left to right. The corresponding ultrasound and MR images are shown along the bottom. Inspection of the images shows good correspondence in shape and location of the lesion. The greatest similarity is between the UST images and MRI. The IDC is seen to be hypoechoic in reflection and has high sound speed and attenuation contrast. An IDC in a heterogeneously dense breast is shown in **Figure 5** This IDC was initially missed by mammography. A large IDC and an intramammary lymph node are shown in **Figure 6**. Note the concordance between the UST images and mammography. **Figure 7** illustrates the chest wall access achievable by UST relative to mammography. Although UST does not access the entire axilla it does visualize the cancer that has invaded the chest wall.

3. MR concordance

UST and MR imaging was performed within weeks of each other. UST imaging was carried out with the SoftVue system (Delphinus Medical Technologies) and the MR exams with a Philips Achieva 3T system. The resulting image sequences were qualitatively and quantitatively to assess imaging performance of UST. As discussed above, UST images correlate best with MR images. Further inspection shows that of the three UST image types, the sound speed image correlates best with MR. **Figure 8** shows a coronal view comparison between UST speed of sound and MR contrast-enhanced fat subtracted images of representative breast parenchyma.

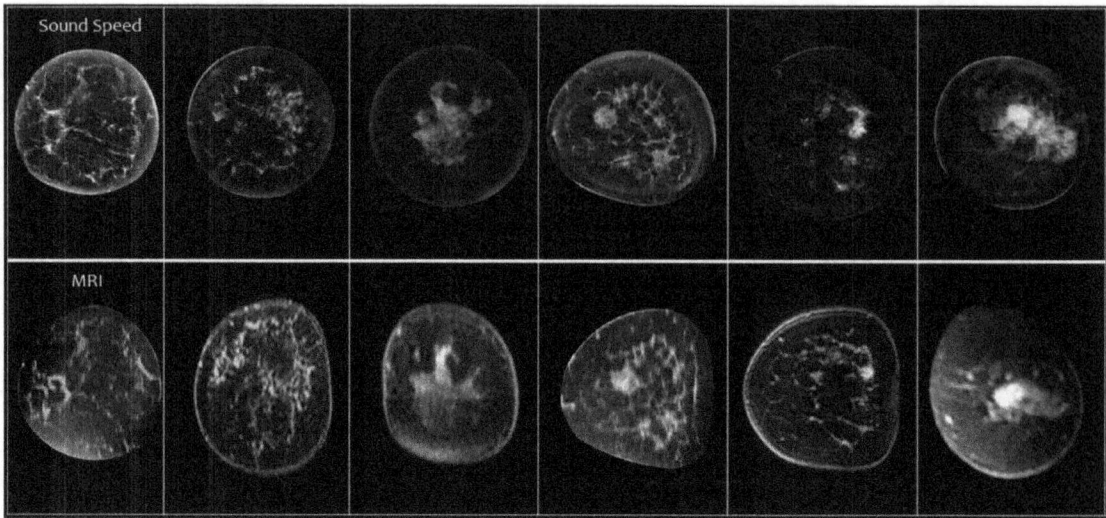

Figure 8. Top: Coronal UST sound speed images for six different patients. Bottom: Corresponding fat subtracted contrast-enhanced MR images.

The parenchymal patterns are very similar with the only major difference relating to the shape of the breast. This difference can be explained by the fact that the SoftVue system utilizes water so that buoyancy foreshortens the breast while with MR, gravity lengthens the breast in the AP dimension (i.e. prone).

As discussed above, UST images correlate best with MR images. Further inspection shows that of the three UST image types, the sound speed image correlates best with MR, as illustrated in **Figure 8**. The parenchymal patterns are very similar with the only major difference relating to the shape of the breast. This difference can be explained by the fact that the SoftVue system utilizes water so that the buoyancy force helps shape the breast while with MR, gravity shapes the breast.

4. Breast volume comparisons

MRI was used as the gold standard for defining the extent of the breast tissue. MRI and UST breast volumes were compared using a paired t-test. In the first step, a k-means segmentation algorithm was applied to T1 breast MR images to automatically separate out the non-tissue background. In the second step, the boundary between the breast tissue and the chest wall was drawn manually and the chest wall removed, leaving behind only breast tissue (**Figure 9**).

In the UST images a semi-automated tool was used to draw a boundary around the breast tissue in each coronal slice and everything outside the boundary removed (water signal). Any slices containing chest wall signal were also removed. The resulting stack of slices then represented the pure breast volume scanned by UST.

The two sets of volumes were plotted against each other as shown in **Figure 10**. The average breast volumes for MRI and UST were compared and the result shown in **Table 2**. As expected, the UST

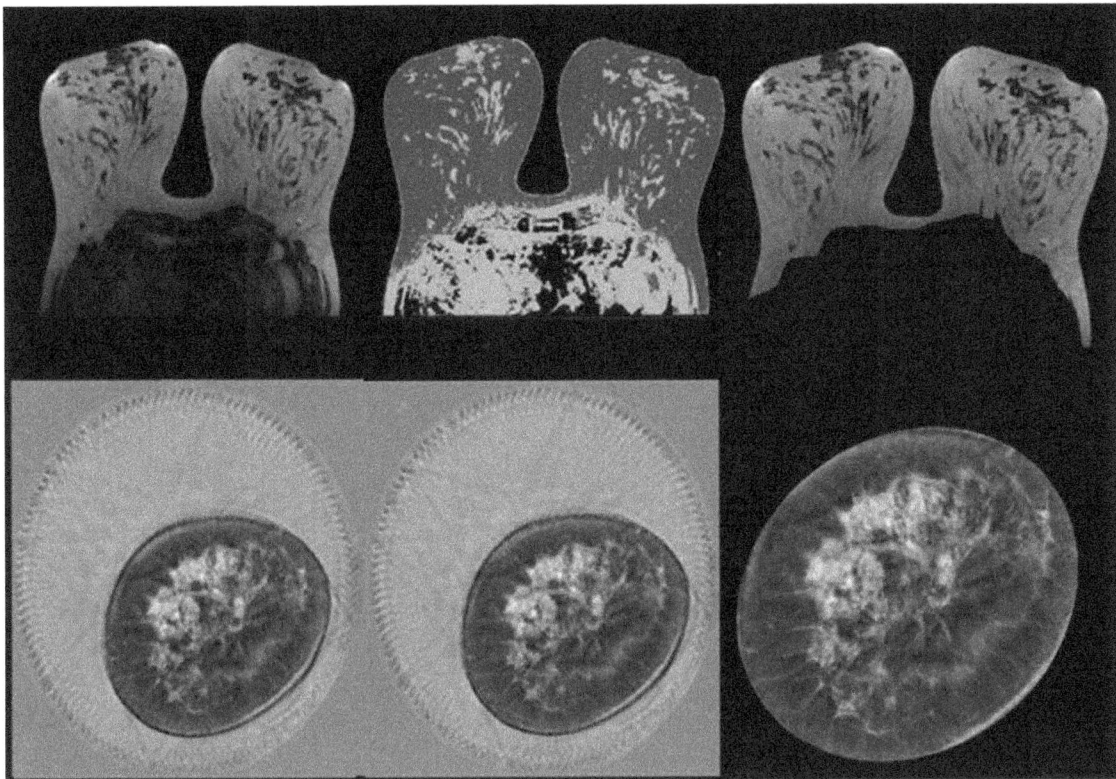

Figure 9. The segmentation process for MR images (top) and UST images (bottom). From left to right, original image, segmentation boundary and the final segmented image.

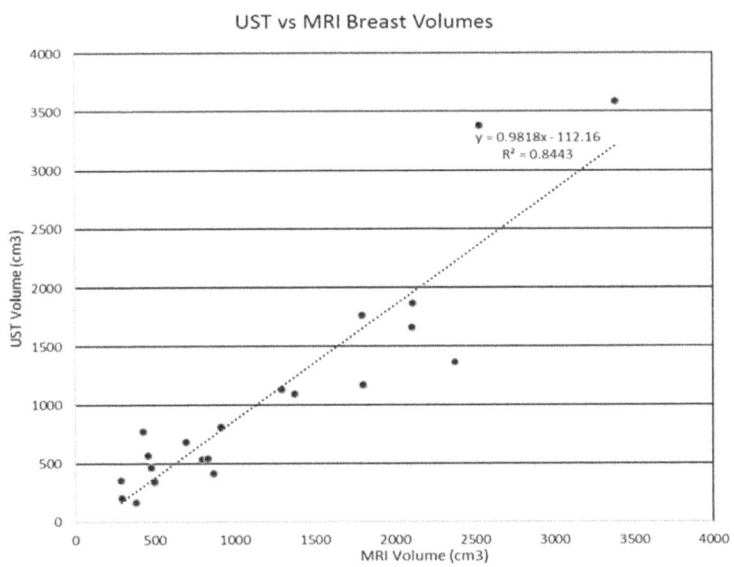

Figure 10. Correlation between UST and MR measured breast volumes.

Mean MRI volume (cm³)	Mean UST volume (cm³)	p Value
1224	1089	0.113

Table 2. Volume comparison.

scanned volume was less than that of MRI and was found to be about 89% of the MRI volume on average. However, a student's paired t-test indicates that this difference is not significant. Since UST cannot fully access the axilla, it is likely that the UST scanned volume is somewhat lower than that of MRI, even though UST generally reaches the pectoralis muscle at the chest wall.

5. Spatial resolution assessment

The spatial resolution of each modality was estimated using profile cuts of thin features using, the full-width, half-maximum criterion as shown in **Figure 11**. The results of the spatial resolution analysis are shown in **Table 3**. The spatial resolution was found to be dependent on the reprojection type for both MRI and with UST outperforming MRI in the coronal plane and MRI outperforming UST in the other projections. (However, MR acquisitions with isotropic voxels would show comparable resolution to UST in the coronal plane). The UST image voxels are not isotropic and data acquisition cannot be readily adjusted like MR, such that UST reconstructed in axial and sagittal planes have resolution that approach the 2.5 mm slice thickness at this time.

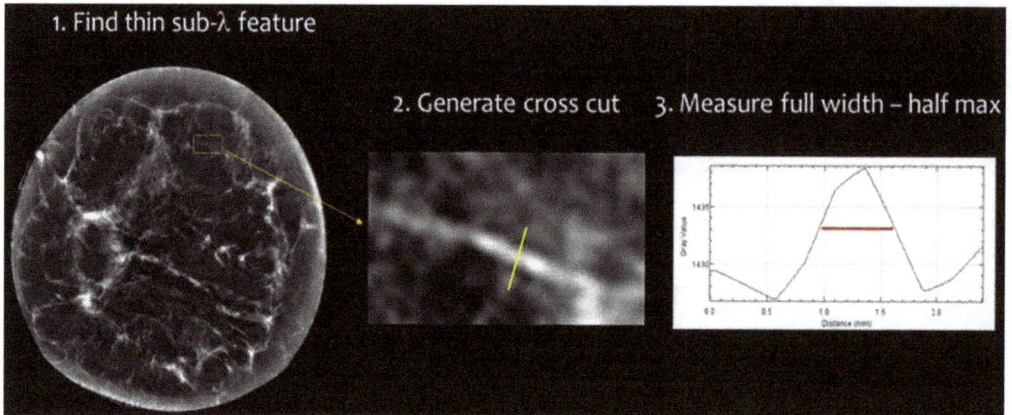

Figure 11. The spatial resolution of each modality was estimated using profile cuts of thin features using, the full-width, half-maximum criterion, as illustrated.

Resolution	UST	MRI
Coronal	0.7 ± 0.1 mm	1.6 ± 0.3 mm
Axial/sagittal	2.5 ± 0.5 mm	0.8 ± 0.1 mm

Table 3. Spatial resolution comparison.

6. Lesion characterization

Ultrasound breast imaging reporting and data system (US-BI-RADS) criteria are predominantly devoted to assessment of tumor shape, margins and interaction with adjacent tissue. However, criteria such as shadowing or enhanced through transmission are not applicable to UST's circular geometry. In addition, UST, operating at 3 MHz, appears more sensitive to the specular reflectors of benign mass capsules, or the spiculations and/or architectural distortions of many cancers. Therefore, we developed a 5-point scale that combined US-BI-RADS criteria for tumor margins, as well as possibilities for peritumoral tissue interaction (**Figure 12**).

Masses were characterized by a (i) Margin Boundary score, (ii) reflectivity, (iii) quantitative SS evaluation and (iv) ATT evaluations. A semi-automatic region-of-interest (ROI) tool was used to determine the quantitative properties of each mass. After identifying the mass of interest, a simple elliptical ROI is drawn around the mass. The ROI algorithm then generates 20 radial ellipsoids – 10 inside and 10 outside the mass. Quantitative information was then measured for each of the 20 annuli for subsequent analysis. The region of interest (ROI) analysis was performed on all identified lesions using all three UST image types. Combinations of the ROI generated values were used to characterize all masses in the study.

Ongoing analyses of the ROI tool have not yet led to full evaluation of second and third-order statistics of textural analyses, as well as their impacts upon decision analysis and predictive values. However, our recent RSNA presentation highlighted the significant impacts of first-order statistics such as standard deviation, within the tumoral ROI and comparisons with the surrounding peritumoral region [69]. Scatterplots and box plots of the optimal methods were used to illustrate the characterization potential. The box plot in **Figure 13** shows the differentiation achieved when using the boundary score (**Figure 6**) combined with the first-order statistic of standard deviation, a more crude measure of heterogeneity, based upon tumoral ROI extracted from ATT images, which had only slightly higher significance than SS [69]. These ROIs were again obtained by simply drawing an elliptical ROI around the mass and determining the standard deviation with in the ROI. The box plot was based on taking the average values for 107 benign lesions and 31 cancers [69].

Upon further investigation, it was found that the SS of the peritumoral mass region (defined by an annular area just outside the mass boundary ROI) further separated the benign masses from cancer. A scatter plot based on all of these parameters is shown in **Figure 14**. The scatter plot shows separately the cancers, fibroadenomas and cancers. The cancers are tightly

1	2	3	4	5
>2/3	1/3-2/3	<1/3	Irregular	Spiculation/Distortion

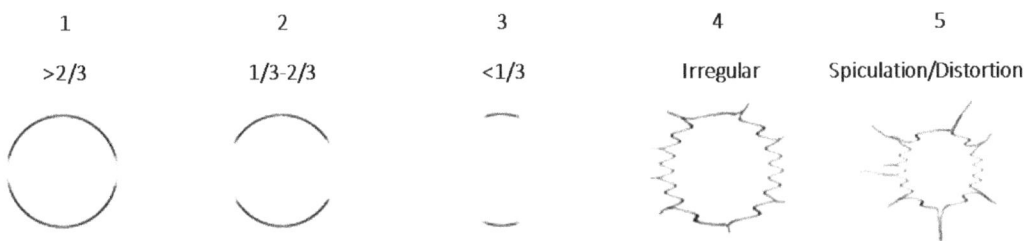

Figure 12. Schematic of shape and margin analysis and associated grading scheme.

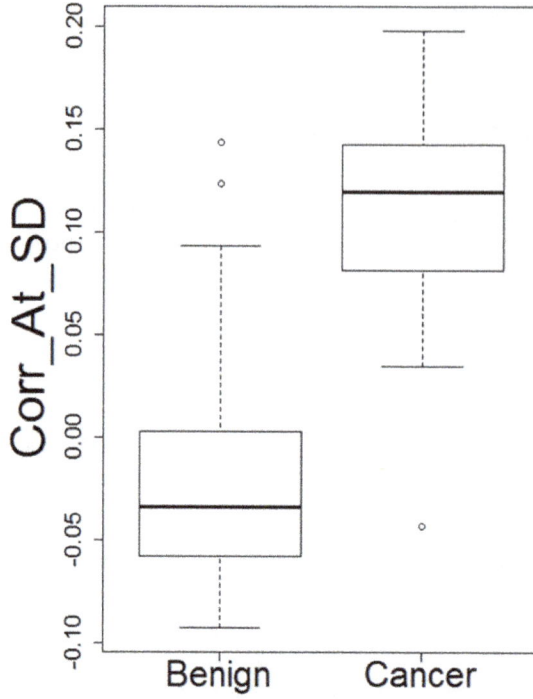

Figure 13. Separation of cancer from benign when using boundary score and hetrogeneity score.

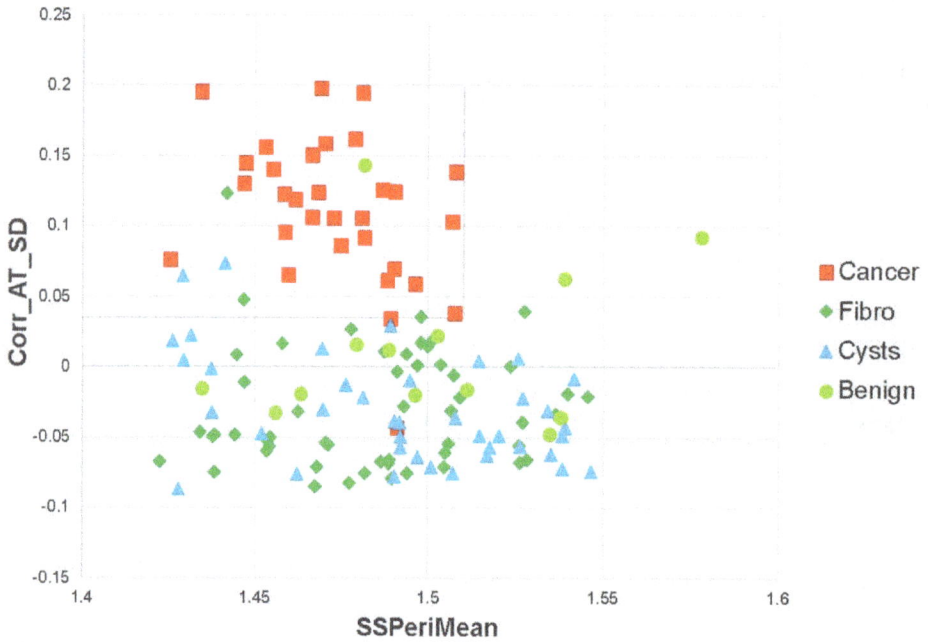

Figure 14. Scatter plot showing the distribution of cancers (squares), Fibroadenomas (diamonds), cysts (triangles) and other benign (circles).

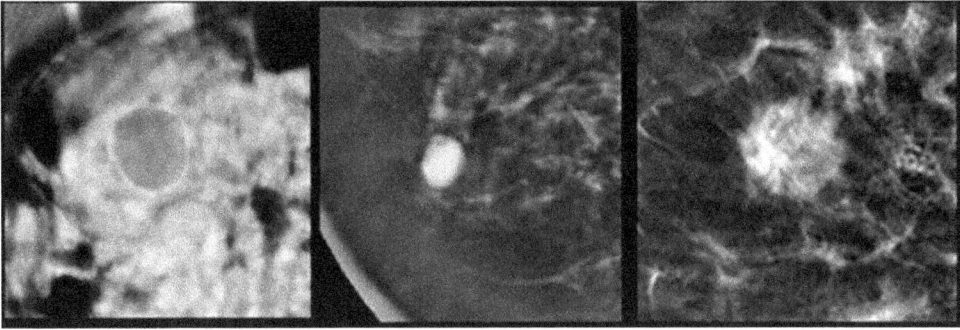

Figure 15. Cyst, fibroadenoma, cancer: Waveform SS images showing well circumscribed margins and smooth internal textures for both the 1.5 cm cyst in dense white breast tissue (left) and the 0.7 cm fibroadenoma (middle) in darker fat. The 1.8 cm cancer (right) has irregular margins, heterogeneous content and subtle peritumoral spiculations.

grouped in the top left corner of the plot indicating high boundary scores, high heterogeneity and lower peritumoral sound speed. By these measures, there was not much separation between cysts and fibroadenomas but significant separation between them and cancer. ROC analysis of the data represented in the scatter plot indicates a PPV of 91% when the sensitivity is 97%. However, this is a subset of data relative to an expanded ongoing study that includes more quantitative margin analyses. The ultimate goal is to generate textural analyses that will be less operator dependent and serve as appropriate diagnostic aids for a detected mass by simply requiring the radiologist to draw an ellipsoidal ROI. This method can also serve as a teaching tool for identifying grossly apparent textural differences within the tumor and surrounding peritumoral region. **Figure 15** shows the basic differences in sound speed texture noted for many cysts, fibroadenomas and cancer.

7. Conclusions

In this study we reviewed the status of breast cancer screening and the potential role that ultrasound tomography (UST) could play in breast imaging. Several results from recent ongoing UST studies were used in this review. The main conclusions from those studies are:

(i)   UST sound speed demonstrated a high degree of correlation of breast tissue structures relative to fat subtracted contrast-enhanced MRI. This correlation of structures was most evident in the coronal plane comparisons.

(ii) UST can scan ~90% of the volume of the breast compared to MRI. With proper positioning UST can image the pectoralis muscle and a portion of the axillary tissue.

(iii) UST demonstrated a spatial resolution of 0.7mm in the coronal plane, similar to MRI.

(iv) Initial clinical results suggest an ability to characterize lesions using margin boundary scores in combination with sound speed and attenuation parameters. These parameters leverage all three imaging modes of UST (reflection, sound speed and attenuation).

UST is a promising new modality that has the potential to complement existing breast imaging methods to aid in lesion detection and characterization. Future larger scale studies will assess UST's role in diagnostic and screening settings.

Acknowledgements

The authors thank Dr. Mark Sak for providing images relating to the MRI comparison study and Mr. Mark Krycia for his help in the statistical analysis of the lesion characterization data. The work presented in this paper was supported by NIH grant 5R44CA165320-05.

Author details

Nebojsa Duric[1]* and Peter Littrup[2]

*Address all correspondence to: duric@karmanos.org

1 Karmanos Cancer Institute, Wayne State University, Detroit, MI, USA

2 Crittenton Hospital, Troy, MI, USA

References

[1] Surveillance, Epidemiology, and End Results Program. Available from: http://seer.cancer.gov/

[2] American Cancer Society. Cancer Prevention & Early Detection Facts & Figures 2009. Atlanta, GA: American Cancer Society; 2009. pp. 34-37

[3] Ernster VL, Barclay J, Kerlikowske K, Wilkie H, Ballard-Barbash R. Mortality among women with ductal carcinoma in situ of the breast in the population-based surveillance, epidemiology and end results program. Archives of Internal Medicine. 2000;**160**(7): 953-958

[4] Chen TH, Yen AM, Fann JC, Gordon P, Chen SL, Chiu SY, Hsu CY, Chang KJ, Lee WC, Yeoh KG, Saito H, Promthet S, Hamashima C, Maidin A, Robinson F, Zhao LZ. Clarifying the debate on population-based screening for breast cancer with mammography: A systematic review of randomized controlled trials on mammography with Bayesian meta-analysis and causal model. Medicine (Baltimore). 2017;**96**:e5684

[5] Boyd NF, Guo H, Martin LJ, Sun L, Stone J, Fishell E, Jong RA, Hislop G, Chiarelli A, Minkin S, et al. Mammographic density and the risk and detection of breast cancer. The New England Journal of Medicine. 2007;**356**:227-236

[6] Chen J, Pee D, Ayyagari R, Graubard B, Schairer C, Byrne C, Benichou J, Gail MH. Projecting absolute invasive breast cancer risk in white women with a model that includes mammographic density. Journal of the National Cancer Institute. 2006;**98**:1215-1226

[7]   Ursin G, Hovanessian-Larsen L, Parisky YR, Pike MC, Wu AH. Greatly increased occurrence of breast cancers in areas of mammographically dense tissue. Breast Cancer Research. 2005;**7**:R605-R608

[8]   Martin LJ, Boyd N. Potential mechanisms of breast cancer risk associated with mammographic density: Hypotheses based on epidemiological evidence. Breast Cancer Research. 2008;**10**:1-14

[9]   Armstrong K, Moye E, Williams S, Berlin JA, Reynolds EE. Screening mammography in women 40 to 49 years of age: A systematic review for the American College of Physicians. Annals of Internal Medicine. 2007;**146**:516-526

[10] Breast Cancer Screening (PDQ®)–Health Professional Version. http://www.cancer.gov/cancertopics/pdq/screening/breast/healthprofessional/page7

[11] Friedewald SM, Rafferty EA, Rose SL, Durand MA, Plecha DM, Greenberg JS, Hayes MK, Copit DS, Carlson KL, Cink TM, Barke LD, Greer LN, Miller DP, Conant EF. Breast cancer screening using tomosynthesis in combination with digital mammography. Journal of the American Medical Association. 2014;**311**(24):2499-2507

[12] Hendrick RE. Radiation doses and cancer risks from breast imaging Radiology. 2010;**257**(1): 246-253

[13] Turnbull LW. Dynamic contrast-enhanced MRI in the diagnosis and management of breast cancer. Journal of Biomolecular NMR. 2008

[14] Jansen SA, Fan X, Karczmar GS, Abe H, Schmidt RA, Newstead GM. Differentiation between benign and malignant breast lesions detected by bilateral dynamic contrast-enhanced MRI: A sensitivity and specificity study. Magnetic Resonance in Medicine. 2008;**59**(4):747. John Wiley & Sons, Ltd

[15] Kuhl CK, Schrading S, Bieling HB, Wardelmann E, Leutner CC, Koenig R, Kuhn W, Schild HH. MRI for diagnosis of pure ductal carcinoma in situ: A prospective observational study. The Lancet. 2007;**370**:485-492

[16] Saslow D, Boetes C, Burke W, Harms S, Leach MO, Lehman CD, Morris E, Pisano E, Schnall M, Sener S, Smith RA, Warner E, Yaffe M, Andrews KS, Russell CA; American Cancer Society Breast Cancer Advisory Group. American Cancer Society guidelines for breast screening with MRI as an adjunct to mammography. CA: A Cancer Journal for Clinicians. 2007;**57**:75-89

[17] Chen JH, et al. MRI evaluation of pathologically complete response and residual tumors in breast cancer after neoadjuvant chemotherapy. Cancer. 2008;**112**(1):17-26

[18] Sharma U, et al. Longitudinal study of the assessment by MRI and diffusion-weighted imaging of tumor response in patients with locally advanced breast cancer undergoing neoadjuvant chemotherapy. NMR in Biomedicine. 2009;**22**(1):104-113

[19] Bando H, et al. Imaging evaluation of pathological response in breast cancer after neoadjuvant chemotherapy by real-time sonoelastography and MRI. European Journal of Cancer-Supplement. 2008;**6**(7):66-66

[20] Bhattacharyya M, et al. Using MRI to plan breast-conserving surgery following neo-adjuvant chemotherapy for early breast cancer. British Journal of Cancer. 2008;**98**(2): 289-293

[21] Partridge S. Recurrence rates after DCE-MRI image guided planning for breast-conserving surgery following neoadjuvant chemotherapy for locally advanced breast cancer patients. Breast Diseases: A Year Book Quarterly. 2008;**19**(1):91-91

[22] Tozaki M. Diagnosis of breast cancer: MDCT versus MRI. Breast Cancer. 2008;**15**(3):205-211

[23] Partridge S, et al. Accuracy of MR imaging for revealing residual breast cancer in patients who have undergone neoadjuvant chemotherapy. American Roentgen Ray Society. 2002;**172**:1193-1199

[24] Brem RF, Tabár L, Duffy SW, Inciardi MF, Guingrich JA, Hashimoto BE, Lander MR, Lapidus RL, Peterson MK, Rapelyea JA, Roux S, Schilling KJ, Shah BA, Torrente J, Wynn RT, Miller DP. Assessing improvement in detection of breast cancer with three-dimensional automated breast US in women with dense breast tissue: The SomoInsight Study. Radiology. 2015 Mar;**274**(3):663-673

[25] Berg WA, Zhang Z, Lehrer D, Jong RA, Pisano ED, Barr RG, Böhm-Vélez M, Mahoney MC, Evans WP 3rd, Larsen LH, Morton MJ, Mendelson EB, Farria DM, Cormack JB, Marques HS, Adams A, Yeh NM, Gabrielli G; ACRIN 6666 Investigators. Detection of breast cancer with addition of annual screening ultrasound or a single screening MRI to mammography in women with elevated breast cancer risk. Journal of the American Medical Association. 2012 Apr 4;**307**(13):1394-1404

[26] Hooley RJ, Greenberg KL, Stackhouse RM, Geisel JL, Butler RS, Philpotts LE. Screening US in patients with mammographically dense breasts: Initial experience with Connecticut Public Act 09-41. Radiology. 2012 Oct;**265**(1):59-69

[27] Kelly KM, Dean J, Comulada WS, Lee SJ. Breast cancer detection using automated whole breast ultrasound and mammography in radiographically dense breasts. European Radiology. 2010 Mar;**20**(3):734-742

[28] Corsetti V, Houssami N, Ferrari A, Ghirardi M, Bellarosa S, Angelini O, Bani C, Sardo P, Remida G, Galligioni E, Ciatto S. Breast screening with ultrasound in women with mammography-negative dense breasts: Evidence on incremental cancer detection and false positives, and associated cost. European Journal of Cancer. 2008 Mar;**44**(4):539-544

[29] Crystal P, Strano SD, Shcharynski S, Koretz MJ. Using sonography to screen women with mammographically dense breasts. American Journal of Roentgenology. 2003 Jul;**181**(1):177-182

[30] Leconte I, Feger C, Galant C, Berlière M, Berg BV, D'Hoore W, Maldague B. Mammography and subsequent whole-breast sonography of non palpable breast cancers: The importance of radiologic breast density. American Journal of Roentgenology. 2003 Jun;**180**(6):1675-1679

[31] Kolb TM, Lichy J, Newhouse JH. Comparison of the performance of screening mammography, physical examination, and breast US and evaluation of factors that influence them: An analysis of 27,825 patient evaluations. Radiology. 2002 Oct;**225**(1):165-175

[32] Kaplan SS. Clinical utility of bilateral whole-breast US in the evaluation of women with dense breast tissue. Radiology. 2001 Dec;**221**(3):641-649

[33] Buchberger W, Niehoff A, Obrist P, DeKoekkoek-Doll P, Dünser M. Clinically and mammographically occult breast lesions: Detection and classification with high-resolution sonography. Seminars in ultrasound, CT, and MR. 2000 Aug;**21**(4):325-336

[34] Gordon PB, Goldenberg SL. Malignant breast masses detected only by ultrasound. A retrospective review. Cancer. 1995 Aug 15;**76**(4):626-630

[35] Ernster VL, Ballard-Barbash R, Barlow WE, Zheng Y, Weaver DL, et al. Detection of ductal carcinoma *in situ* in women undergoing screening mammography. Journal of the National Cancer Institute. 2002;**94**:1546-1554

[36] Johnson S, et al. From laboratory to clinical trials: An odyssey of ultrasound inverse scattering imaging for breast cancer diagnosis. The Journal of the Acoustical Society of America. 2006;**120**:3023

[37] Johnson SA and Tracy ML. Inverse scattering solutions by a sinc basis, multiple source, moment method. Part I: Theory, Ultrasonic Imaging. 1983;**5**:361-375

[38] Schreiman JS, Gisvold JJ, Greenleaf JF, Bahn RC. Ultrasound transmission computed tomography of the breast. Radiology. 1984;**150**:523-530

[39] Natterer FA. Propagation backpropagation method for ultrasound tomography. Inverse Problems. 1995;**11**:1225-1232

[40] Carson PL, Meyer CR, Scherzinger AL, Oughton TV. Breast imaging in coronal planes with simultaneous pulse echo and transmission ultrasound. Science. 1981 Dec 4;**214**(4525): 1141-1143

[41] Andre MP, Janee HS, Martin PJ, Otto GP, Spivey BA, Palmer DA. High-speed data acquisition in a diffraction tomography system employing large-scale toroidal arrays. International Journal of Imaging Systems and Technology. 1997;**8**:137-147

[42] Johnson SA, Borup DT, Wiskin JW, Natterer F, Wuebbling F, Zhang Y, Olsen C. Apparatus and Method for Imaging with Wavefields using Inverse Scattering Techniques. United States Patent 6,005,916; 1999

[43] Marmarelis VZ, Kim T, Shehada RE. Proceedings of the SPIE: Medical Imaging 2003; San Diego, California; Feb 23-28, 2002. Ultrasonic Imaging and Signal Processing – Paper 5035-6

[44] Liu DL, Waag RC. Propagation and backpropagation for ultrasonic wavefront design. IEEE Transactions on Ultrasonics, Ferroelectrics, and Frequency Control. 1997;**44**(1):1-13

[45] Liu D, Waag R. Harmonic amplitude distribution in a wideband ultrasonic wavefront after propagation through human abdominal wall and breast specimens. The Journal of the Acoustical Society of America. 1997;**101**:1172

[46] Duric N, Littrup PJ, Poulo L, et al. Detection of breast cancer with ultrasound tomography: First results with the computed Ultrasound Risk Evaluation (UST) prototype. Medical Physics. 2007;**34**:773-785

[47] Boyd NF, et al. Breast tissue composition and susceptibility to breast cancer. JNCI: Journal of the National Cancer Institute (0027-8874). 2010;**102**(16):1224. (Review Article)

[48] Glide C, Duric N, Littrup P. Novel approach to evaluating breast density utilizing ultrasound tomography. Medical Physics. 2007;**34**(2):744-753

[49] Glide-Hurst CK, Duric N, Littrup P. Volumetric breast density evaluation from ultrasound tomography images. Medical Physics. 2008;**35**(9):3988-3997

[50] Myc L, Duric N, Littrup P, Li C, Ranger B, Lupinacci J, Schmidt S, et al. Volumetric breast density evaluation by Ultrasound Tomography and Magnetic Resonance Imaging: A preliminary comparative study. Proceedings of SPIE. 2010;**7629**:76290N

[51] Li C, Duric N, Huang L. Clinical breast imaging using sound-speed reconstructions of ultrasound tomography data. Proceedings of SPIE. 2008;**6920**:6920-69309

[52] Li C, Duric N, Huang L. Comparison of ultrasound attenuation tomography techniques for breast cancer diagnosis. Proceedings of SPIE. 2008;**6920**:6920-6949

[53] Li C, Huang L, Duric N, Zhang H, Rowe C. An improved automatic time-of-flight picker for medical ultrasound tomography. Ultrasonics. (Accepted)

[54] Duric N, Littrup P, Li C, Rama O, Bey-Knight L, Schmidt S, Lupinacci J. Detection and characterization of breast masses with ultrasound tomography: Clinical results. Proceedings of SPIE: Medical Imaging. 2009;**7265**:72651G-1-8

[55] Simonetti F, Huang L, Duric N. A multiscale approach to diffraction tomography of complex three-dimensional objects. Applied Physics Letters (0003-6951). 2009;**95**(6):061904

[56] Simonetti F, Huang L, Duric N, Littrup P. Diffraction and coherence in breast ultrasound tomography: A study with a toroidal array. Medical Physics. 2009;**36**(7):2955-2965

[57] Duric N, Littrup P, Chandiwala-Mody P, Li C, Schmidt S, et al. In-vivo imaging results with ultrasound tomography: Report on an ongoing study at the Karmanos Cancer Institute. Proceedings of SPIE. 2010;**7629**:76290M

[58] Ranger B, Littrup P, Duric N, Li C, Lupinacci J, Myc L, Rama O, Bey-Knight L. Breast imaging with acoustic tomography: A comparative study with MRI. Proceedings of SPIE: Medical Imaging. 2009;**7265**:726510-1-8

[59] Ranger B, Littrup P, Duric N, Li C, Schmidt S, et al. Breast imaging with ultrasound tomography: A comparative study with MRI. Proceedings of SPIE. 2010;**7629**:76291C

[60] Ranger B, Littrup PJ, Duric N, Chandiwala-Mody P, Li C, Schmidt S, Lupinacci J. Breast ultrasound tomography versus magnetic resonance imaging for clinical display of anatomy and tumor rendering: Preliminary results. American Journal of Roentgenology. 2012;**198**(1):233

[61] Schmidt S, Huang Z, Duric N, Li C, Roy O. Modification of Kirchhoff migration with variable sound speed and attenuation for acoustic imaging of media and application to tomographic imaging of the breast. Medical Physics. 2011;**38**:998

[62] Entrekin RR, Porter BA, Sillesen HH, Wong AD, Cooperberg PL, Fix CH. Real-time spatial compound imaging application to breast, vascular, and musculoskeletal ultrasound. Seminars in Ultrasound, CT, and MR. 2001;**22**:50-64

[63] Stavros AT, Thickman D, Rapp CL, Dennis MA, Parker SH, Sisney G. Solid breast nodules: Use of sonography to distinguish between benign and malignant lesions. Radiology. 1995;**196**(1):123-134

[64] Greenleaf JF, Johnson SA, Bahn RC, Rajagopalan B. Quantitative cross-sectional imaging of ultrasound parameters. 1977 Ultrasonics Symposium Proc., IEEE Cat. # 77CH1264-1SU; 1977. pp. 989-995

[65] Goss SA, Johnston RL and Dunn F. Comprehensive compilation of empirical ultrasonic properties of mammalian tissues. The Journal of the Acoustical Society of America. 1978;**64**:423-457

[66] Duck FA. Physical Properties of Tissue. London: Academic Press; 1990

[67] Edmonds PD, Mortensen CL, Hill JR, Holland SK, Jensen JF, Schattner P, Valdes AD. Ultrasound tissue characterization of breast biopsy specimens. Ultrasound Imaging. 1991;**13**:162-185

[68] Weiwad W, Heinig A, Goetz L, Hartmann H, Lampe D, Buchman J, et al. Direct measurement of sound velocity in various specimens of breast tissue. Investigative Radiology. 2000;**35**:721-726

[69] Littrup PJ, Duric N, Brem RF, Yamashita MW. Improving specificity of whole breast ultrasound using tomographic techniques. Paper SSA02-05. Presented at Radiology Society of North America, Nov 27, 2016

5

Incorporating Breast Asymmetry Studies into CADx Systems

José María Celaya Padilla,
Cesar Humberto Guzmán Valdivia,
Jorge Issac Galván Tejada, Carlos Eric Galván Tejada,
Hamurabi Gamboa Rosales,
Juan Rubén Delgado Contreras,
Antonio Martinez-Torteya, Roberto Olivera Reyna,
Jorge Roberto Manjarrez Sánchez,
Francisco Javier Martinez Ruiz, Idalia Garza-Veloz,
Margarita L. Martinez-Fierro, Victor Treviño and
Jose Gerardo Tamez-Peña

Abstract

Breast cancer is one of the global leading causes of death among women, and an early detection is of uttermost importance to reduce mortality rates. Screening mammograms, in which radiologists rely only on their eyesight, are one of the most used early detection methods. However, characteristics, such as the asymmetry between breasts, a feature that could be very difficult to visually quantize, is key to breast cancer detection. Due to the highly heterogeneous and deformable structure of the breast itself, incorporating asymmetry measurements into an automated detection system is still a challenge. In this study, we proposed the use of a bilateral registration algorithm as an effective way to automatically measure mirror asymmetry. Furthermore, this information was fed to a machine learning algorithm to improve the accuracy of the model. In this study, 449 subjects (197 with calcifications, 207 with masses, and 45 healthy subjects) from a public database were used to train and evaluate the proposed methodology. Using this procedure, we were able to independently identify subjects with calcifications (accuracy = 0.825, AUC = 0.882) and masses (accuracy = 0.698, AUC = 0.807) from healthy subjects.

Keywords: breast cancer, asymmetry, bilateral registration, CAD

1. Introduction

Cancer is one of the leading causes of death worldwide. In 2008, nearly 13% (7.6 million) of all deaths were cancer related. Among all types of cancer, lung, liver, colon, breast, and cervical are the most frequent ones. Recent studies predict 13.1 million cancer deaths for 2030 [1]. Among women, breast cancer is the deadliest type of cancer. Nearly 1.8% of all worldwide deaths are breast cancer related [2].

Till today, there is no cure for breast cancer, and since the trigger to develop any type of cancer is still a mystery, there is not an effective way to prevent the occurrence. Early detection of breast cancer plays a key role in a positive prognosis. There are several imaging technologies that might be used by specialists for the early detection of breast cancer, such as magnetic resonance imaging, ultrasound, and X-ray mammogram. The last technique is the primary tool used to diagnose and detect breast cancer worldwide, and it has been proved to be the best cost-effective tool to diagnose the disease [3].

In clinical practice, mammography allows for the detection of early signs of tumors before they become apparent [3]. Common signs of early cancer inside the breast tissue are micro-calcifications, architectural distortions, and masses [4]. During the screening procedure, radiologists use those signs to generate a standardized evaluation of the risk of cancer in a given patient, called Breast Imaging-Reporting and Data System (BI-RADS). This report helps oncologists to decide a course of action among women at risk of developing breast cancer [5].

The broad use of mammogram has driven the development of computer-aided detection (CADe) and computer-aided diagnosis (CADx) systems. While both approaches aim to assist radiologists to detect and diagnose breast cancer as early as possible, CADx systems are used as a second opinion [6] and CADe ones aim to improve visualization of the lesions (with up to 35% improvement in detection rate [7]). However, although it has been shown that CADe systems have helped radiologists to better interpret findings [8], it has also been demonstrated that in some cases they may make interpreting the images more difficult, reducing the accuracy of early cancer detection [7]. Furthermore, these systems also may increase the workload of the radiologists [8].

A typical CADe system, whose workflow is shown in **Figure 1**, consists of two algorithms applied sequentially, one to detect suspicious regions or regions of interest (ROI), and one to refine such regions. The former includes the preprocessing of the images, segmentation of

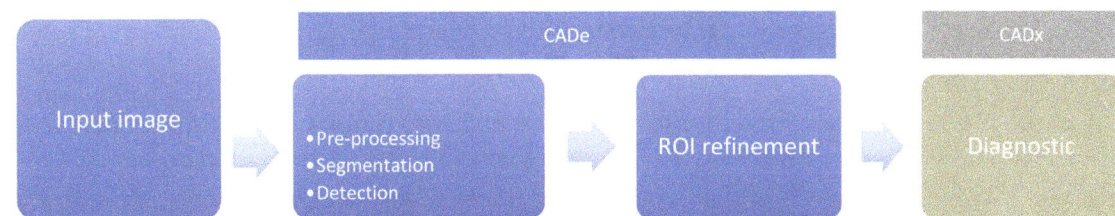

Figure 1. Typical workflow of a CADe/CADx system, adapted from Chen g et al. [13].

the breast tissue, and the detection of the ROI itself. The latter process is performed to reduce the number of false positives [8], and usually relies on machine learning techniques [9–11]. Lastly, the results are presented to the radiologist, highlighting in the original mammography the regions that the analysis deemed highly suspicious. As seen in the same image, CADx systems follow the same workflow as CADe ones. However, besides highlighting areas of higher risk to the radiologist, additional algorithms are used to analyze each ROI and generate a computer-based diagnosis. It is important to mention that, currently, few CADe and CADx commercial systems have been approved by the Food and Drug Administration of the United States of America [12].

Many methodologies used by CADx systems analyze only one breast, or even just a subregion of the breast, at a time. That is, they evaluate the left and right breasts as independent objects, unlike radiologists, who analyze images of both breasts simultaneously to evaluate their asymmetry. Radiologists do so because asymmetry is related to early signs of breast cancer (i.e. parenchymal distortion, bright spots, masses, etc.) [14, 15] and it may be used to reduce the rate of false positive detection of masses [16, 17]. Asymmetry can refer to either a longitudinal study, where current and prior mammograms are compared, or a bilateral study, where differences between the left and right breast are analyzed.

A few CADx systems have already tried to incorporate asymmetry studies to enhance diagnosis [14, 18–20]. Some researchers have studied the use of a feature-based asymmetry analysis, where the mammograms are processed individually and the differences between the individual analyses are used as a mean to quantify asymmetry [21]. This approach has also been used to characterize risk factors, such as breast density, and predict near-term breast cancer [14].

Another method that evaluates asymmetry, this one trying to mimic the approach used by radiologists, is the mammogram subtraction. In this approach, differences between mammograms are enhanced by performing a rigid registration (alignment) of the images. However, this methodology was originally employed only in longitudinal studies [22], comparing the same breast at two different times, since the highly heterogeneous and deformable tissue of the breast has hindered the inclusion of subtraction approaches in bilateral asymmetry studies [19].

Miller et al. [23] proposed a technique for the detection of bilateral symmetry using a semi-automated texture-based procedure that segments the glandular tissue, measuring the shape between views, and thus detecting the occurrence of asymmetries. The algorithm obtained an accuracy of 0.867 on a validation dataset of 30 screening mammogram pairs. Later, Miller et al. [24] presented a method for the detection of bilateral asymmetry based on measures of shape, topology, and distribution of brightness. This method was tested on 104 mammogram pairs, yielding a classification accuracy of 0.74.

Lau et al. [25] proposed a method for the detection of breast tumors that extracted measures of brightness, roughness, and directionality, and was based on localized asymmetry. This method was evaluated using 10 pairs of mammograms where asymmetry was a significant factor in the radiologist's diagnosis. A sensitivity of 0.92 was obtained, with 4.9 false positives per mammogram. However, the alignment was tuned manually using control points.

Ferrari et al. [26] characterized asymmetry as variations in oriented textural patterns, obtained using directional filtering with Gabor wavelets at different orientations and scales. Using a database with 80 images resulted in a classification accuracy of up to 0.744.

Rodriguez-Rojas et al. [21] presented a CADx system targeted to detect high-risk cancer patients. To do so, automated breast tissue segmentations were performed on 200 Mexican subjects labeled as either low- or high-risk according to their BI-RADS score. Then, 50 features were extracted, and bilateral differences between mammograms were defined by subtracting corresponding features in both mammograms. Finally, a genetic algorithm selected a predictive combination of features. Using this methodology, they were able to classify low-risk and high-risk cases with an area under the receiver operating characteristic (ROC) curve (AUC) of 0.88 on a 150-fold cross-validation set. The features included in the model were associated with the differences in signal distribution and tissue shape.

In summary, and as presented, most asymmetry detection methods are either feature-based, rely on simple bilateral subtraction techniques [14, 27], or depend on an ROI provided by a radiologist [24, 25]. Thus, in order to efficiently measure asymmetry, a better and automatic registration must be performed [28]. To do so, alignment has been improved by using the nipple as a reference point [29] and by co-registering both breasts using a robust point matching approach [22]. Nevertheless, none of those works include a fully automated bilateral registration. In this chapter, a methodology that incorporates an automatic asymmetry analysis with both a feature-based and a pixel-wise bilateral subtraction into a CADx system is presented.

2. Methodology

The proposed methodology follows the CADx workflow presented in the previous section. However, asymmetry measurements are used to aid in the diagnosis. To obtain such measurements, two additional stages are incorporated into the workflow: registration and pixel-wise subtraction. Additionally, a series of image transformations are incorporated to enhance different characteristics of the breast in the mammograms. This work is based on and follows previous efforts [30–32].

Figure 2 shows how the bilateral asymmetry information was incorporated into the CADx system. Briefly, soft tissue is first segmented, the image of the left breast is then registered to its right counterpart and a bilateral subtraction of the co-registered images is performed;

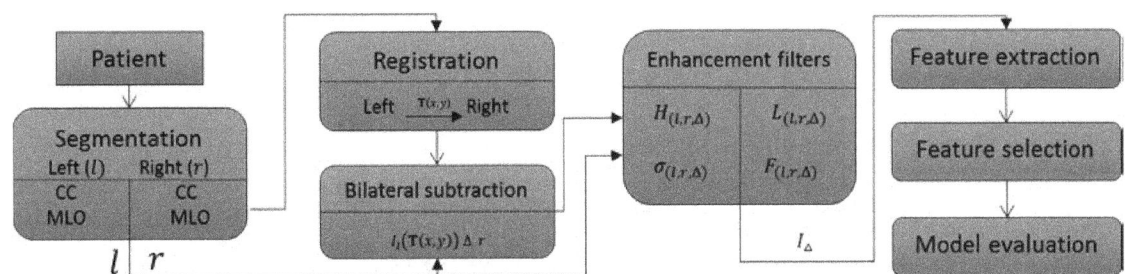

Figure 2. Workflow of the proposed methodology.

images are then filtered and features are extracted; a multivariate model is selected using a train set; and finally, the model is evaluated on a validation set. A detailed explanation of each stage is presented in the following sections.

2.1. Materials

A total of 1796 digitalized film mammograms from 449 different subjects were used. From those, 45 were classified as healthy subjects (HS) (mean age of 59.3 and standard deviation (SD) of 9.8 years), 197 as subjects with malignant calcifications (CS) (mean age of 58 and SD of 10.9 years), and 207 as subjects with malignant masses (MS) (mean age of 64.1 and SD of 10.1 years). Each subject had the four standard mammograms taken, namely, left and right craniocaudal (CC), and left and right mediolateral oblique (MLO) projections.

In order to avoid problems associated with intra-scanner variability [17, 22, 33], all mammograms in this study were obtained from the Howtek dataset of the Digital Database for Screening Mammography public database [34], in which all mammograms were digitalized using a Howtek 960 scanner using a sampling rate of 43.5 micrometers per pixel and a 12-bit depth.

2.2. Segmentation

Segmentation, also called categorization by computer vision definitions, allows delimiting one or several parts of a given image assigning one class label (e.g. bone, muscle, fat, skin, calcification, and mass). This process is defined by the division or segmentation of the image into several homogeneous regions disjointed from their surroundings. A commonly used automatic segmentation of the breast tissue is based on the estimation of the background noise. For this study, an initial segmentation mask was created by estimating the background noise in the image and discarding all pixels below five standard deviations of the noise level. Then, holes were removed by applying closing morphological operations with a 3×3 supporting region, as described by Eq. (1):

$$S(A) = (A(x,y) \oplus B(x,y)) \ominus B(x,y) \tag{1}$$

where $\oplus$ and $\ominus$ are the grayscale dilation and erosion morphological operations, respectively. $B(x,y)$ is a 3×3 structural element. $A(x,y)$ is the image being segmented and $S(A)$ is the resulting segmentation of the $A(x,y)$ image. The largest connected region is used as the segmentation mask while all other high-intensity regions are removed from the images. **Figure 3** shows an example of the results of the segmentation procedure.

2.3. Registration

Image registration can be defined as the intensity and spatial mapping between two images [35]. Given two input images F and M, image registration can be expressed as $R' = g[T(F)]$, where T is a spatial transformation function, g an intensity transformation function, and R' the registered image. The transformation function is not always necessary; a lookup table can be used to pinpoint intensities. A visual example of image registration is presented in **Figure 4**, where an image M is being registered to match image F.

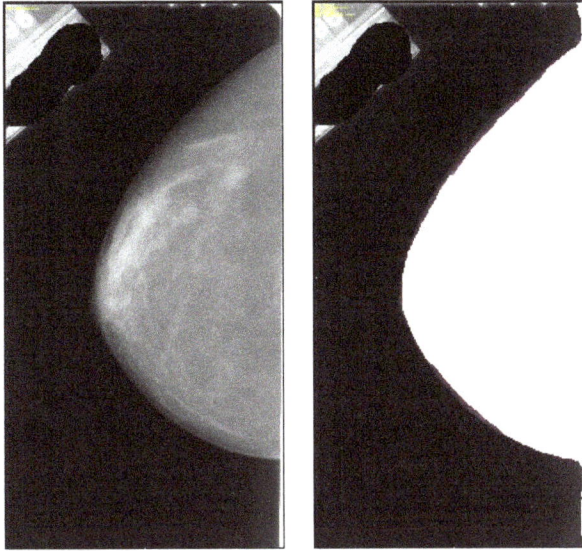

Figure 3. Segmentation of breast tissue. The image on the left is the original CC mammogram and the image on the right shows the superimposed segmentation mask in white (image from Ref. [32]).

Image registration has been widely used in medical applications [28, 36, 37]. However, the soft nature of the breast tissue makes them highly deformable, and rigid registration procedures, in which only rotation, translation, and scaling functions are used, are not sufficient. Therefore, nonrigid registration methods are necessary [38, 39]. There are many approaches to deal with medical imaging registration, the most recent comparison of algorithms based on a retrospective evaluation was published by West et al. [40], but it was constrained to do intra-patient rigid registration. Also recently, Diez et al. [28] and Celaya-Padilla et al. [30] compared registration algorithms with breast images as a source, and both concluded that the B-Splines approach was the most consistent.

Breast image registration based on a B-Splines transformation is defined as follows: given two input images (F = target image, M = image being registered), M is deformed by modifying a mesh of control points following a maximization of a similarity measure based on steepest descent gradient [6, 15]. The deformed image is compared to F using a similarity metric. If the images are similar enough, the process stops. Otherwise, the process reiterates.

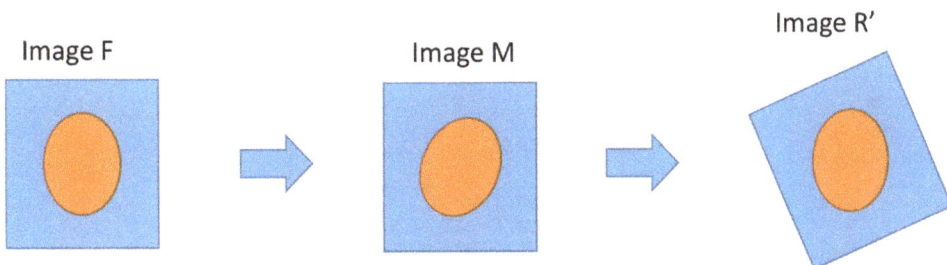

Figure 4. Basic example of an image registration procedure. F is the target image, M is the image to be registered, and R' is the registered image.

Figure 5 shows a multi-resolution pyramid approach [41] for the B-Spline implementation. There, the images are first registered using low-resolution images, the B-Spline transformation parameters are moved into the next higher resolution and parameter optimization is run again, and so on. This often avoids issues with local minima in the parameter search space and reduces computational time [15].

For this study, the image to be registered was first horizontally flipped. Then, both the moving image and the target image were resampled into a lower resolution image. Next, the pyramids for the multi-resolution were generated. Afterwards, the registration process detailed in **Figure 5** was carried out. And finally, the original moving image was deformed using the final parameters of the registration. For this implementation, mutual information [39] was used as the similarity metric. In **Figure 6**, the checkerboard of an example result from the B-Spline registration procedure is presented. There, it can be seen that the registered image was successfully aligned with its counterpart.

2.4. Image subtraction

Once the images were co-registered, a pixel-wise absolute difference was computed between the left and right images, as defined by Eq. (2) as follows:

$$I_{\triangle}(x, y) \; = \; \left| I_r(x, y) - I_l(T(x, y)) \right| \tag{2}$$

where $I_r(x, y)$ represents the right image, $I_l(T(x, y))$ represents the left image registered to the right image space, and $I_{\triangle}(x, y)$ represents the map of absolute differences. **Figure 7** shows an example of the differential image for two given input images.

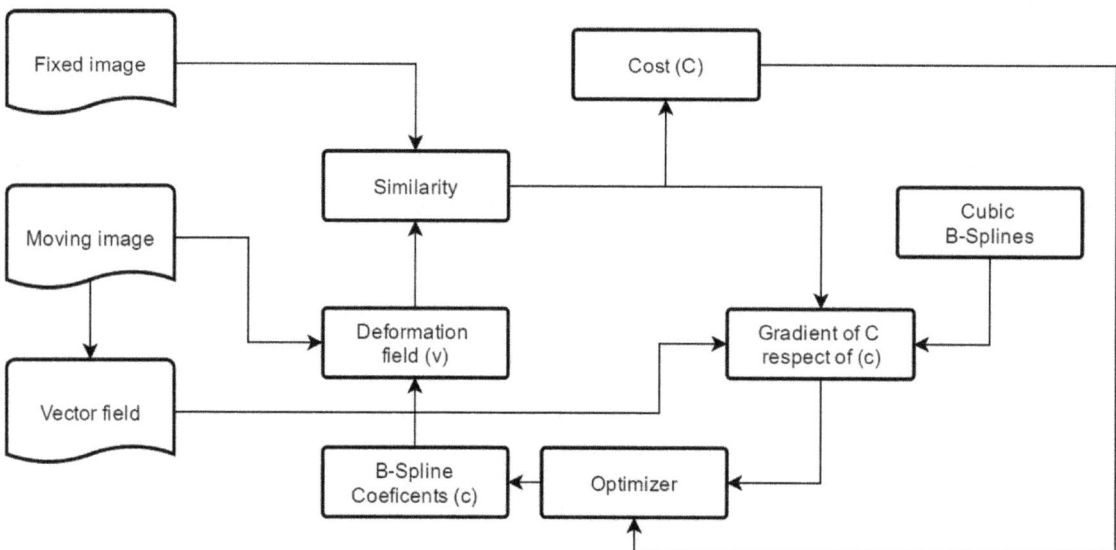

Figure 5. B-Spline registration typical framework.

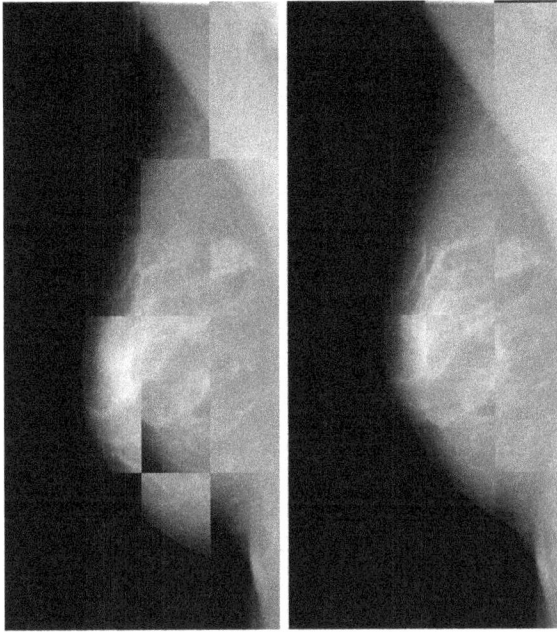

Figure 6. Checkerboard comparison of images *pre* and *post* B-Spline registration. The image in the left shows a comparison between a left and horizontally flipped right breast before registration, and the right image shows the results of the registering process.

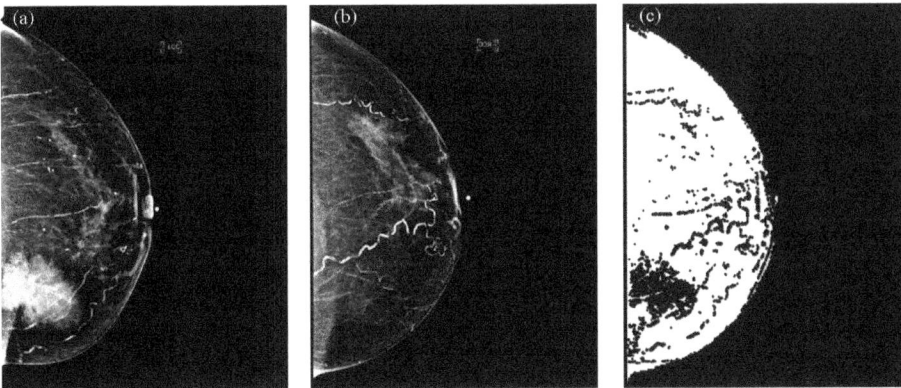

Figure 7. Image subtraction example. Left: unaltered CC view of left breast, middle: horizontally flipped CC view of right breast, and right: color map of the subtraction image I_Δ. White and black pixels inside the breast tissue represent small and large intensity differences, respectively.

2.5. Image enhancement

To study the appearance of the architectural distortions, two enhancing filters were applied to the images: a morphological high-frequency enhancement filter (H) designed to enhance fiber-like tissues, and a Laplacian of Gaussian filter (L) that enhances high-frequency patterns inside the breast tissue. Additionally, since the texture between normal and abnormal tissues is different [42], two texture maps were created. The first map computed the local standard deviation (σ) of the mammograms, and the second map computed the local fractal dimension (F). All image processing was implemented in C++ using Insight Segmentation and Registration Toolkit (ITK) libraries for image manipulation following previous efforts [32, 43].

2.6. Feature extraction

There are several features that may be quantified when aiming to detect early signs of cancer. For this analysis, 43 features were extracted from each image. These features can be grouped in three main categories: shape (i.e. area, perimeter, compactness, elongation, region centroid, region scatter), signal (i.e. mean, median, energy, variance, standard deviation, dynamic range, z mean, entropy, skewness, kurtosis, z range, fraction greater than z deviations, fraction lower than z deviations, value at fraction, 5% trimmed mean, 5% trimmed standard deviation, 5% trimmed z Mean), and morphology (i.e. total signal, signal centroid, signal scatter, and signal surface). Details of the full feature extraction procedure can be found in Ref. [32].

The enhancement filters and texture maps presented in Section 2.5 were applied to the four screening mammograms (i.e. left and right CC, and left and right MLO) and to the two bilateral subtraction images (CC and MLO), yielding a set of 15 images for both the CC and the MLO views: I, I_l, I_Δ, H_r, H_l, H_Δ, L_r, L_l, L_Δ, σ_r, σ_l, σ_Δ, F_r, F_l, and F_Δ, where I is the raw image, H, L, σ, and F are the enhanced images described in Section 2.5, and r, l, and Δ, stand for the right, left, and bilateral subtraction images, respectively. Features were then extracted from this set of images. Additionally, to study the feature-based asymmetry analysis, the average and absolute difference of each left-right pair of measurements was also analyzed, resulting in 860 additional features, resulting in a total of 2150 features per subject.

2.7. Feature selection

The first step of the feature selection process consisted discarding highly correlated to avoid redundancy. For any pair of features with a Spearman correlation coefficient larger than 0.96, one feature was randomly selected to be kept, and the other removed from the selection. The dataset was normalized using the empirical distribution of the healthy subjects and a z-normalization was performed using the rank-based inverse normal transformation [44].

In order to select the most accurate and compact set of features from each dataset, the least absolute shrinkage and selection operator (LASSO) method was used [45]. The shrinkage and selection method minimizes the sum of squared errors and penalizes the regression coefficients, as described by Eq. (3) as follows:

$$\hat{\beta}^{lasso} = \text{argmin} \sum_{i=1}^{N} \left(y_i - \beta_0 - \sum_{j=1}^{p} x_{ij} \beta_j \right)^2 \text{ subject to:} \sum_{j=1}^{p} |\beta| \leq t \qquad (3)$$

Given a set of input measurements $x_1 \ldots x_n$ and an outcome y, the lasso method fits a linear model where x_i is the covariate vector for the ith case and y_i is the outcome, t is a tuning parameter that determines the amount of regularization, and N is the number of cases.

The multivariate search was performed using a class balanced data sample of 100 subjects for training and the remaining subjects as a blind test set. The models were calibrated using a leave-one-out cross-validation strategy, training the models at every split using $N - 1$ subjects and evaluating the model using the remaining subjects [46]. The final reported performance was obtained by applying the final model gathered on the training stage and evaluating it in the blind test set.

3. Results

A total of 1796 mammograms were successfully segmented. The image sets of nine subjects had to be removed from the experiment due to problems with the registration process, six were from MS, two from CS, and one from HS. All the remaining subjects were included in the subsequent stages of the analysis. The 2150 extracted features were filtered by the correlation process, removing 826 features.

Table 1 shows the features that were selected for each model: the CS versus HS ($n = 12$), and the MS versus HS ($n = 16$). The former achieved an accuracy of 0.825 with an AUC of 0.882 and the latter an accuracy of 0.698 with an AUC of 0.807. **Figure 8** shows the ROC curves for both the models.

#	CS versus HS			MS versus HS		
	View	Image	Feature	View	Image	Feature
1	CC	H_Δ	27	CC	L_Δ	40
2	CC	F_Δ	13	CC	I_r	29
3	CC	I_r	29	CC	L_l	40
4	CC	H_l	29	CC	F_r	6
5	CC	H_l	6	MLO	H_l	11
6	MLO	I_l	28	CC	$L_{\Delta avg}$	29
7	MLO	H_l	11	CC	$I_{\Delta s}$	28
8	MLO	H_l	21	CC	$\sigma_{\Delta s}$	38
9	CC	$I_{\Delta s}$	28	CC	$F_{\Delta avg}$	12
10	CC	$\sigma_{\Delta s}$	38	MLO	$I_{\Delta s}$	40
11	MLO	$L_{\Delta avg}$	27	MLO	$I_{\Delta s}$	28
12	CC	H_Δ	27	MLO	$I_{\Delta s}$	29
13				MLO	$H_{\Delta s}$	31
14				MLO	$H_{\Delta s}$	7
15				MLO	$L_{\Delta avg}$	39
16				MLO	$L_{\Delta avg}$	27

Note: Features are grouped by dataset, symmetric features are denoted with:
$$I_{\Delta avg} = \frac{I_r + I_l}{2}, H_{\Delta avg} = \frac{H_r + H_l}{2}, L_{\Delta avg} = \frac{L_r + L_l}{2}, \sigma_{\Delta avg} = \frac{\sigma_r + \sigma_l}{2}, F_{\Delta avg} = \frac{\sigma_r + \sigma_l}{2},$$
$$I_{\Delta s} = |I_r - I_l|, H_{\Delta s} = |H_r - H_l|, L_{\Delta s} = |H_r - H_l|, \sigma_{\Delta s} = |H_r - H_l|, F_{\Delta s} = |H_r - H_l|.$$

Table 1. Features of the proposed models.

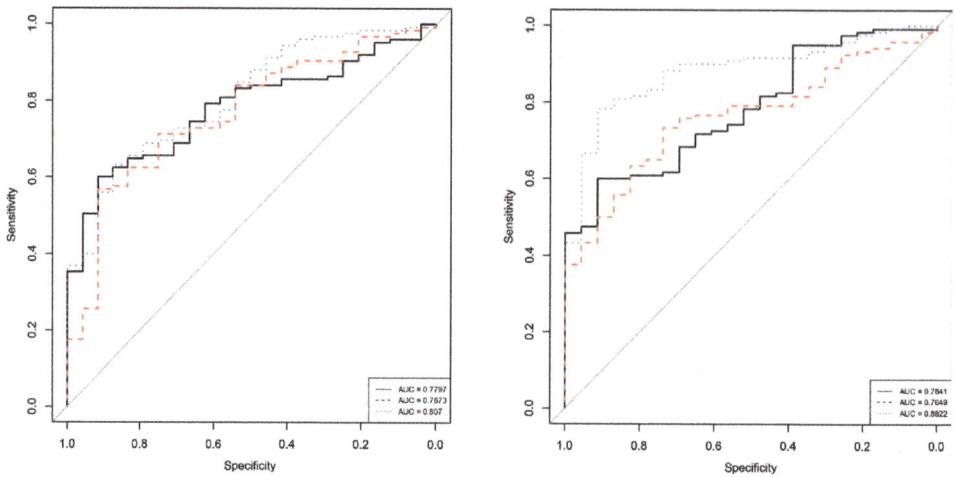

Figure 8. ROC curves for the classification models. Left: MS versus HS, right: CS versus HS. The dashed line represents the model with the features from only the difference images, the solid line the one with features from only the raw images, and the dotted line the one with the features from all images (from Ref. [32]).

4. Discussion

The proposed methodology is fully automated and does not require manual intervention as previous proposals [16, 17]. Although the approach is similar to others [22], we did not attempt to remove the pectoral muscle from the segmentation mask, since the presence of abnormal axillary lymph in this area is an indicator of occult breast carcinoma [47]. However, from the computational point of view, the feature extraction process may be affected if the region processed is not well focused [48].

The proposed registration process achieved a good performance having only 2.0% of the subjects that had to be discarded due to registration issues. This performance is remarkable when considering the amount of deformation undergoing in a mammography procedure. The B-spline deformation is an improvement over rigid or affine co-registration methods [33]. The advantage of the deformable registration has been recognized as a key element in breast analysis and has been successfully used in longitudinal studies [22]. Regarding digital subtraction, the differences in the X-ray projection, and image acquisition and digitizing artifacts may affect the detection of asymmetric patterns. Our results indicate that even in the presence of registration artifacts, the digital subtraction added information that was successfully incorporated during the feature selection process.

The B-Spline transformation algorithm, proposed for the bilateral mammogram registration presented, shows a clear improvement after the registration. Due to lack of temporal mammograms, temporal registration was not tested. Nevertheless, the methodology could be implemented in such task. However, the temporal registration should be re-optimized using a new set of parameters.

The enhanced images and texture maps enriched the feature set providing a four-fold increase in extracting features per patient, which were also incorporated in the final classification models. Regarding symmetry, the strategy of exploring bilateral symmetry has been explored by other researchers where a series of features (signal, texture, breast density, etc.) were computed from each mammogram and the absolute difference between both breasts was obtained to measure breast tissue asymmetry, and used it to predict the likelihood of developing cancer [19]. We extended this idea by registering the left and right images using a deformable transformation, which increased the number of features per patient by 25%.

This study shows that healthy subjects, subjects with calcifications, and subjects with masses can accurately be classified through models generated via mammography registration and a feature selection methodology. The analysis of the feature selection strategy demonstrated that even when using a different approach for the feature selection strategy, the proposed methodology achieved similar results as the previously presented ones. Therefore, we can say that the methodology is robust to the feature selection strategy.

The methodology demonstrated that the image subtraction of registered images generates information that aids in the identification of subjects with lesions, such as malignant masses and calcifications. The methodology also incorporated the use of feature-based asymmetry into the CADx system. The combination performance achieved has the potential to be used to queue cases with a high chance of malignant findings, or may have the practical use of triaging mammograms in developing countries where there is a deficiency of expert readers.

Author details

José María Celaya Padilla[1*], Cesar Humberto Guzmán Valdivia[1], Jorge Issac Galván Tejada[2], Carlos Eric Galván Tejada[2], Hamurabi Gamboa Rosales[2], Juan Rubén Delgado Contreras[3], Antonio Martinez-Torteya[4], Roberto Olivera Reyna[2], Jorge Roberto Manjarrez Sánchez[5], Francisco Javier Martinez Ruiz[2], Idalia Garza-Veloz[6], Margarita L. Martinez-Fierro[6], Victor Treviño[7] and Jose Gerardo Tamez-Peña[7]

*Address all correspondence to: jose.celaya@uaz.edu.mx

1 Autonomous University of Zacatecas/ CONACyT – Universidad Autónoma de Zacatecas (CONACyT – UAZ), Jardín Juarez, Centro, Zacatecas, Zacatecas, Mexico

2 Electric Engineering Department, Autonomous University of Zacatecas (UAZ), Jardín Juarez, Centro, Zacatecas, Zacatecas, Mexico

3 Superior Technical Institute of Zacatecas South (ITSZaS), Las lomitas, Tlaltenango, Zacatecas, Mexico

4 Engineering Department, Monterrey University (UdeM), Morones Prieto Pte, Jesús M. Garza, San Pedro Garza García, Nuevo Leon, Mexico

5 Computer Engineering Systems Department, Superior Technical Institute of Jerez (ITSJ) Libramiento Fresnillo-Tepetongo, Fracc. Los Cardos, Jerez de García Salinas, Zacatecas, Mexico

6 Health Sciences Department ,Human Medical School, Autonomous University of Zacatecas (UAZ), Jardín Juarez, Centro, Zacatecas, Zacatecas, Mexico

7 Bioinformatic group, Medical School, Monterrey Institute of Technology (ITESM), Eugenio Garza Sada, Monterrey, Nuevo Leon, Mexico

References

[1] World-Health. Cancer Fact sheet No. 297 [Internet]. 2015. Available from: http://www.who.int/mediacentre/factsheets/fs297/en/index.html [Accessed: 09/02/2015]

[2] DeSantis C, Ma J, Bryan L, Jemal A. Breast cancer statistics, 2013. CA: A Cancer Journal for Clinicians. 2014;**64**(1):52-62

[3] Ng K, Muttarak M. Advances in mammography have improved early detection of breast cancer. Honk Kong College or Radiologist. 2003;**6**(3):126-131

[4] Chan H-P, et al. Computer-aided classification of mammographic masses and normal tissue: Linear discriminant analysis in texture feature space. Physics in Medicine and Biology. 1995;**40**(5):857-876

[5] D'orsi C, Bassett L, Berg W, Feig S, Jackson V, Kopans D. Breast Imaging Reporting and Data System: ACR BI-RADS-Mammography. Reston: American College of Radiology (ACR); 2003

[6] Doi K. Current status and future potential of computer-aided diagnosis in medical imaging. The British Journal of Radiology. 2005;**78**(1):S3-S19

[7] Sampat MP, Markey MK, Bovik AC, et al. Computer-aided detection and diagnosis in mammography. Handbook of Image and Video Processing. 2005;**2**(1):1195-1217

[8] Dromain C, Boyer B, Ferre R, Canale S, Delaloge S, Balleyguier C. Computed-aided diagnosis (CAD) in the detection of breast cancer. European Journal of Radiology. 2013;**82**(3):417-423

[9] Ramos-Pollán R, et al. Discovering mammography-based machine learning classifiers for breast cancer diagnosis. Journal of Medical Systems. 2012;**36**(4):2259-2269

[10] Li M, Zhou Z-H. Improve computer-aided diagnosis with machine learning techniques using undiagnosed samples. IEEE Transactions on Systems, Man and Cybernetics, Part A: Systems and Humans. 2007;**37**(6):1088-1098

[11] Doi K. Computer-aided diagnosis in medical imaging: historical review, current status and future potential. Computerized Medical Imaging and Graphics. 2007;**31**(4-5):198-211

[12] Eadie LH, Taylor P, Gibson AP. A systematic review of computer-assisted diagnosis in diagnostic cancer imaging. European Journal of Radiology. 2012;**81**(1):e70-e76

[13] Cheng H-D, Cai X, Chen X, Hu L, Lou X. Computer-aided detection and classification of microcalcifications in mammograms: A survey. Pattern Recognition. 2003;**36**(12):2967-2991

[14] Zheng B, Sumkin JH, Zuley ML, Wang X, Klym AH, Gur D. Bilateral mammographic density asymmetry and breast cancer risk: A preliminary assessment. European Journal of Radiology. 2012;**81**(11):3222-3228

[15] Scutt D, Lancaster GA, Manning JT. Breast asymmetry and predisposition to breast cancer. Breast Cancer Research. 2006;**8**(2):R14

[16] Giger ML, Yin FF, Vyborny CJ. Comparison of bilateral-subtraction and single-image processing techniques in the computerized detection of mammographic masses. Investigative Radiology. 1993;**28**(6):473-481

[17] Yin FF, Giger ML, Doi K, Metz CE, Vyborny CJ, Schmidt RA. Computerized detection of masses in digital mammograms: Analysis of bilateral subtraction images. Medical Physics. 1991;**18**(5):955-963

[18] Tan M, Zheng B, Ramalingam P, Gur D. Prediction of near-term breast cancer risk based on bilateral mammographic feature asymmetry. Academic Rradiology. 2013;**20**(12):1542-1550

[19] Wang X, Lederman D, Tan J, Wang XH, Zheng B. Computerized prediction of risk for developing breast cancer based on bilateral mammographic breast tissue asymmetry. Medical Engineering & Physics. 2011;**33**(8):934-942

[20] Wang X, Lederman D, Tan J, Wang XH, Zheng B. Computerized detection of breast tissue asymmetry depicted on bilateral mammograms: A preliminary study of breast risk stratification. Academic Radiology. 2010;**17**(10):1234-1241

[21] Rodriguez-Rojas J, Garza-Montemayor M, Trevino-Alvarado V, Tamez-Pena JG. Predictive features of breast cancer on Mexican screening mammography patients. In: Spie Medical Imaging. International Society for Optics and Photonics; Florida, USA. 2013, pp. 867023-867023-9

[22] Martí R, Díez Y, Oliver A, Tortajada M, Zwiggelaar R, Lladó X. Detecting abnormal mammographic cases in temporal studies using image registration features. In: Breast Imaging. Springer; Gifu, Japan. 2014. pp. 612-619

[23] Miller P, Astley SM. Detection of breast asymmetry using anatomical features. In: IS&T/ SPIE's Symposium on Electronic Imaging: Science and Technology. International Society for Optics and Photonics; Los Ángeles California, USA. 1993. pp. 433-442

[24] Miller P, Astley S. Automated detection of breast asymmetry using anatomical features. State of the Art in Digital Mammographic Image Analysis, Series in Machine Perception and Artificial Intelligence. 1994;**9**:247-261

[25] Lau TK, Bischof WF. Automated detection of breast tumors using the asymmetry approach. Computers and Biomedical Research. 1991;**24**(3):273-295

[26] Ferrari RJ, Rangayyan RM, Desautels JL, Frère AF. Analysis of asymmetry in mammograms via directional filtering with Gabor wavelets. IEEE Transactions on Medical Imaging. 2001;**20**(9):953-964

[27] Suri JS, Rangayyan RM. Recent Advances in Breast Imaging, Mammography, and Computer-Aided Diagnosis of Breast Cancer. SPIE press; Washington, USA. 2006. pp. 488-525

[28] Diez Y, et al. Revisiting intensity-based image registration applied to mammography. IEEE Transactions on Information Technology in Biomedicine. 2011;**15**(5):716-725

[29] Mendez AJ, Tahoces PG, Lado MJ, Souto M, Correa JL, Vidal JJ. Computer-aided diagnosis: Automatic detection of malignant masses in digitized mammograms. Medical
Physics. 1998;**25**:957

[30] Celaya-Padilla JM, Rodriguez-Rojas J, Trevino V, Tamez-Pena JG. Local image registration a comparison for bilateral registration mammography. In: Presented at the
International Seminar on Medical Image Processing and Analysis; Mexico, DF; 2013

[31] Celaya-Padilla JM, Rodriguez-Rojas J, Galván-Tejada JI, Martínez-Torteya A, Treviño V,
Tamez-Peña JG. Bilateral image subtraction features for multivariate automated classification of breast cancer risk. In: SPIE Medical Imaging. International Society for Optics
and Photonics; San Diego, CA, USA. 2014. pp. 90351T-90351T-7

[32] Celaya-Padilla J, Martinez-Torteya A, Rodriguez-Rojas J, Galvan-Tejada J, Treviño V,
Tamez-Peña J. Bilateral image subtraction and multivariate models for the automated
triaging of screening mammograms. BioMed Research International. 2015;**2015**:1-12

[33] Yin FF, Giger ML, Doi K, Vyborny CJ, Schmidt RA. Computerized detection of masses in
digital mammograms: Automated alignment of breast images and its effect on bilateral-
subtraction technique. Medical Physics. 1994;**21**(3):445-452

[34] Heath M, Bowyer K, Kopans D, Moore R, Kegelmeyer P. The digital database for
screening mammography. In Proceedings of the 5th International Workshop on Digital
Mammography. San Diego, CA, USA. 2000. pp. 212-218

[35] Guo Y, Suri J, Sivaramakrishna R. Image registration for breast imaging: A review. In:
27th Annual International Conference of the IEEE Engineering in Medicine and Biology
Society, 2005. IEEE-EMBS 2005. IEEE; Toronto, Canada. 2006. pp. 3379-3382

[36] Marias K, Behrenbruch C, Parbhoo S, Seifalian A, Brady M. A registration framework
for the comparison of mammogram sequences. IEEE Transactions on Medical Imaging.
2005;**24**(6):782-790

[37] Kok-Wiles SL, Brady M, Highnam R. Comparing mammogram pairs for the detection of
lesions. In Digital Mammography. Springer; Nijmegen, Netherlands. 1998. pp. 103-110

[38] Hill DL, Hawkes DJ. Across-modality registration using intensity-based cost functions.
In Handbook of Medical Imaging. Academic Press, Inc; Orlando, FL, USA. 2000. pp.
537-553

[39] Mattes D, Haynor DR, Vesselle H, Lewellyn TK, Eubank W. Nonrigid multimodality image registration. In: Medical Imaging 2001. International Society for Optics and
Photonics; San Diego, CA, USA. 2001. pp. 1609-1620

[40] West J, et al. Comparison and evaluation of retrospective intermodality brain image registration techniques. Journal of Computer Assisted Tomography. 1997;**21**(4):554-568

[41] Rosenfeld A. Multiresolution Image Processing and Aanalysis. Springer Science & Business
Media; Heidelberg, Germany. 2013

[42] Rangayyan RM, Banik S, Desautels JL. Computer-aided detection of architectural distortion
in prior mammograms of interval cancer. Journal of Digital Imaging. 2010;**23**(5):611-631

[43] Ibanez L, Schroeder W, Ng L, Cates J. The ITK Software Guide. Kitware; New York, USA. 2003

[44] Beasley TM, Erickson S, Allison DB. Rank-based inverse normal transformations are increasingly used, but are they merited? Behavior Genetics. 2009;**39**(5):580-595

[45] Tibshirani R. Regression shrinkage and selection via the lasso. Journal of the Royal Statistical Society. Series B (Methodological). 1996;**58**:267-288

[46] Friedman J, Hastie T, Tibshirani R, Regularization Paths for Generalized Linear Models via Coordinate Descent. Journal of Statistical Software, Innsbruck, Austria, 2010;**33**(1):1-22

[47] Ganesan K, Acharya UR, Chua KC, Min LC, Abraham KT. Pectoral muscle segmentation: A review. Computer Methods and Programs in Biomedicine. 2013;**110**(1):48-57

[48] Raba D, Oliver A, Martí J, Peracaula M, Espunya J. Breast segmentation with pectoral muscle suppression on digital mammograms. In: Pattern Recognition and Image Analysis. Springer; Berlin, Heidelberg, Germany. 2005. pp. 471-478

6

Breast Imaging and Translation into Targeted Oncoplastic Breast Surgery

Michael Friedrich and Stefan Kraemer

Abstract

Preoperative staging of breast cancer based on breast imaging is mandatory. Breast imaging encompasses mammography, breast sonography and MR-mammography. Earlier diagnosis of breast cancer results in a favourable oncological outcome. Limitations and influences on operative procedures of MR-mammography in diagnosis and staging of breast cancer have to be discussed. Different interventional procedures have been developed. The histological results of interventional procedures guided by ultrasound, stereotactic mammography or magnetic resonance have to be integrated in planning surgical resection margins in oncoplastic breast-conserving surgery. Image-guided wire markings are an important tool for planning these surgical resection margins. This chapter summarises the results of breast imaging, interventional procedures and wire markings for the breast-conserving therapy of breast cancer. Breast imaging and interventional procedures are the basis for a concept of targeted oncoplastic breast surgery.

Keywords: breast cancer, breast imaging, mammography, breast ultrasound, magnetic resonance mammography, oncoplastic surgery, interventional breast diagnostics

1. Breast imaging

Earlier diagnosis of breast cancer results in a favourable outcome. Tumour size at diagnosis and the lymph node stage are the best predictive factors of outcome. As a result, the current strategy for reducing breast cancer mortality is to diagnose the disease as early as possible. Breast imaging is fundamental for the early diagnosis of breast cancer when symptoms occur or during screening programs.

Breast imaging is a general term that encompasses mammography, breast sonography, breast magnetic resonance imaging (MRI) and other technologies. To provide uniformity in the assessment of breast imaging findings, the American College of Radiologists (ACR) established final assessment classifications [Breast Imaging Reporting and Data System (BI-RADS)] [1–3]. The final assessment categories are as follows: BI-RADS 1, negative; BI-RADS 2, benign; BI-RADS 3, probably benign (risk of malignancy <2%); BI-RADS 4, suspicious abnormality (biopsy should be considered); BI-RADS 5, highly suggestive of malignancy.

BI-RADS 4 and 5 assessments indicate abnormalities that require tissue biopsy for diagnosis. These categories represent a wide range (3–100%) of breast cancer risk.

2. Mammography

Mammography has been the basis of breast imaging for more than 30 years. The sensitivity of mammography for breast cancer is age dependent. The denser the breast, the less effective this method is for detecting early signs of breast cancer. In younger women, breast density tends to be higher, and increased density inhibits the detection of early signs of breast cancer [4]. The sensitivity of mammography for breast cancer in women over 60 years of age is about 95%, while mammography can be expected to detect less than 50% of breast cancers in women under 40 years of age [5]. Mammography is based on X-rays. Consensus is that the benefits of mammography in women over the age of 40 years are likely to far outweigh any oncogenic effects of repeated exposure. Screening of women over the age of 50 by mammography is accepted practice. However, in symptomatic patients with a palpable nodule in the breast, there is even an indication for performing mammography in women under the age of 35 when there is a strong clinical suspicion of malignancy. Practice is changing, and ultrasound is being increasingly used for the assessment of women with focal breast symptoms in this age range. Mammography is performed every 2 years in all women in the screening age group (50 years of age – 69 years of age) attending symptomatic patients who have not had a screening mammogram in the past year. Film/screen mammography has been refined over the years and has now reached the limits of this technology [6]. Film/screen mammography is a difficult technique to maintain at the quality levels required for optimal diagnosis because labour-intensive quality control measures are necessary to maintain the diagnostic standards. Today, digital mammography is the new standard. Major benefits have been predicted from acquiring mammograms in a direct digital format [7]. Compared with conventional mammography, the predicted benefits of full-field digital mammography include better imaging of the dense breast, the application of computer-aided detection and a number of logistical advantages providing potential for more efficient mammography services. The much wider dynamic range of digital mammography means that visualization of the entire breast density range on a single image is easily achievable. In the clinical setting, comparative studies have shown that digital mammography performs as well as film/screen mammography [8–11].

Recent preoperative mammographic evaluation is necessary to determine patient's eligibility for breast-conserving therapy. Mammography defines the extent of a patient's disease, the presence or absence of multicentricity and other factors (extent of microcalcifications) that might influence the treatment decision, and evaluates the contralateral breast. If the mass is associated with microcalcifications, an assessment of the extent of the calcifications is performed. Magnification mammography is important for further characterisation of microcalcifications.

Mammography is the basis for stereotactic-guided breast biopsy. Stereotactic biopsy can be carried out using a prone biopsy table or by using an add-on device to a conventional upright mammography unit. This technique is used for biopsy of clinically occult lesions that are not detectable by ultrasound (e.g. microcalcifications) [12].

3. Ultrasound

High-frequency (≥7.5 MHz) ultrasound is a very effective diagnostic tool for the investigation of focal breast symptoms. It has a high sensitivity for breast lesions and also a very high negative predictive value. High-resolution ultrasound easily distinguishes between most solid and cystic lesions and can differentiate benign from malignant lesions with a high accuracy. Ultrasound is the technique of choice for the further investigation of focal symptomatic breast lesions at all ages. Under 35 years of age, when the risk of breast cancer is very low, it is usually the preferred imaging technique. Over 35 years of age, when the risk of breast cancer begins to increase, it is often used in conjunction with mammography. Ultrasound is less sensitive than mammography for the early signs of breast cancer and is therefore not used for population-based screening. However, ultrasound increases the detection of small breast cancer in women with a dense background tissue on mammography [13–15]. In the screening setting, there is currently insufficient evidence of any mortality benefit even in women with dense mammograms. Ultrasound is the preferred technique to guide biopsy of both palpable and impalpable breast lesions visible on scanning [16]. Ultrasound is being increasingly used to assess the axilla in women with breast cancer. Axillary nodes that show abnormal morphology can be accurately sampled by needle core biopsy.

Doppler ultrasound adds additional accuracy to breast diagnosis and is widely used. Three-dimensional ultrasound of the breast also increases the accuracy of biopsy and the detection of multifocal disease but is not widely available [17, 18]. Elastography is a new application of ultrasound technology that allows the accurate assessment of the stiffness of the breast tissue. It is being evaluated at present and may prove to be a useful tool in excluding significant abnormalities, for instance, in assessment of asymptomatic abnormalities detected by ultrasound.

4. Magnetic resonance mammography

Magnetic resonance imaging (MRI) is widely available and used in breast cancer diagnosis. Magnetic resonance mammography (MRM) requires dedicated breast coils. In order to image the breast, the patient is scanned prone, and injection of intravenous contrast (Gd-DTPA) is required. A variety of possible clinical indications for contrast-enhanced MRM have been reported. These include screening for breast cancer, determining the local extent of malignant disease, identifying an occult primary, assessing response to neoadjuvant chemotherapy, identifying local recurrences after breast-conserving therapy, breast imaging after implant reconstruction or breast augmentation, and the detection of ipsilateral breast cancer in patients presented with axillary lymph node metastases (CUP-syndrome) [19–23].

MRM is the most sensitive technique for detection of breast cancer, approaching 100% for invasive cancer and 60–70% for ductal carcinoma in situ (DCIS), but it has a high false-positive rate [24–28]. Rapid acquisition of images facilitates assessment of signal enhancement curves that can be helpful in distinguishing benign and malignant disease. Breast lesions seen on MRM that are larger than 10 mm can be seen on ultrasound if they are clinically significant (second-look ultrasound). MRM is likely to prove the best method for screening younger women (under 40 years) at increased risk of breast cancer but it is unlikely to be used for general population screening. MRM is the best technique for imaging women with breast implants. It is also of benefit in identifying recurrent breast cancer after breast-conserving therapy where conventional imaging has failed to exclude recurrence. Performed more than 12 months after surgery, MRM will accurately distinguish between tumour recurrence and scars [29, 30]. MRM is being increasingly used to examine women for multifocal or multicentric disease prior to conservation surgery, especially in patients with invasive lobular breast cancer. MRI of the axilla will demonstrate axillary metastatic disease but its sensitivity is not sufficient for it to replace surgical staging of the axilla.

Many questions surrounding the use of MRM of the breast in patients with breast cancer remain unanswered. Just because MRM can detect additional areas of cancer, does it really matter clinically? Should surgical treatment be altered because MRM detects additional foci of cancer, especially in those cases when these areas represent foci of DCIS? Would these additional areas of cancer identified on MRM be successfully treated with postoperative radiation therapy? The rate of MRM-detected multifocal disease, which ranges from 16–37%, is clearly much higher than the rate of in-breast recurrence after breast-conserving therapy, with reported rates in two studies with a 20-year follow-up of 8.8% and 14.3%, respectively [31, 32]. This strongly suggests that in some, and perhaps many cases, the additional foci of cancer identified only on MRM, especially those that prove to be in situ disease, would likely be successfully treated with postoperative radiation. Which MRM-detected multifocal or multicentric cancer would be successfully treated with postoperative radiation and which would not, later presenting as a local "recurrence"? In those cases when MRM detects an invasive cancer that is clearly separate from the primary cancer, either in the same or a different quadrant, should mastectomy be recommended, based on the historical treatment of clinically or mammographically detected multifocal or multicentric cancer, or is the patient still eligible for breast-conserving therapy if the lesion can be successfully excised with negative margins [33]? There are additional questions concerning patient selection. Which are the patients at the highest risk for having multifocal or multicentric cancer who would benefit most from MRM (young patients, patients with dense breasts, patients with lobular cancer)? Based on the current success of breast-conserving surgery, it is unlikely that MRM of the breast is warranted in all patients with newly diagnosed breast cancer [20, 34]. Clinical investigation continues in an effort to find answers to these questions (**Figure 1**).

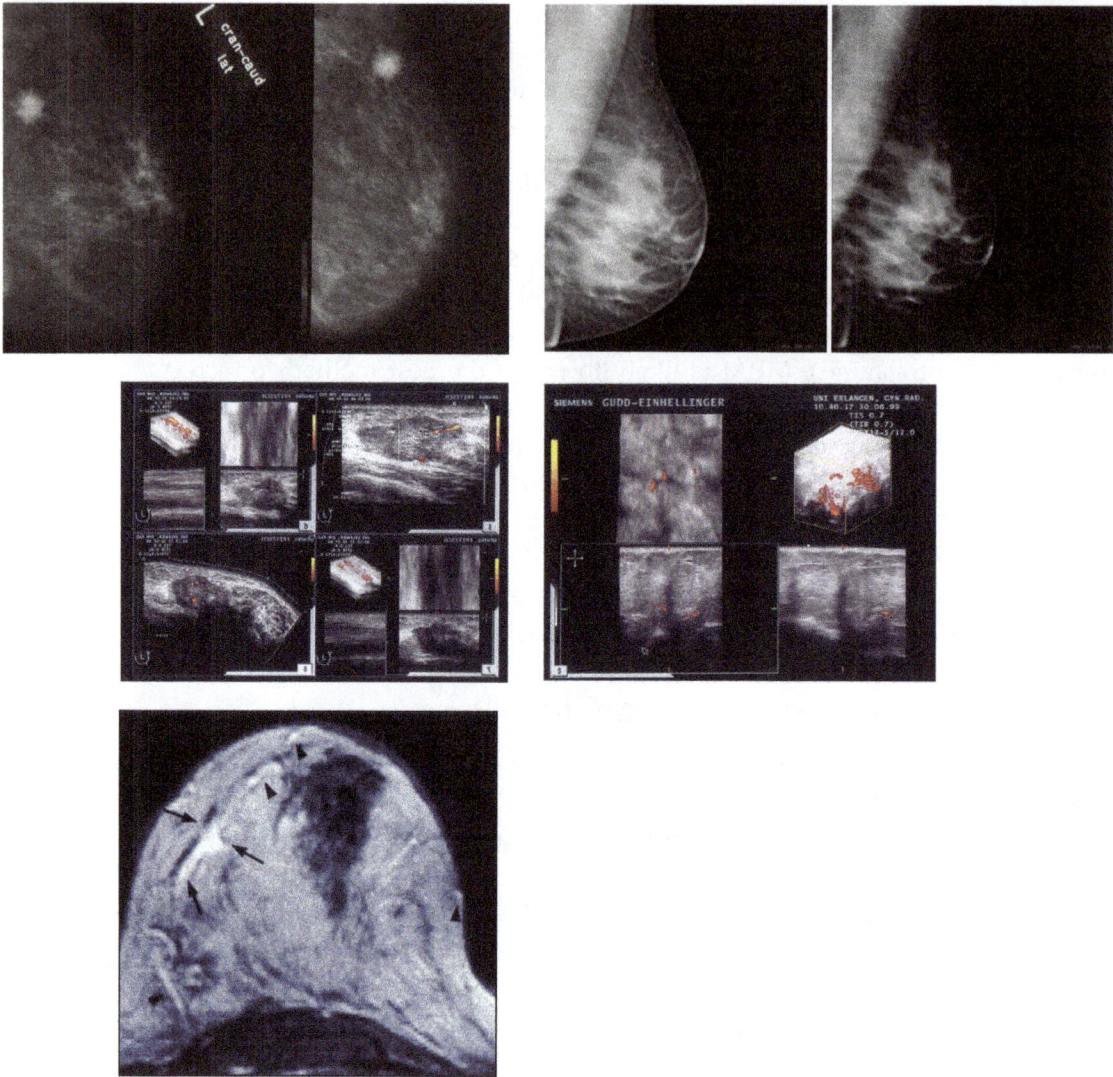

Figure 1. Complementary breast imaging.

5. Breast cancer screening

The aim of breast cancer screening is to reduce mortality through early detection. Randomised controlled trials and case–control studies demonstrated that population screening by mammography can be expected to reduce overall breast cancer mortality by around 25%. [35, 36]. The validity of these trials was questioned, but subsequent reviews have reaffirmed the mortality benefit of mammographic screening and determined that criticisms of the mammographic screening trials were unjustified [37, 38]. The mortality benefit of screening is greatest in women aged 50–70 years. Screening of women under the age of 40 has not been shown to provide any mortality benefit [39–41].

The screening method is two-view mammography. Clinical examination of the breast and breast self-examination have not been shown to contribute to mortality reduction through early detection.

Women at increased risk of developing breast cancer due to a proven inherited predisposing genetic mutation, family history, previous radiotherapy or benign risk lesions may be selected for screening at young age [42, 43]. There is evidence that MRM is the most sensitive method of imaging young women [44]. The specificity of MRM is low and the rate of false-positive results is high—these circumstances have been extensively discussed. Second-look and targeted ultrasound and preoperative MRI-guided biopsy can increase the low specificity of MRM.

6. Image-guided breast biopsy

Needle biopsy is highly accurate in determining the nature of most breast lesions classified as BI-RADS 4 or 5. Patients with benign conditions avoid unnecessary surgery. Carrying out open surgical biopsy for diagnosis should be regarded as a failure of the diagnostic process. For patients who prove to have breast cancer, needle biopsy provides accurate understanding of the type and extent of disease, so ensuring that patients and the doctors treating them are able to make informed treatment choice. Needle biopsy not only provides information on the nature of malignant disease, such as histological type and grade, but also enables pretreatment analyses of prognostic and predictive factors to characterise the immunohistochemical phenotype and the tumour biology (hormone-receptors, HER-2 receptor, genetic profiling, etc.) [45, 46].

Breast needle biopsies of nonpalpable lesions require imaging to guide needle placement. Imaging guidance can be performed with ultrasonography, stereotactic mammography or MRM. Ultrasound guidance is the technique of choice; it is less costly and easy to perform. Ultrasound provides real-time visualisation of the biopsy procedure and visual confirmation of adequate sampling. Between 80 and 90% of breast abnormalities will be clearly visible on ultrasound [47]. For impalpable abnormalities not visible on ultrasound, stereotactic-guided biopsy is required. A few lesions are only visible on MRM and require magnetic resonance-guided biopsy.

Most lesions selected for ultrasound-guided biopsy are solid masses that can be sampled with 14-gauge core needles. The technical aspects involved in performing ultrasound-guided procedures with a free-hand approach have been described previously [48]. The technique used consists of the following steps: imaging the lesion, finding the needle in the longitudinal plane through the breast, maximally visualising the needle tip and placing the needle in the lesion. Development of good hand-eye coordination is crucial to a successful lesion sampling (**Figure 2**) [49].

Using the 14-gauge needle, multiple core biopsy samples are necessary to ensure accurate sampling of different areas of the lesion. In most cases, accurate lesion sampling can be achieved by obtaining 3–5 core samples for masses and 5–10 core samples for microcalcifications [50, 51].

To improve sampling of microcalcifications using digital, stereotactic mammography guidance, the vacuum-assisted biopsy instrument with probes coming in 11-gauge size has been developed [12]. In contrast to the automated biopsy gun devices, the directional, vacuum-assisted biopsy instrument is inserted once and rotated while in the breast to obtain samples from different areas of the lesion. A vacuum is used to pull tissue samples into the sample notch, where it is cut and transported back through the needle and out to the collection chamber. Multiple tissue samples are collected without removing the needle from the breast (**Figure 3**).

Studies have shown improved sampling of microcalcifications with the vacuum-assisted biopsy instrument [52, 53]. For calcifications, it is imperative that there is a proof of representative

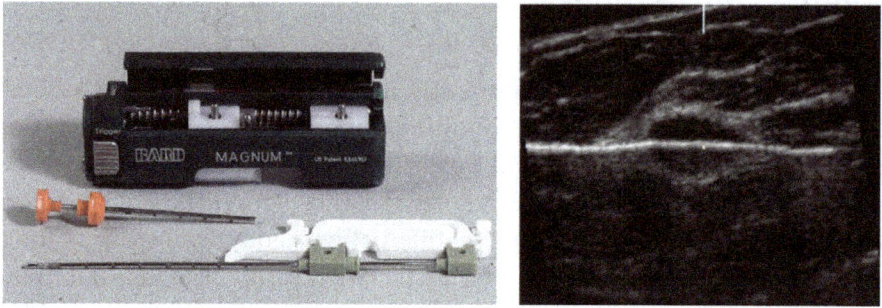

Figure 2. US-guided breast core biopsy (14-gauge).

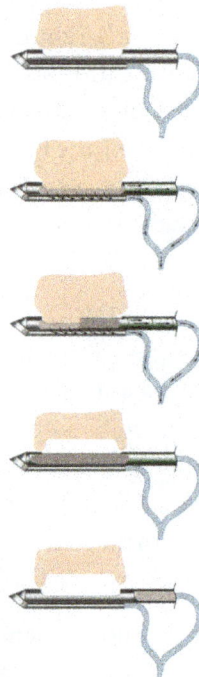

Figure 3. Vacuum-assisted core biopsy (11-gauge).

sampling with specimen radiography. If calcification is not demonstrated on the specimen radiography and the histology is benign, then management cannot be based on this result as there is a high risk of sampling error; the procedure must either be repeated or open surgical biopsy carried out [54–60].

An 8-gauge vacuum-assisted biopsy probe is preferred for therapeutic removal of breast lesions such as fibroadenomas [61–64].

The low specificity of MRM requires the ability to perform MRI-guided biopsies, which require an additional specialised MRI biopsy coil and MRI-compatible wires and needles for localisation and core biopsies [65–67]. Centres that cannot perform MRI-guided localisation and biopsy lack the ability to manage lesions visible only with MRI and are at a clear disadvantage.

The technical aspects of MRI-guided localisation and biopsy are similar to those for stereotactic biopsies in that the patient is prone during the procedure, the breast is held in compression, and the needle plane is guided into the tissue parallel to the chest wall. Needle placement is performed with the patient outside the bore of the magnet using an MRI-compatible needle, often made of titanium. The patient is then returned to the magnet, and confirmation of adequate needle placement is obtained. After sufficient core samples are obtained outside of the bore of the magnet, a clip is placed marking the biopsy cavity. In our practice, patients with MRM-detected indeterminate or suspect lesions are first scheduled for targeted second-look ultrasonography because often these lesions can be visualised after discovery on MRM.

In cases of complete radiological removal of small occult breast lesions with needle biopsies, clip marking with the possibility for re-localisation in cases of necessary therapeutic open surgical resection is mandatory. Core needle and vacuum-assisted biopsy is extremely useful in the evaluation of patients with multiple suspect lesions.

It is important that the result of needle breast biopsy is always correlated with the clinical and imaging findings before clinical management is discussed with the patient. This is best achieved by reviewing each case at prospective multidisciplinary meetings. The results of image-guided breast biopsies are translated in the planning process of targeted oncoplastic breast surgery when malignancy is diagnosed. Breast surgery is directly based on breast imaging and interventional diagnosis. Multidisciplinary coworking between radiology, pathology and breast surgery is mandatory.

7. Wire-guided surgical excision

The number of impalpable, clinically occult breast lesions is increasing. Accurate localisation techniques are required to facilitate their surgical excision as the therapeutic part of a planned oncoplastic breast-conserving procedure [68]. The hooked wire is the most commonly employed technique and has proved very reliable. There are various designs of localisation wire in common use. All have some form of anchoring device such as a hook with a splayed

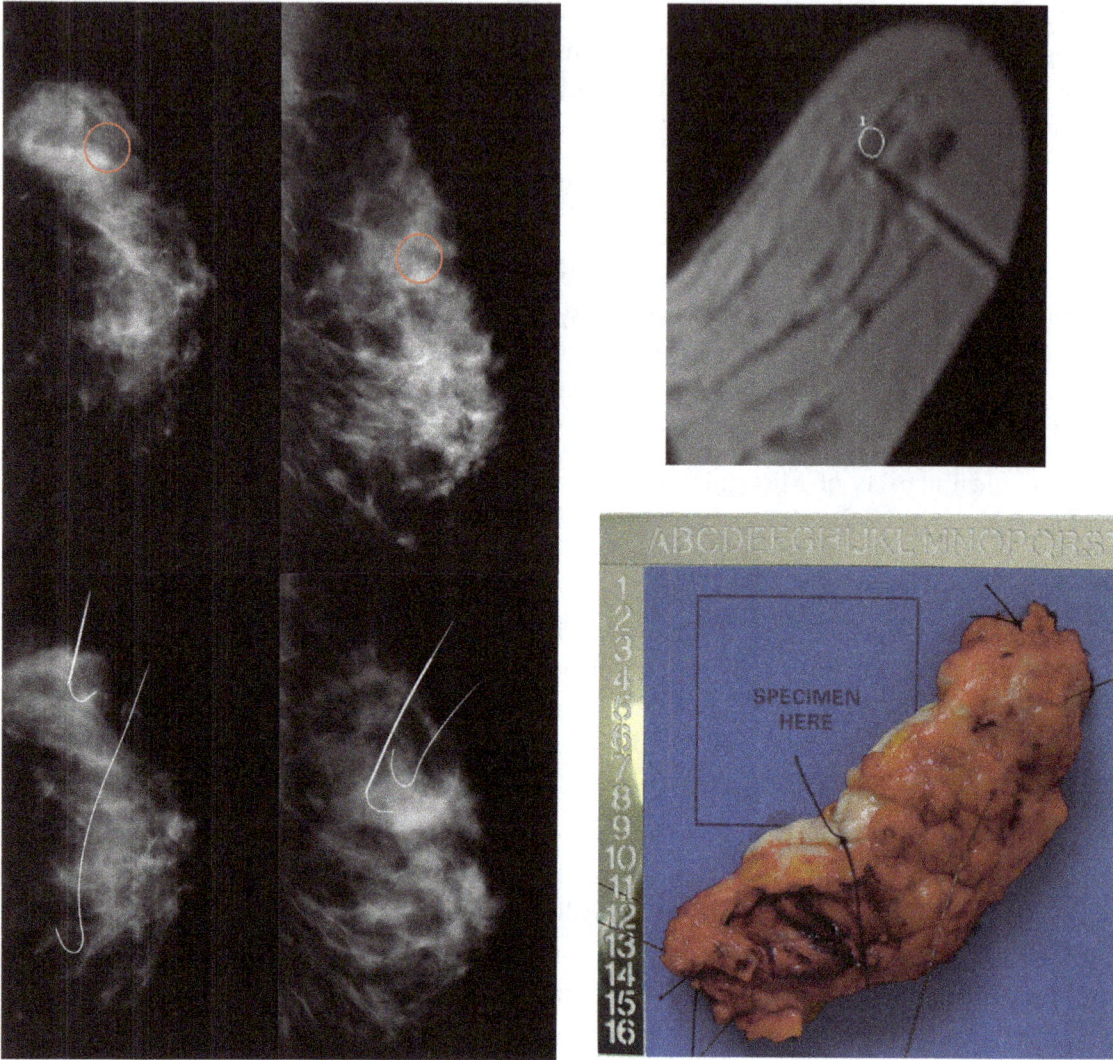

Figure 4. Wire-guided (mammography and MRI) segmental excision.

or barbed tip. The wire is placed under ultrasound, stereotactic or MRI guidance (for MRM lesions only) within a rigid over-sheath cannula, which is then removed once positioning is satisfactory. Most wires are very flexible, and when the cannula is removed, the wire may assume a quite circuitous course. Care must be taken to avoid displacing the wire.

Procedures that can be surgically more challenging are wide local excisions (segmental resection) for DCIS with no mass lesion. In such cases, where the distribution of disease is often more eccentric, careful three-dimensional excision planning especially in oncoplastic procedures is necessary. Inserting more than one wire and even bracketing and framing the lesion with two or three can occasionally be useful (**Figure 4**).

If the procedure is being performed to establish a diagnosis (diagnostic segmentectomy), a representative portion of the lesion is excised through a small incision, thus leaving a satisfactory cosmetic result if the lesion proves to be benign. In the therapeutic situation, the marked lesion should be completely excised. Intraoperative specimen radiography is essential, both to check that the lesion has been removed and, if cancer has been diagnosed, to ensure that adequate radiological resection margins have been achieved. We have to consider that especially in DCIS, the proved radiological resection margin (specimen radiography) sometimes differs from the histological resection margin [68–71].

8. Translation of breast imaging into targeted breast surgery

Advances in breast imaging have led some to question whether whole-breast ultrasound or MRM should be part of the standard preoperative evaluation of a patient with breast cancer. Golshan et al. [72] reviewed the impact of ipsilateral whole-breast ultrasound on the surgical management of 426 patients with clinical stage I and II cancer. Seventy-five of the 426 patients (18%) had additional lesions identified by ultrasound, but only 12 were malignant. The role of ultrasound as a diagnostic tool for the evaluation of breast masses is well established (as is its role in defining lesions that are poorly seen on mammogram or are mammographically occult), and the available data support its use as a routine tool when evaluating patients for breast-conserving therapy.

Tillmann et al. [73] reported the results of a similar study of the impact of MRM on the management of 207 women with DCIS and stage I and II breast cancer. The MRM findings affected clinical management in 20% of cases. In 6%, MRM had an unfavourable effect due to false-positive findings that resulted in unnecessary mastectomy or additional breast biopsies.

The work of Holland et al. [33] indicated that microscopic foci of invasive and non-invasive cancer are present at a distance from apparently localised primary tumours in a significant number of patients. Only 39% of specimens showed no evidence of cancer beyond the reference tumour, while in 20%, additional cancer was found within 2 cm of the reference tumour. Forty-one per cent of patients had residual cancer more than 2 cm from the reference tumour. The percentage of patients with residual cancer more than 2 cm from the reference tumour corresponds well to the rate of local recurrences reported in patients treated with breast-conserving surgery alone without postoperative radiotherapy. Radiotherapy is effective in controlling the majority of these occult foci of carcinoma.

The ability of MRM and ultrasound to identify these tumour foci raises the possibility that significant numbers of women who could be treated with breast-conserving therapy will be subject to unnecessary mastectomy. Histologic subtype other than invasive ductal carcinoma does not appear to be associated with an increased risk of recurrence. If the tumour is not diffuse in the breast and can be completely excised with negative margins, patients with invasive lobular carcinoma are candidates for breast-conserving therapy. However, because of the increased incidence of multicentricity, invasive lobular cancer associated with increased mammographic density is an accepted indication for preoperative MRM before breast-conserving therapy.

9. Conclusion

The translation of breast imaging, interventional procedures and wire-guided surgical excision into a concept of targeted oncoplastic breast-conserving surgery is mandatory, and an interdisciplinary task for the breast radiologist and the breast surgeon to achieve the best oncological and aesthetic outcomes for patients with breast cancer is also mandatory.

Acknowledgements

Version 2.0 after incorporation of the mentioned comments of the review. Dr. Krämer was senior author and writing author of the article in Breast Care, He is a well-known co-developer of the translation concept of breast imaging into Targeted Oncoplastic Breast Surgery.

Author details

Michael Friedrich[1]* and Stefan Kraemer[1,2]

*Address all correspondence to: michael.friedrich@helios-kliniken.de

1 Department of Obstetrics and Gynecology, HELIOS Medical Center, Krefeld, Germany

2 Breast Unit, HELIOS Hospital, Lutherplatz, Krefeld, Germany

References

[1] Balleyguier C, Ayadi S, Van Nguyen K, Banel D, Dromain C, Sigal R BIRADS. Classification in mammography. European Journal of Radiology. 2007;**61**:192-194

[2] Levy L, Suissa M, Chiche JF, Teman G, Martin B. BIRADS ultrasonography. European Journal of Radiology. 2007;**61**:202-211

[3] Tardivon AA, Athansiou A, Thibault F, El Khoury C. Breast imgaging and reporting data system (BIRADS): Magnetic resonance imaging. European Journal of Radiology. 2007;**61**:212-215

[4] Fasching PA, Heusinger K, Loehberg CR, Wenkel E, Lux MP, Schrauder M, Koscheck T, Bautz W, Schulz-Wendtland R, Beckmann MW, Bani MR. influence of mammographic density on the diagnostic accuracy of tumor size – Assessment and association with breast cancer tumor characteristics. European Journal of Radiology. 2006;**60**:398-404

[5] Kopans DB. The positive predictive value of mammography. American Journal of Roentgenology. 1992;**158**:521-526

[6]   Kopans DB. The accuracy of mammographic interpretation. The New England Journal of Medicine. 1994;**331**:1521-1522

[7]   Schulz-Wendtland R, Hermann KP, Bautz W. Clinical results of digital mammography. Radiologe. 2005;**45**:255-263

[8]   James JJ. The current status of digital mammography. Clinical Radiology. 2004;**59**:1-10

[9]   Säbel M, Aichinger U, Schulz-Wendtland R, Bautz W. Digital full field mammography. Röntgenpraxis. 1999;**52**:171-177

[10] Lewin JM, D'Orsi CJ, Hendrick RE. Clinical comparison of full-field digital mammography with screen-film mammography for detection of breast cancer. American Journal of Roentgenology. 2002;**179**:671-677

[11] Schulz-Wendtland R, Lell M, Wenkel E, Aichinger U, Imhoff K, Bautz W. Experimental investigations at the new digital mammographic system. RöFo Journal. 2003;**175**:1564-1566

[12] Schulz-Wendtland R, Aichinger U, Krämer S. Interventionelle mammographisch gestützte Techniken. In: Duda V, Schulz-Wendtland R, editors. Mammadiagnostik – Komplementärer Einsatz aller Verfahren. Springer Verlag; 2004

[13] Stavros AT, Thickman D, Rapp CL. Solid breast nodules: Use of sonography to distinguish between benign and malignant lesions. Radiology. 1995;**196**:123-134

[14] Madjar H, Mundinger A, Degenhardt F, Duda V, Hackelöer BJ, Osmers R. Quaitätskontrolle in der Mamma-Sonographie. Ultraschall in der Medizin. 2003;**24**:190-194

[15] Duda VF, Bock K, Ipsen A, Schulz KD. Sonographisches Mehrstufenkonzept in der Mammadiagnostik. RöFo Journal. 2001;**173**:54-55

[16] Schulz-Wendtland R, Krämer S, Döinghaus K, Mitze M, Lang N. Sonographisch gesteuerte Mikrobiopsie der Brust: Eine neue interventionelle Technik. Gynäkologie. 1997;**2**:50-56

[17] Krämer S, Schulz-Wendtland R, Aichinger U, Bautz W, Lang N. Panorama-Sonographie (Siescape 3D) der Brust – Planung der brusterhaltenden Therapie beim Mammakarzinom. Ultraschall in der Medizin. 1999;**20**:104

[18] Watermann DO, Földi M, Hanjalic-Beck A, Hasenburg A, Lüghausen A, Prömpeler H, Gitsch G, Stickeler E. Three-dimensional ultrasound for the assessment of breast lesions. Ultrasound in Obstetrics & Gynecology. 2005;**25**:592-598

[19] Liberman L, Morris EA, Kim CMMR. Imaging findings in the contralateral breast of women with recently diagnosed breast cancer. American Journal of Roentgenology. 2003;**180**:333-341

[20] Krämer S, Schulz-Wendtland R, Hagedorn K, Bautz W, Lang N. Magnetic resonance imaging and its role in the diagnosis of multicentric breast cancer. Anticancer Research. 1998;**18**:2163-2164

[21] Krämer S, Schulz-Wendtland R, Hagedorn K. Magnetic resonance imaging in the diag-
     nosis of local recurrences in breast cancer. Anticancer Research. 1998;**18**:2159

[22] Rieber A, Brambs HJ, Gabelmann A, Breast MRI. For monitoring response of primary
     breast cancer to neo-adjuvant chemotherapy. European Radiology. 2002;**12**:1711

[23] Schulz-Wendtland R, Aichinger U, Krämer S, Lang N, Bautz W. Scars and local recur-
     rences – The role of the MRI. European Radiology. 2000;**10**:41-43

[24] Kaiser WA, Zeitler EMR. Imaging of the breast: Fast imaging sequences with and with-
     out Gd-DTPA: Preliminary observations. Radiology. 1989;**170**:681-686

[25] Heywang SH, Wolf A, Pruss EMR. Imaging of the breast with Gd-DTPA: Use and limita-
     tions. Radiology. 1989;**171**:95-103

[26] Sittek H, Kessler M, Bredl T. Lebeau A, Bohmert H, Reiser MF. Breast malignancies:
     Dynamic FLASH 3D MR-mammography versus mammography. Radiology. 1994;**193**:121

[27] Orel SG, Schnall MD, LiVolsi VA. MR imaging of the breast with rotating delivery of
     excitation off resonance: Clinical experience with pathologic correlation. Radiology.
     1993;**187**:493-501

[28] Orel SG, Mendonca MH, Reynolds C. MR imaging of ductal carcinoma in situ. Radiology.
     1997;**202**:413-420

[29] Schulz-Wendtland R, Aichinger U, Krämer S, Wilhelmi U, Lell M, Lang N, Bautz
     W. Follow-up after breast-conserving therapy: Comparison of conventional imaging
     methods with MRI. Geburtsh Frauenheilk. 2001;**61**:396-399

[30] Aichinger U, Schulz-Wendtland R, Dobritz M, Lell M, Krämer S, Lang N, Bautz W. Scar
     or recurrence – Comparison of MRI and color-coded ultrasound with echo signal ampli-
     fiers. Fortschr Röntgenstr. 2002;**174**:395-1401

[31] Veronesi U, Cascinelli N, Mariani L. Twenty-year follow-up of a randomized study com-
     paring breast-conserving surgery with radical mastectomy for early breast cancer. The
     New England Journal of Medicine. 2002;**347**:1227-1232

[32] Fisher B, Anderson S, Bryant J. Twenty-year follow-up of a randomized trial comparing
     total mastectomy, lumpectomy, and lumpectomy plus irradiation for the treatment of
     invasive breast cancer. The New England Journal of Medicine. 2002;**347**:1233-1241

[33] Holland R, Connolly J, Gelman R. Histologic multifocality of Tis, T1-2 breast carcino-
     mas: Implications for clinical trials of breast-conserving treatment. Cancer. 1985;**56**:979

[34] Fischer U, Kopka L, Grabbe E. Breast carcinoma: Effect of preoperative contrast-enhanced
     MR imaging on the therapeutic approach. Radiology. 1999;**213**:881-888

[35] Skaane P, Young K, Skjennald A. Comparison of film-screen mammography and full-
     field mammography with soft-copy reading in a population-based screening program:
     The Oslo II study. Radiology. 2002;**225**:267

[36] Tabar L, Fagerberg CJ, Gad A, Baldetorp I, Holmberg LH, Grontoft O, Ljungquist U, Lundstrom B, Manson JC, Eklund G. Reduction in mortality from breast cancer after mass screening with mammography. Lancet 1985;I:829-832

[37] Olsen O, Gotzsche PC. Cochrane review on screening for breast cancer with mammography. Lancet. 2001;**358**:1340-1342

[38] Nystrom L, Andersson I, Bjurstam N. Long-term effects of mammographic screening: Update overview of the Swedish randomised trials. Lancet. 2002;**359**:909-919

[39] Schulz-Wendtland R, Becker N, Bock K, Anders K, Bautz W. Mammography screening. Radiologe. 2007;**47**:359-369

[40] Schulz-Wendtland R, Krämer S, Döinghaus K, Säbel M, Lang N, Bautz W, Die Bedeutung d. Röntgen-Mammographie für das Mammakarzinomscreening. Röntgenpraxis. 1997;**50**: 103-109

[41] Tabar L, Vitak B, Tony HH. Beyond randomised controlled trials: Organised mammographic screening substantially reduces breast carcinoma mortality. Cancer. 2001;**91**:1724-1731

[42] Beckmann MW, Fasching RA, Gall C, Bani M, Brumm C, Krämer S. Genetic risk factors in breast cancer. Gynakologe. 2002;**35**:527-536

[43] Beckmann MW, Bani MR, Fasching PA, Strick R, Lux MP. Risk and risk assessment for breast cancer: Molecular and clinical aspects. Maturitas. 2007;**57**:56-60

[44] Kuhl CK, Schmutzler RK, Leutner CC, Breast MR. Imaging screening in 192 women proved or suspected to be carriers of a breast cancer susceptibility gene: Preliminary results. Radiology. 2000;**215**:267-279

[45] Fersis N, Smyczek-Gargya B, Krainick U, Mielke G, Müller-Schimpfle M, Kiesel L, Wallwiener D. Clinical experience with large-core needle biopsies of the breast and evaluation of histopathology. Zentralbl Gynäkol. 2001;**123**:132-135

[46] Schulz-Wendtland R, Krämer S, Lang N, Bautz W. Ultrasonic guided microbiopsy in mammary diagnosis: Indications, technique and results. Anticancer Research. 1998;**18**: 2145-2146

[47] Parker SH, Jobe WE, Dennis MA. US-guided automated large-core breast biopsy. Radiology. 1993;**187**:507

[48] Schulz-Wendtland R, Krämer S, Döinghaus K, Mitze M, Lang N. Interventionelle Techniken in der Mammadiagnostik: sonographisch gezielte Stanzbiopsie. Akt Radiology. 1997;**7**:30-34

[49] Sickles EA, Parker SH. Appropriate role of core biopsy in the management of probably benign lesions. Radiology. 1994;**190**:313

[50] Schulz-Wendtland R, Aichinger U, Krämer S, Tartsch M, Kuchar I, Magener A, Bautz W. Sonographical breast biopsy: How many core biopsy specimens are needed ? Fortschr Röntgenstr 2003;**173**:94-98

[51] Liberman L, Feng TL, Dershaw DD. US-guided core breast biopsy: Use and cost-effectiveness. Radiology. 1998;**208**:717-723

[52] Kettritz U, Rotter K, Murauer M. Stereotaxic vacuum biopsy in 2874 patients: A multi-center study. Cancer. 2004;**100**:245-251

[53] Heywang-Koebrunner SH, Schaumloeffel U, Viehweg P. Minimally invasive stereotaxic vacuum core breast biopsy. European Radiology. 1998;**8**:377-338

[54] Azavedo E, Svane G, Auer G. Stereotaxic fine needle biopsy in 2594 mammographically detected nonpalpable lesions. Lancet. 1989;**1**:1033

[55] Parker SH, Lovin JD, Jobe WE. Nonpalpable breast lesions: Stereotactic automated large core biopsies. Radiology. 1991;**180**:403

[56] Liberman L, Dershaw DD, Rosen PP. Stereotaxic 14-gauge breast biopsy: How many core biopsy specimens are needed? Radiology. 1994;**192**:793

[57] Burbank F. Mammographic findings after 14 gauge automated needle and 14 gauge directional vacuum assisted stereotactic breast biopsy. Radiology. 1997;**204**:153

[58] Liberman L, Dershaw D, Morris EA. Clip placement after stereotactic vacuum-assisted breast biopsy. Radiology. 1997;**205**:417

[59] Krämer S, Schulz-Wendtland R, Lang N. Qualitätssicherung bei der stereotaktischen Stanzbiopsie durch Einsatz eines Phantoms. Akt Radiology. 1996;**6**:153-155

[60] Schulz-Wendtland R, Heywang-Köbrunner S, Aichinger U, Krämer S, Wenkel E, Bautz W. Do tissue marker clips after sonographically or stereotactically guided breast biopsy improve follow-up of small breast lesions and localisation of breast cancer after chemotherapy ? Fortschr Röntgenstr. 2002;**174**:620-624

[61] Parker SH, Klaus AJ, McWey M. Sonographically guided directional vacuum-assisted breast biopsy using a handheld device. American Journal of Roentgenology. 2001;**177**:405-408

[62] Schulz-Wendtland R, Krämer S, Bautz W. First experiences with a new vacuum-assisted device for breast biopsy. Fortschr Röntgenstr. 2003;**173**:1496-1499

[63] Krainick-Strobel U, Majer I, Huber B, Gall C, Krämer B, Gruber I, Fehm T, Huober J, Hierlemann H, Doser M, Meyberg-Solomayer G, Hoffmann J, Wallwiener D, Hahn M. Development of a gel-simulation model and generation of standard tables for the complete extirpation of benign breast lesions with vacuum assisted biopsy under ultrasound guidance. Ultrasound in Medicine & Biology. 2006;**32**:1539-1544

[64] Krämer S, Schulz-Wendtland R, Bautz W, Lang N. Neue Aspekte in der interventionellen Mammdiagnostik und Brustchirurgie – ABBI (Advanced Breast Biopsy Instrumentation) in der Diagnostik und minimal invasiven Mammachirurgie. In: Waclawiczek HW, editor. Die interdisziplinäre kurative Behandlung des Mammakarzinoms. Heidelberg: Johann Ambrosius Barth Verlag; 1998

[65] Kuhl CK, Elevelt A, Leutner CC. Interventional breast MR imaging: Clinical use of ste-reotactic localization and biopsy device. Radiology. 1997;**204**:667-675

[66] Heywang-Koebrunner SH, Schaumlöffel-Schulze U, Heinig A. MR-guided percutaneous vacuum biopsy of breast lesions: Experience with 100 lesions. Radiology. 1999;**213**:289

[67] Fischer U, Vosshenrich R, Döler W, Hamadeh A, Oestmann JW, Grabbe E. MR-imaging-guided breast intervention: Experience with two systems. Radiology. 1995;**195**:533-538

[68] Krämer S, Jäger W, Lang N, Beckmann MW. Surgical treatment of breast cancer in the elderly. Journal of Menopausal Medicine. 2004;**2**:9-15

[69] Meyer JE, Kopans DB, Stomper PC. Occult breast abnormalities: Percutaneous preopera-tive needle localization. Radiology. 1984;**150**:335-337

[70] Schulz-Wendtland R, Bauer M, Krämer S, Büttner A, Lang N. Stereotaxie – Eine Methode zur Punktion, Stanzbiopsie und Markierung kleinster mammographischer Herdbefunde. Chirurgische Praxis. 1995;**49**:123-136

[71] Orel SG, Schnall MD, Newman RW. MR imaging-guided localization and biopsy of breast lesions: Initial experience. Radiology. 1994;**193**:97-102

[72] Golshan M, Fung BB, Wolfman J. The effect of ipsilateral whole breast ultrasound on the surgical management of breast carcinoma. American Journal of Surgery. 2003;**186**:391

[73] Tillman GF, Orel SG, Schnall MD. Effect of breast magnetic resonance imaging on the clinical management of women with early-stage breast carcinoma. Journal of Clinical Oncology. 2002;**20**:3413

7

A Case of an Invasive Lobular Carcinoma with Extracellular Mucin: Radio-Pathological Correlation

Shinya Tajima, Keiko Kishimoto,
Yoshihide Kanemaki, Ichiro Maeda, Akira Endo,
Motohiro Chosokabe, Takafumi Ono,
Koichiro Tsugawa and Masayuki Takagi

Abstract

A case of 77-year-old female with an invasive lobular carcinoma with extracellular mucin is presented. She felt palpable mass in her left breast. Then, she came to our hospital for further examination. Mammography of right in full view revealed architectural distortion in left upper portion. And ultrasonography demonstrated low-echoic mass about 2 cm in diameter and invasion of the fat tissue was observed. Hence, malignancy was suspected and magnetic resonance imaging (MRI) was performed. MRI findings showed irregular shaped and margined mass with small T2-high-signal intensity. These findings suggested invasive carcinoma with mucin. Because the cancer lesion was not large, partial mastectomy was performed. Interestingly, pathological diagnosis was invasive lobular carcinoma with extracellular mucin. Extracellular mucinous lesion was concordant with small T2-high-signal intensity. This type of carcinoma was previously reported only in three cases, and rare but important, because the treatment and prognosis might change by histological subtypes. We suggest one of the MRI special features of our case is not only irregular shaped and margined mass but also small T2-high-signal intensity. These MR findings might be one of the valuable findings for the diagnosis and differentiation between this type of carcinoma from other tumors.

Keywords: magnetic resonance imaging, breast, invasive lobular carcinoma, extracellular mucin, E-cadherin

1. Introduction

To discriminate between invasive lobular carcinoma and invasive ductal carcinoma is a big theme for both radiologically and pathologically. The limitation of radiologic imaging in the detection and evaluation of invasive lobular carcinoma have been recognized for a long time. Whereas, advances in breast radiologic imaging present opportunities to improve the diagnosis of invasive lobular carcinoma.

On mammography, invasive lobular carcinoma is not likely to form calcifications. However, calcifications may be present in benign proliferative lesions such as sclerosing adenosis [1]. The most common manifestations of invasive lobular carcinoma are asymmetric density, irregular, or spiculated mass on mammography [2–4].

On ultrasonography, 60.5% of invasive lobular carcinomas produced "a heterogeneous low-echoic mass with angular or irregular margins and posterior acoustic shadowing." The remaining tumors had various other sonographic characteristics, including 12% that were "ultrasonographically invisible." The sensitivity of ultrasonography for tumors measuring less than 1 cm was 85.7%. Invasive lobular carcinoma of common type tended to produce "focal shadowing without a discrete mass," whereas tumors with pleomorphic histology were seen as "a shadowing mass." Tumors of the alveolar, solid, and signet-ring variant of invasive lobular carcinoma were most often manifested as a "lobulated, well circumscribed mass" [5]. Ultrasonography is useful and more accurate than mammography in diagnosing invasive lobular carcinoma [5]. However, it is difficult to narrow down the diagnosis of invasive lobular carcinoma.

Breast magnetic resonance imaging (MRI) has an overall sensitivity of 93% for detecting invasive lobular carcinoma, similar to the detection of breast cancers overall (90%). On MRI, tumor of smooth margin, or absence of smooth margin and the distribution of nonmass-like enhancement are the features of invasive lobular carcinoma. Invasive lobular carcinoma may present as ductal, segmental, regional, or diffuse patterns [6]. MR imaging is considered to be a useful tool for detecting invasive lobular carcinoma on radiologically.

Pathologically, the invasive lobular carcinoma includes not only classical type (Foote and Stewart advocated in 1946 [7]) but also variants of solid, alveolar, pleomorphic, tubulolobular, signet-ring, trabecular, and mixed types [8].

We encountered a tumor of invasive carcinoma coexisting with mucinous carcinoma-like lesion. At first, the differential diagnoses of this tumor are (i) mixed mucinous-ductal carcinoma, (ii) mucinous carcinoma with neuroendocrine feature, (iii) mucinous papillary neoplasms, and (iv) carcinoma of mixed type (lobular and ductal carcinoma). Lobular carcinoma has been considered a variant of mucin-secreting carcinoma with only intracytoplasmic mucin [9–11]. In common practice, a diagnosis of mucinous carcinoma or ductal carcinoma with mucinous features is often made in the presence of extracellular mucin, without immunohistochemical confirmation of the ductal phenotype [10]. However, final diagnosis was "invasive lobular carcinoma with extracellular mucin" which has been reported only in three cases in the English medical literature [9–11]. Accordingly, the current report is the fourth documented case in pathology, and in the viewpoint of radiology, this is the first case.

Taking into consideration of the above information, we will discuss the unique variant of "invasive lobular carcinoma with extracellular mucin" with radiopathological correlation.

2. Materials and methods

2.1. MR imaging protocol

MR imaging was performed using a 1.5T MR system (Achieva 1.5T, Philips Healthcare Nederland, Eindhoven, Netherland), and a synergy breast coil. Routine breast MR images were acquired as follows in the prone position: axial T2-weighted turbo spin echo (TSE) with STIR images (repetition time (TR)/echo time (TE) = 5175/60 ms, section thickness = 5 mm, FOV = 280 mm, matrix = 480 × 480), and axial diffusion-weighted (DW) images using a single-shot EPI (FOV = 280 mm, matrix = 128 × 128), with MPG pulse applied along three directions (x, y, and z axes) with TR/TE of 5532/80 ms and b-factors of 0, 1000, and 2000 s/mm^2. Apparent diffusion coefficient (ADC)-maps were automatically generated on a postprocessing workstation. After axial T1-weighted SE images, [TR/TE = 468.8/12 ms, flip angle = 90, section thickness = 5 mm, FOV = 280 mm, matrix = 128 × 128] were obtained, axial 3D dynamic contrast enhanced T1-weighted images with SPAIR using eTHRIVE sequence [TR/TE = 5.9/2.8 ms, flip angle = 10, section thickness = 5 mm, FOV = 280 mm, matrix = 512 × 512] were performed in precontrast, double arterial phase, and delayed phase.

2.2. Image interpretation

For image interpretation of mammography, ultrasonography, and magnetic resonance imaging, we used the breast imaging and reporting data system (BI-RADS) lexicon and associated report of Tozaki et al. [12, 13].

2.3. Hematoxylin and eosin staining

Operation samples obtained from the partial mastectomy were fixed at least 8 h in 10% neutral phosphate buffered formalin, then, embedded in paraffin, and sectioned at 3–4 μm. The paraffin-embedded specimens were stained with hematoxylin and eosin (HE) for light microscopic examination.

2.4. Immunohistochemistry

Paraffin-embedded sections measuring 3–4 μm thick were deparaffinized. Antigen retrieval was then performed for 20–40 min in boiling water (95°C) containing citric acid solution (pH 6.0) or Target Retrieval Solution (pH 9.0; cat. no. 415211; Nichirei, Tokyo, Japan), and (pH 6.0; cat. no. S2031; Dako, Glostrup, Denmark). Sections were pretreated with 0.3% peroxide and reacted with primary monoclonal antibodies against estrogen receptor (ER), progesterone receptor (PgR), HER2, Ki67, E-cadherin, Synaptophysin, MUC1, and MUC3 are shown in **Table 1**. Subsequently, specimens were incubated with a secondary antibody (Histofine simple stain MAX-PO; cat. no. 424154; Nichirei). The chromogenic substrate was 3,3'-diaminobenzidine (DAB), and the slides were counterstained with hematoxylin.

Antibody	Clone	Source	Activation	Dilution
ER	EP1	DAKO	Heat pH 9.0/40 min	1:2
PgR	PgR636	DAKO	Heat pH 6.0/40 min	1:2
HER2	Rabbit poly	DAKO	Heat pH 6.0/40 min	1:1
Ki-67	MIB-1	DAKO	Heat pH 6.0/40 min	1:200
E-cadherin	35B5	Leica	Heat pH 6.0/40 min	1:2
Synaptophysin	27G12	NICHIREI	Heat pH 9.0/40 min	1:2
MUC1	Ma552	Leica	Heat pH 6.0/40 min	1:100
MUC3	1143/B7	Lab Vision	Heat pH 6.0/40 min	1:100

Table 1. Primary monoclonal antibodies against ER, PgR, HER2, Ki67, E-cadherin, synaptophysin, MUC1, and MUC3.

3. Results

A case of 77-year-old female is presented. She felt palpable mass in her left breast since 1 month and came to our hospital for further examination.

Physical examination revealed a 2.7 cm palpable mass in left upper inner and outer quadrants without nipple discharge and lymphadenopathy. No familial history of breast cancer was confirmed.

On mammography, the breast appeared dense. However, mediolateral oblique (MLO) view of the mammography demonstrated architectural distortion in left upper portion (**Figure 1**). Hence, this lesion was of four categories. Right MLO view revealed no evidence of malignancy.

Ultrasonography revealed a low-echoic mass about 2 cm in diameter with posterior acoustic shadowing, and disruption of the anterior border line (the anterior border line means boundary line between fat tissue layer and breast parenchymal layer) of the mass was observed in her left breast (**Figure 2**). There was no lesion suggesting malignancy in her right breast. No lymph node swelling was seen.

These findings suggested the possibility of malignancy. Therefore, magnetic resonance imaging (MRI) of 1.5T (Philips) was performed. On MRI, diffusion-weighted image of b-value 1000 s/mm^2 showed mass-like lesion with high signal intensity (**Figure 3A**). Apparent diffusion coefficient (ADC)-map revealed diffusion limitation of the water molecule (**Figure 3B**). Dynamic contrast-enhanced T1 weighted images demonstrated early enhancement and delayed washout pattern of irregular shaped and margined mass about

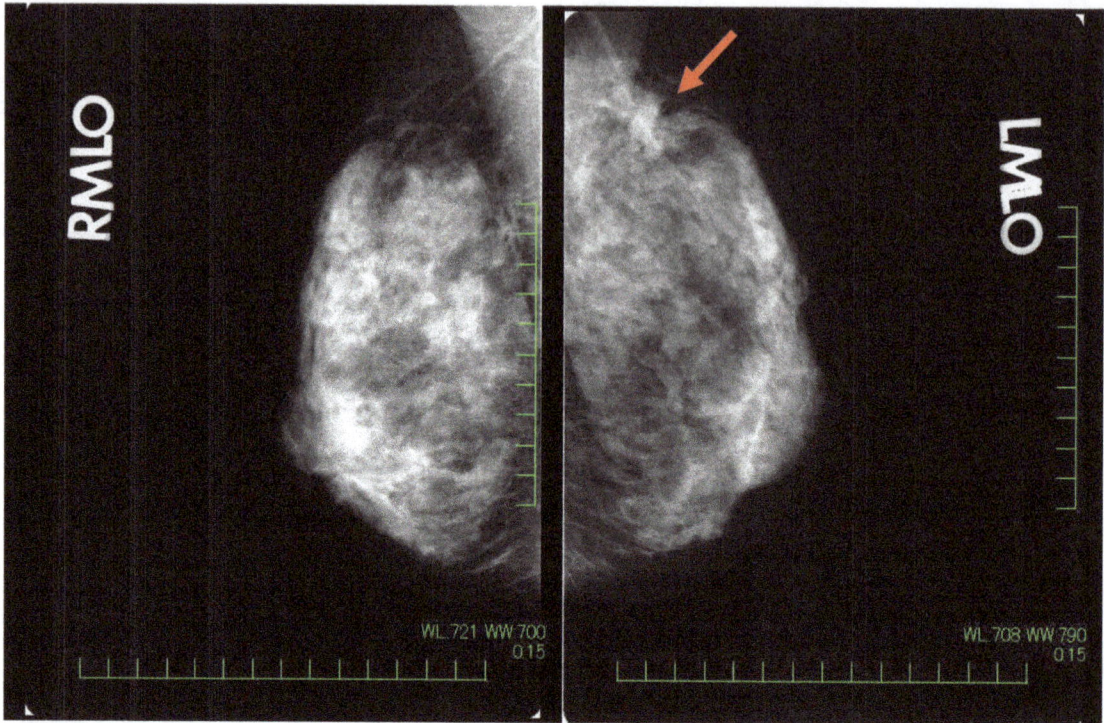

Figure 1. MLO view of the mammography demonstrates architectural distortion in left upper portion (arrow).

2 cm in diameter (**Figure 3C** and **D**). The mass included a small high signal intensity area on fat-saturated T2 weighted image, which was confirmed pathologically as extracellular mucin. (**Figure 3E**). Dynamic-curve of the contrast-enhanced MRI showed rapid wash-out pattern (**Figure 3F**). ADC value was 0.577×10^{-3} mm^2/s; hence, the existence of water restriction was suggested.

Neoadjuvant chemotherapy was not performed. Then, partial mastectomy was performed because of the imaging findings. Sentinel lymph node was negative for metastatic cancer lesion. Further, axillary lymph node resection was not performed. Histopathological findings revealed low-grade tumor with little or no nuclear atypia and inconspicuous nucleoli. Besides, the tumor was composed of single cell with moderate pleomorphism and lack of cohesion. The neoplastic cells were arranged in files or cords infiltrating the stroma. Partially, trabecular type lesion was observed (**Figure 4A**). Within the tumor, there were areas showing signet-ring cells floating in a pool of mucin (**Figure 4B**). The presence of the extracellular mucin is not a characteristic of lobular carcinomas. Therefore, immunohistochemical stain for E-cadherin was performed. However, the lesions were negative for E-cadherin immunostaining (**Figure 4C**). Besides, neuroendocrine marker of synaptophysin was completely negative. MIB1 (Ki67)-index was about 10%. Estrogen receptor (ER), progesterone receptor (PgR), and human epidermal growth factor receptor 2 (HER2) status were 99, 0%, and negative, respectively. Additionally, special stainings for mucin as MUC1 and MUC3 were performed, and both stainings were positive of both infiltrating cells and signet-ring cells floating in a pool of mucin (**Figure 4D** and **E**).

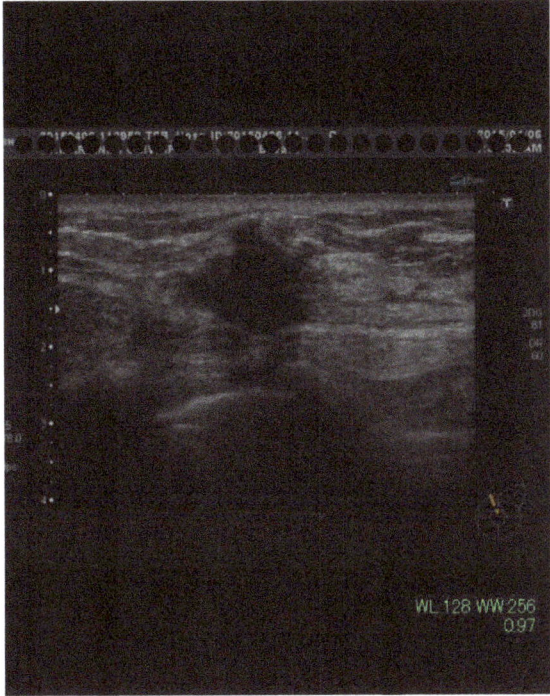

Figure 2. Ultrasonography reveals a low-echoic mass, posterior acoustic shadowing, and disruption of the anterior border line is observed.

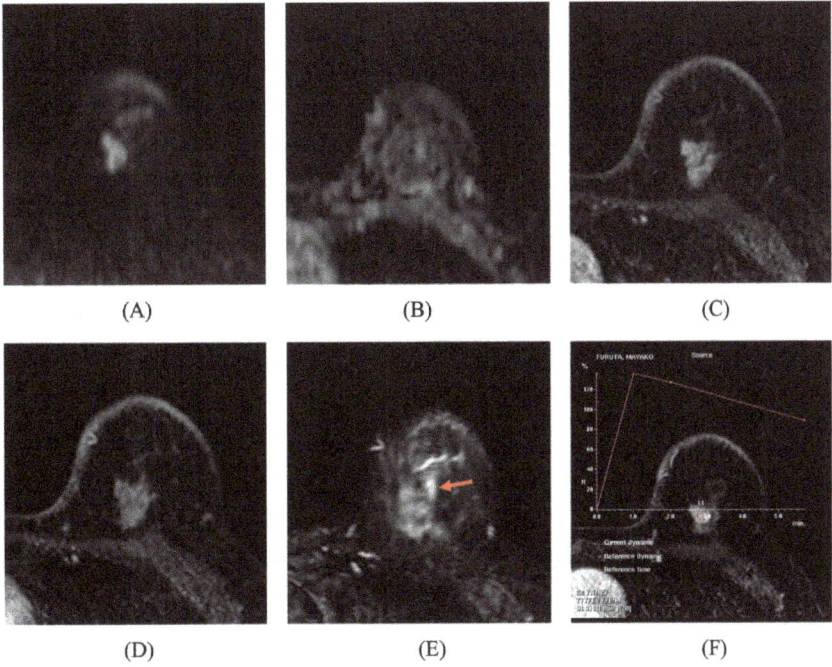

(A)   (B)   (C)

(D)   (E)   (F)

Figure 3. (A) Diffusion-weighted image of b-1000 shows mass like high signal intensity. (B) Apparent diffusion coefficient (ADC)-map reveals diffusion limitation of the water molecule. (C) Contrast-enhanced T1 weighted images demonstrate early enhancement and (D) delayed washout pattern. (E) The mass included a small high-signal intensity on fat-saturated T2 weighted image, which is confirmed pathologically as extracellular mucin (arrow). (F) Dynamic-curve of the MRI shows rapid washout pattern.

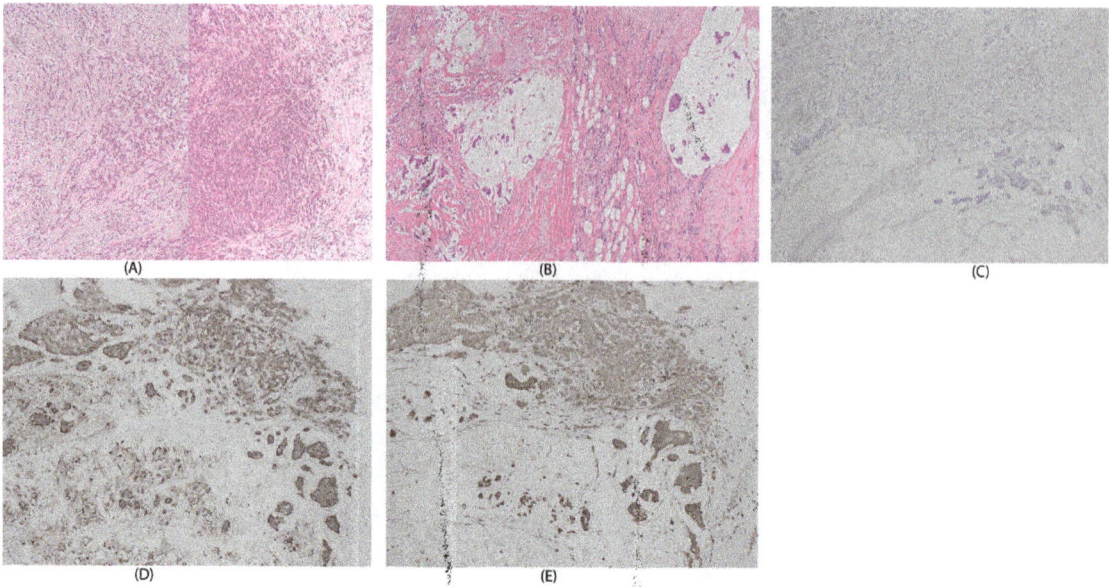

Figure 4. (A) The neoplastic cells are arranged in files or cords infiltrating the stroma. Partially, trabecular type lesion is observed. (B) Within the tumor, there are areas showing atypical cells floating in a pool of mucin. (C) All the tumor cells are negative for E-cadherin immunostaining. (D) All the tumor cells and extracellular mucin are MUC1 positive. (E) All the tumor cells and extracellular mucin are MUC3 positive.

4. Discussion

The major types of invasive carcinomas are categorized as ductal carcinoma. Invasive lobular carcinoma is the second most common histological type of breast carcinoma, accounting for about 5–15% of all invasive breast cancers [14, 15]. Hence, accurate diagnosis of invasive lobular carcinoma is thought to be important. We will discuss about general radiological findings of invasive lobular carcinoma and correlation of our case.

In mammography, Berg et al. [16] examined the performance of mammography as a function of both tumor type and breast density. Mammographic sensitivity was 81% for invasive ductal carcinoma compared with 34% for invasive lobular carcinoma; when only those patients with dense breast tissue were considered, sensitivities decreased dramatically to 60 and 11%, respectively [16]. Because of these diagnostic interests, it is crucial for breast radiologists to be aware of the asymmetric and subtle mammographic features of invasive lobular carcinoma.

A high-density spiculated or irregular margined mass on mammography means invasive carcinoma. Spicula or irregular margin is thought to be invasion of the breast fat tissue and stromal reaction that disrupts normal breast parenchymal architecture. common mammographic manifestations of invasive lobular carcinoma include spiculated or irregular margined mass or asymmetric density. In our case, these findings are not observed. Apart from spiculated, irregular margined masses and asymmetric densities, the most common mammographic manifestation of invasive lobular carcinoma is architectural distortion, which accounts for about 14–25% of cases of mammographically detected invasive lobular carcinoma [3, 17, 18].

Similarly, our case demonstrated architectural distortion on left upper portion in MLO view. We think distortion on mammography means stromal reaction and malignancy.

Ultrasonography of the breast is used primarily as a diagnostic imaging tool. The most common sonographic appearance of invasive lobular carcinoma is a low-echoic mass with posterior acoustic shadowing occurring in up to 60% of cases, however, posterior acoustic shadowing may be lacking in up to 20% of cases [19]. The present case of ultrasonographical findings is thought to be concordant with report of Karen et al. [19].

Here, we will discuss correlation between MRI findings and pathological findings. Our case of mammographic and ultrasonographic findings suggested the possibility of malignancy. Therefore, magnetic resonance imaging (MRI) of 1.5T (Philips) was performed. On MRI, diffusion-weighted image of b-value 1000 s/mm^2 showed mass-like high signal intensity. Apparent diffusion coefficient (ADC)-map revealed diffusion limitation of the water molecule. Besides, irregular shaped and margined mass was observed in T1 weighted image. These findings suggest malignancy in our case. Furthermore, this finding is similar to the report of Mann et al. of invasive lobular carcinoma [6]. Fat-saturated T2 weighted image of the mass showed small high signal intensity area within the mass. This finding suggests the tumor associated mucinous lesion or coexistence of mucinous carcinoma. However, Rosa et al. [9] reported signet-ring cells floating in a pool of mucinous areas (extracellular mucinous lesion) represented at the most 20% of the tumor. We think this extracellular mucin area is not so large but a small area. If invasive carcinoma and mucinous carcinoma are coexisted as collision tumor, the mucinous area which shows very high signal intensity on T2 weighted image would be larger. In our case, extracellular mucin area was approximately 10% of the tumor. This small area of high signal intensity on T2 weighted image might be one of the specific features of invasive lobular carcinoma with extracellular mucin. Dynamic-curve of the contrast-enhanced MRI showed rapid washout pattern. Rapid washout pattern is also seen in invasive ductal or lobular carcinoma. ADC value was 0.577×10^{-3} mm^2/s, hence the existence of water restriction was suggested. From these findings, dynamic-curve, diffusion-weighted image, and ADC-map were suggestive for malignant tumor. And contrast-enhanced T1 weighted image of irregular shaped and margined mass was indicative of invasive carcinoma such as invasive ductal carcinoma or invasive lobular carcinoma. T2 weighted image of small high signal intensity area is thought to be mucinous carcinoma or mucin production. And mucin production is known to be associated with neuroendocrine differentiation. Taking these findings into consideration, other differential diagnoses of this tumor were (i) mixed mucinous-ductal carcinoma, (ii) mucinous carcinoma with neuroendocrine feature, (iii) mucinous papillary neoplasms, and (iv) carcinoma of mixed type (lobular and ductal carcinoma). However, histopathological findings revealed the tumor was composed of single cell with moderate pleomorphism and lack of cohesion. The neoplastic cells were arranged in files or cords infiltrating the stroma. In situ lesion of the invasive lobular carcinoma was not observed. The multifocality of cancer lesion was not demonstrated. Within the tumor, there were areas showing signet-ring cells floating in a pool of mucin. The presence of extracellular mucin is not characteristic of lobular carcinomas. Therefore, immunohistochemical stain for E-cadherin was performed. However, the lesions were completely negative for E-cadherin immunostaining. E-cadherin, a cell-cohesion protein encoded by a gene on chromosome 16q22.1, is the current marker of choice to help discriminate between lobular and ductal carcinoma [11]. Neuroendocrine marker of synaptophysin immunostaining was also negative. Hence, final diagnosis of our tumor is invasive ductal carcinoma with extracellular mucin. From the results of MRI findings, irregular shaped and margined mass with small area of fat-saturated T2 high signal intensity might be one of the special feature of invasive lobular carcinoma with extracellular mucin. Our case is the fourth case in the English literature. Because the number of cases of these tumors is limited, it is difficult to comment on the biological behavior and molecular profiles. However, this diagnosis is important for prognosis and management, and further examination is needed.

In our case, estrogen receptor (ER), progesterone receptor (PgR), and human epidermal growth factor receptor 2 (HER2) status were 99, 0%, and negative, respectively. Invasive lobular carcinoma is known to be more commonly estrogen receptor-positive and HER2-negative, in other words, invasive lobular carcinoma is usually categorized as luminal subtype. The previous reports of Rosa et al. and Haltas et al. [9, 11] are ER positive of luminal subtype. Our case is concordant with their results. However, the results of Yu et al. [10] were not only ER-positive but also HER2 strongly positive. They thought that this type of HER2 status demonstrate various features.

The spectrum of breast lesions that demonstrate extracellular mucin includes fibrocystic change with luminal mucin, mucocele-like lesions, papillary lesions with mucin secretion, and mucinous carcinoma among others [9]. In contrast, lobular neoplasia and invasive lobular carcinoma demonstrate intracytoplasmic mucin, and no cases of lobular carcinoma with extracellular mucin have been found except previous three reports [9–11, 20].

Invasive lobular carcinoma comprises 5–15% of invasive breast tumors [14, 15]. They can occur at any age. The median age at diagnosis is between 45 and 56 years and there is a tendency to affect older patients compared with ductal carcinoma [8, 9], similar to our results of the 77-year-old. The presenting symptom in most cases is a mass with irregular margins or a breast thickening with diffuse nodularity [8, 9]. The clinical features of invasive lobular carcinoma are also different from that of ductal carcinomas. Invasive lobular carcinomas tend to be more often multifocal and bilateral [8, 9], with a distinct metastatic pattern and a higher frequency of bone, gastrointestinal tract, uterus, meninges, and diffuse serosal involvement [21]. Hence, discrimination between lobular carcinoma and ductal carcinoma is important clinically, radiologically, and pathologically. In our case, multifocality of the tumor was not observed similarly to the reports of Rosa et al. and Yu et al. [9, 10]. However, the case of Haltas et al. [11] indicated multifocality. We think this is because the variant of invasive lobular carcinoma with extracellular mucin might present different behavior compared with classical invasive lobular carcinoma.

Mucin has been classified as membrane-bound mucin, which mediates signal transduction, and secretary mucin, which are directly secreted into extracellular spaces. In the MUC immunostaining family, the membrane-bound mucins include MUC1, MUC3, MUC4, and the secretary mucins include MUC2, MUC5AC, MUC6 [22]. In our current case, MUC4, MUC5AC, and MUC6 were negative; however, all the tumor cells revealed cytoplasmic expression of MUC1. Molecular and biochemical studies have demonstrated that MUC1 is involved in the inhibition of E-cadherin mediated -cell and cell-matrix adhesion [10, 22–25]. The cytoplasmic domain of MUC1 molecule has been shown to inhibit the formation of E-cadherin-β-catenin complex [10, 24]. Therefore MUC1 may play a role in tumor invasion and metastases by disrupting cell adhesions [10]. Similarly, our case of tumor invasion may correlate with the MUC1 cytoplasmic expression.

Additionally, our case of all the tumor cells was positive for MUC3 immunostaining. Rakha et al. and Furuya et al. [26, 27] reported that MUC3 immunostaining is useful for distinguishing between benign lesion and malignant lesion of the breast carcinoma. Our case is concordant with their reports, and membrane-bound mucin of MUC3 may mediate signal transduction correlate with malignancy. Furthermore, Rakha et al. [26] indicated that most breast carcinomas express MUC1, MUC3, and MUC4; however, MUC1 and MUC3 are potential prognostic indicators. Hence, diagnosing invasive lobular carcinoma with extracellular mucin is important on not only pathologically but also radiologically.

Early genomic studies revealed very little overall difference in genomic profiles between low-grade invasive ductal carcinoma and classical invasive lobular carcinoma, implying that classical invasive lobular carcinoma might represent a subtype of low-grade invasive ductal carcinoma [10]. Recent gene expression studies comparing invasive lobular carcinoma and invasive ductal carcinoma have identified two subsets of invasive lobular carcinoma with distinct transcription patterns [10]. Approximately, half of the invasive lobular carcinomas differs from invasive ductal carcinomas in gene expression profiles ("typical" invasive lobular carcinomas), while the remaining invasive lobular carcinomas closely resemble invasive ductal carcinomas in transcription patterns. ("ductal-like" invasive lobular carcinomas) [10]. On the other hand, a recent study on grade- and molecular subtype-matched invasive lobular carcinomas and invasive ductal carcinomas of no special type demonstrated that invasive lobular carcinomas had different transcriptomic profiles in the genes related to cell-to-cell adhesion and signaling, as well as actin cytoskeleton signaling, when compared with grade- and molecular subtype-matched invasive ductal carcinomas [10]. This finding suggested that even though invasive lobular carcinomas and invasive ductal carcinomas might present as a spectrum or form of a family [10]. Taking into consideration of the above Yu et al. reported case, our current case might be in the middle stage of the spectrum between lobular carcinoma and ductal carcinoma. We think existence of extracellular mucin is not definitive for ductal phenotype not only histologically but also genetically.

5. Conclusion

We encountered the distinct variant of invasive lobular carcinoma with extracellular mucin. We described the correlation of its radiological and pathological interest. Radiological findings of invasive lobular carcinoma with extracellular mucin are documented in English literature for the first time. We suggest one of the MRI special features of our case is not only irregular shaped and margined mass but also small T2-high-signal intensity. These findings by the knowledge from radiopathological correlation might be one of the specific features of invasive lobular carcinoma with extracellular mucin. Further examinations are needed to clarify this lesion.

Acknowledgements

We thank Shigeko Ohnuma and Manabu Kubota department of the St. Marianna University of pathology for their technical assistance and advices.

Author details

Shinya Tajima[1,2]*, Keiko Kishimoto[2], Yoshihide Kanemaki[2], Ichiro Maeda[1], Akira Endo[1], Motohiro Chosokabe[1], Takafumi Ono[2], Koichiro Tsugawa[3] and Masayuki Takagi[1]

*Address all correspondence to: stajima0829@gmail.com

1 Department of Pathology and Radiology, St. Marianna University School of Medicine, Kawasaki City, Kanagawa, Japan

2 Department of Radiology, St. Marianna University School of Medicine, Kawasaki City, Kanagawa, Japan

3 Department of Breast and Endocrine Surgery, St. Marianna University School of Medicine, Kawasaki City, Kanagawa, Japan

References

[1] Mendelson EB, Harris KM, Doshi N, et al. Infiltrating lobulacarcinoma: Mammographic patteforrns with pathologic correlation. American Journal of Radiology. 1989;**153**:265-271

[2] Helvie MA, Paramagul C, Oberman HA, et al. Invasive lobular carcinoma imaging features and clinical detection. Investigative Radiology. 1993;**28**:202-207

[3] Le GM, Ollivier L, Asselain B, et al. Mammographic features of 455 invasive lobular carcinomas. Radiology. 1992;**185**:705-708

[4] White JR, Gustafson GS, Wimbish K, et al. Conservative surgery and radiation therapy for infiltrating lobular carcinoma of the breast. The role of preoperative mammograms in guiding treatment. Cancer. 1994;**74**:640-647

[5] Butler RS, Venta LA, Wiley EL, et al. Sonographic evaluation of infiltrating lobular carcinoma. American Journal of Roentgenology. 1999;**172**:325-330

[6] Mann RM, Hoogeveen YL, Blickman JG, et al. MRI compared to conventional diagnostic work-up in the detection and evaluation of invasive lobular carcinoma of the breast: A review of existing literature. Breast Cancer Research and Treatment. 2008;**107**:1-14

[7] Foote FW Jr, Stewart FW. A histologic classification of carcinoma of the breast. Surgery. 1946;**19**:74-99

[8]   Rosen PP. Invasive lobular carcinoma. In: Rosen's Breast Pathology. 3rd ed. Philadelphia, PA: Lippincott Williams and Wilkins; 2001. pp. 690-705

[9]   Rosa M, Mohammadi A, Masood S. Lobular carcinoma of the breast with extracellular mucin: New variant of mucin-producing carcinoma? Pathology International. 2009;**59**:405-409

[10] Yu J, Bhargava R, Dabbs DJ. Invasive lobular carcinoma with extracellular mucin production and HER-2 overexpression: A case report and further case studies. Diagnostic Pathology. 2010;**5**:36

[11] Haltas H, Bayrak R, Yenidunya S, et al. Invasive lobular carcinoma with extracellular mucin as a distinct variant of lobular carcinoma: A case report. Diagnostic Pathology. 2012;**7**:91

[12] D'Orsi CJ, Sickles EA, Mendelson EB, et al, editors. ACR BI-RADS Atlas Breast Imaging Reporting and Data System. 5th ed. Reston, VA: American College of Radiology; 2013

[13] Tozaki M, Fukuma E. MR spectroscopy and diffusion weighted imaging of the breast: Are they useful tools for characterizing breast lesions before biopsy?. American Journal of Roentgenology. 2009;**193**:840-809

[14] Sastre-Garau X, Jouve M, Asselain B, et al. Infiltrating lobular carcinoma of the breast. Clinicopathologic analysis of 975 cases with reference to data on conservative therapy and metastatic patterns. Cancer. 1996;**77**:113-120

[15] Borst MJ, Ingold JA. Metastatic patterns of invasive lobular versus invasive ductal carcinoma of the breast. Surgery. 1993;**144**:637-641

[16] Berg WA, Gutierrez L, NessAiver MS, et al. Diagnostic accuracy of mammography, clinical examination, US, and MR imaging in preoperative assessment of breast cancer. Radiology. 2004;**233**:830-849

[17] Hilleren DJ, Andersson IT, Lindholm K, et al. Invasive lobular carcinoma: Mammographic findings in a 10-year experience. Radiology. 1991;**178**:149-154

[18] Krecke KN, Gisvold JJ. Invasive lobular carcinoma of the breast: Mammographic findings and extent of disease at diagnosis in 184 patients. American Journal of Roentgenology. 1993;**161**:957-960

[19] Karen J, Deba S, Shelley EH. Lobular breast cancer series: imaging. Breast Cancer Research. 2015;**17**:94

[20] Tan PH, Tse GM, Bay BH. Mucinous breast lesions: Diagnostic challenges. Journal of Clinical Pathology. 2008;**61**:11-19

[21] Ellis OI, Schnitt SJ, Sastre-Garau X, et al. Invasive breast carcinoma. In: Tavassoli FA, Devillee P, editors. Tumours of the Breast and Female Genital Organs. Lyon: IARC Press; 2003. pp. 23-25, 48-49

[22] Singh PK, Hollingsworth MA. Cell surface-associated mucins in signal transduction. Trends in Cell Biology. 2006;**16**:467-476

[23] Rahn JJ, Dabbagh L, Pasdar M, et al. The importance of MUC1 cellular localization in patients with breast carcinoma: An immunohistologic study of 71 patients and review of the literature. Cancer. 2001;**91**:1973-1982

[24] Kondo K, Kohno N, Yokoyama A, et al. Decreased MUC1 expression induces E-cadherin-mediated cell adhesion of breast cancer cell lines. Cancer Research. 1998;**58**:2014-2019

[25] Wesseling J, van der Valk SW, Hilkens J. A mechanism for inhibition of E-cadherin-mediated cell-cell adhesion by the membrane-associated mucin episialin/MUC1. Molecular Biology of the Cell. 1996;**7**:565-577

[26] Rakha EA, Boyce RWG, El-Rehim DA, et al. Expression of mucins (MUC1, MUC2, MUC3, MUC4, MUC5AC and MUC6) and their prognostic significance in human breast cancer. Modern Pathology. 2005;**18**:1295-1304

[27] Furuya C, Kawano H, Yamanouchi T, et al. Combined evaluation of CK5/6, ER, p63, and MUC3 for distinguishing breast intraductal papilloma from ductal carcinoma in situ. Pathology International. 2012;**62**:381-390

8

High-Risk Breast Lesions

Azlena Ali Beegan and Gozie Offiah

Abstract

It is well known that certain types of pre-malignant lesions can predispose some women to increased risk of breast cancer. These certain types of pre-malignant lesions are generally classified as high-risk breast lesions. These lesions become invasive cancers in about 15% of patients and hence the management and treatment of these lesions warrant a significant discussion. There are several categories of these lesions, to include atypical hyperplasia of the breast (atypical ductal hyperplasia and atypical lobular hyperplasia); carcinoma in situ (ductal carcinoma in situ and lobular carcinoma in situ); columnar cell pre-malignant lesions; lobular intraepithelial neoplasia (LIN III); radial scar/complex sclerosing lesion; sclerosing adenosis and papillary lesions of the breast. These lesions are morphologically, radiologically, histologically and clinically heterogeneous and early identification can help to prevent progression to invasive cancers. The management of these lesions has been debated internationally for years by experts as to the best treatment modality with surgical excision of the lesion often not considered necessary. It is thus important to evaluate each patient on an individual case-by-case basis. The characteristics of these high-risk breast lesions are further discussed in this chapter.

Keywords: breast cancer, in-situ carcinoma, atypical hyperplasia, pre-malignant, breast lesions, mammogram, breast ultrasound

1. Introduction

Breast cancer is the most common cancer diagnosed in women worldwide [1]. It is the fifth most common cause of death from cancer worldwide but is the second most common cause of death in developed countries [1]. The mortality rates up to 5 years after diagnosis is higher in the less developed countries compared to more developed countries specifically in Europe and North America [1]. Breast lesions can be divided into benign or non-proliferative, high risk or pre-malignant and invasive or infiltrating breast lesions [2]. Benign or non-proliferative breast lesions are non-cancerous breast lesions that can occur in any anatomical structure of the breast and can present symptomatically or as an incidental finding on imaging or histological findings [3]. Types of benign breast lesions include mammary duct ectasia, mastitis, fat necrosis, benign cysts, breast abscess, epithelial-related calcifications, non-sclerosing adenosis, benign intraductal papilloma, breast haematoma, lipoma, fibroadenoma, periductal fibrosis and gynaecomastia (in men) [3]. Invasive breast cancers are a group of heterogeneous malignant breast lesions that originate from breast epithelial cells and invade surrounding breast tissue as well as having the potential to metastasise via lymphatics and blood to distant sites [4]. Invasive or infiltrating breast cancers tend to commonly involve the ducts and lobules of the breast [4]. These include the invasive ductal carcinoma (IDC) and invasive lobular carcinoma (ILC), which comprise of around 80 and 10% of the total invasive carcinoma types respectively [2]. The other less common types of invasive breast carcinomas (~10% of all breast cancers) include medullary, mucinous, tubular, inflammatory, papillary, adenoid cystic, apocrine, lymphoma, sarcoma, phyllodes and Paget's disease of the nipple [2].

This chapter will primarily focus on high-risk or pre-malignant breast lesions. High-risk or pre-malignant breast lesions are breast lesions that have the potential to become malignant but the risk and time to progression is variable in each lesion [5]. These lesions are usually asymptomatic and are detected incidentally on breast imaging in the majority of cases [6]. Some of the more proliferative lesions (e.g. DCIS) may present with symptoms [6]. Types of high-risk breast lesions include atypical ductal hyperplasia (ADH), atypical columnar cell hyperplasia/columnar alteration with prominent apical snouts and secretions (CAPSS), ductal carcinoma in situ (DCIS), atypical lobular hyperplasia (ALH), lobular intraepithelial neoplasia (LIN III), lobular carcinoma in situ (LCIS), radial scar/complex sclerosing lesion, sclerosing adenosis, papillary lesions of the breast and flat epithelial atypia [5, 7].

In an attempt to classify breast lesions to determine the lesions that have a high relative risk of becoming malignant, Page categorised breast lesions based on morphological features into four categories [20]. The first category included non-proliferative lesions (no increased risk) such as florid adenosis, apocrine change, mild epithelial hyperplasia of usual type and duct ectasia [20]. The second category included epithelial proliferative lesions without atypia (1.5–2 times increased risk) such as moderate/florid hyperplasia of usual type or papillomatosis [20]. The third category consists of atypical hyperplastic lesions (4–5 times increased risk) such as ADH and ALH [20]. Finally the fourth category is lesions considered to be carcinoma in situ and high-risk lesions (8–10 times increased risk), which include DCIS and LCIS [20]. This criterion is still referred to by pathologists to classify breast lesions based on their histology.

2. Types of high-risk breast lesions

2.1. Atypical hyperplasia of the breast (ADH and ALH)

2.1.1. Atypical ductal hyperplasia (ADH)

Atypical ductal hyperplasia (ADH) is a pre-malignant lesion of the breast that carries a four to five times increased risk of developing carcinoma of the breast in the general population [8].

Several previous studies showed that the cumulative risk for developing invasive breast cancer is approximately 13% over a duration of up to 25 years post diagnosis of ADH [9–11]. This risk is doubled in women with a family history of breast cancer in a first-degree relative [8]. Over half of the breast cancers that develop from ADH are moderate or high grade and usually involve the ducts on histology [11]. Of the invasive breast cancers, 25% tend to be node-positive and over 80% being oestrogen receptor (ER) positive [11]. These cancers are also more likely to develop on the same breast that had ADH as opposed to the contralateral side [11]. Menopausal status of patients with ADH was also considered in determining the risk of developing invasive cancer. Some authors report that the risk is greater in premenopausal women with atypical hyperplasia [12]; while others suggested that this may only be relevant in ALH but not in ADH and that this risk was modified once the patient approaches menopause [13]. A more recent study done in 2017 showed a reduction of the cumulative risk to two times the risk of developing invasive breast cancer 10 years after the diagnosis of ADH [14]. This study was performed on a cohort of 955,331 women of which 2785 were diagnosed with ADH following either a core needle biopsy (CNB) or excisional breast biopsy (EBB) [14]. The results from this study showed a reduction in the risk of developing invasive breast cancer at 10 years following an ADH diagnosis to 5.7–6.7% [14].

It has been shown that ADH and DCIS have very similar characteristics histologically. Often it has been difficult to distinguish between ADH and DCIS especially on smaller tissue samples such as those obtained from fine needle aspiration cytology (FNAC) or core needle biopsy (CNB) [15]. Hence, the most accurate method for diagnosis is by excisional biopsy of the entire lesion [15]. ADH is described histologically as lesions with structurally complex patterns formed from the expansion and filling of breast ducts with the proliferation of monotonous epithelial cells and the presence of secondary lumens [16]. Its features are very similar to DCIS on radiological investigation and can be difficult to distinguish using imaging and CNB only [16]. On mammography, a cluster of calcifications may represent ADH [17]. Atypical hyperplasia diagnosis is confirmed in up to 10% of all the CNB performed on these calcifications [17]. Its features are similar to DCIS on ultrasonography and appears as a mildly hypoechoic microlobulated mass with normal acoustic transmission [18]. There is also a higher rate for an inaccurate diagnosis by using only an ultrasound-guided CNB instead of an excisional biopsy [19]. Studies have shown that more than half of the ADH diagnosed using this technique yielded a malignant pathology on surgical excision [19].

Page had previously categorised breast lesions based on morphological features into four categories based on the risk of developing malignancy [20]. To assess if these categories of diagnosing pre-malignant breast lesions are reproducible, a study was performed evaluating the inter-observer variation in the diagnosis of various pre-malignant ductal breast lesions including non-atypical ductal hyperplasia, ADH and DCIS [21]. Pathologists in the study followed strictly to Page's standardised criteria [20]. The study concluded that there were no significant inter-observer differences in forming the diagnosis of these lesions and if adhered to, the standardised diagnosis criteria can be a useful tool [20, 21]. However, despite these classifications, some pathologists argue that the interpretation of ADH and DCIS lesions are still subjective as histologically these lesion are very similar despite being quantitatively different as ADH involve less than two ducts in the breast [22].

ADH is usually diagnosed with a CNB; however, due to the small quantity of samples obtained, a DCIS or invasive carcinoma are unable to be excluded as previous studies have shown that ADH may exist alongside DCIS and invasive cancer [23]. A study done by Gadzala et al. confirmed this notion as they found in 36 patients that had a diagnosis of ADH on stereotactic CNB, 17 patients (47%) were confirmed to have DCIS or IDC after EBB was performed [23]. Therefore, excisional breast biopsy (EBB) was found to be the best option to confirm the ADH diagnosis and outrule ductal carcinoma [23]. In contrary, some researchers believed that it was unwarranted to perform EBB when the more improved techniques of CNB used larger gauge needles (9-, 11- or 14-gauge) and has the potential to diagnose as well as treat ADH without the need for EBB [24]. They suggested that ADH with fewer than three foci and the complete removal of calcifications on biopsy was adequate and prevented the need for EBB in some patients, which has some cosmetic deformity consequences as well as the unnecessary risk of undergoing a surgical procedure [24]. Nevertheless, the clinical recommendation for the definitive management of ADH still remains as EBB despite the improved CNB techniques as the percentage of underestimation of cancer after an ADH diagnosis can carry a risk of over 10% [11, 15].

2.1.2. Atypical lobular hyperplasia (ALH)

Another type of atypia that can be found in the breast is atypical lobular hyperplasia (ALH). Similar to ADH, its risk of developing future breast cancer is high (4–5 increased risk compared to women with no atypia), hence ALH is also categorised as a pre-malignant breast cancer [8]. Page et al. had previously reported that the high risk may be due to the involvement of ducts in some ALH lesions; however, if there is no ductal involvement, the risk is reduced to 2.7 [25]. The risk of developing breast cancer with a prior ALH lesion is higher in pre and perimenopausal women (aged 46–55) and reduced in the postmenopausal cohort, conversely, menopausal status has no bearing on ADH risk of breast cancer as both pre and post menopausal women have similar risk scores [13]. The cumulative risk for developing invasive breast cancer is approximately 18% over a duration of up to 25 years post the diagnosis of ALH, which is higher than the risk seen with ADH [9–11]. Previous studies have also shown that ALH tend to develop into moderate or high grade breast cancers and has an increased risk when associated with a strong positive family history of breast cancer as similarly observed in patients with ADH diagnosis [11]. ALH has not only been associated with the occurrence of future ipsilateral breast cancer but also with contralateral breast cancers [26].

ALH is usually asymptomatic and may be found incidentally using breast imaging; however, the majority of ALH are found as an association to mass lesions like fibroadenomas, radial scars, ADH, intraductal papillomas, pleomorphic LCIS or DCIS following a CNB [26]. If seen solitarily, these lesions appear as clustered calcifications and can be difficult to diagnose using the imaging modality alone as its characteristics on a mammogram are similar to other pre-malignant breast conditions [26].

ALH and LCIS have morphologically similar findings and have been termed collectively as lobular neoplasia (LN); however, they differ primarily based on the filling of the lobular unit and the degree of proliferation [27]. The histology of ALH obtained from either a CNB or EBB (if associated to another mass lesion) shows the filling of the acini in the lobular unit with monotonous, small, round, cuboidal or polygonal cells with a loss of acinar lumens [16]. The diagnosis of ALH can be obtained following Page's criteria based on the morphology of breast lesions [20]. ALH falls into the third category, which also consists of ADH [20].

Multiple studies have been carried out to determine the most suitable management option for ALH. The diagnosis of ALH was made using stereotactic CNB or EBB if another pre-malignant lesion was present [16]. The perplexing issue with ALH is whether the need for management via a surgical excision is justified when it presents on its own in a CNB specimen or if it presents alongside a benign lesion on an EBB sample. The management of ALH diagnosed on CNB has remained controversial as there are conflicting opinions. A study performed by Bauer et al. divided the diagnosis of LN observed into three groups coexisting with other breast pathologies, which comprised of DCIS or invasive cancer (Group 1), ADH, phyllodes tumour, radial scar or intraductal papilloma (Group 2) and benign fibrocystic changes (Group 3) [28]. They concluded that LN in the absence of breast cancer or pre-malignant conditions (Group 1 and 2) do not need EBB [28]. Other authors had similar recommendations as patients with ALH alone or in association with benign breast disease were not associated with breast carcinoma (<8% associated with cancer) and were not deemed high risk; hence, the residual microcalcifications did not require a further EBB [29]. In addition to this, it was suggested that if strict radiographic-pathologic correlation and histologic criteria are adhered to, then the patients who do not require EBB, should be closely monitored with regular clinical follow-up and breast imaging (mammogram, ultrasound, MRI breast) [26, 30]. Another study contradicted this recommendation as they found that 17% of the patients with LN developed either DCIS or invasive carcinoma [31]. Of the ALH cohort of 20 patients, 2 developed DCIS, hence only the LCIS cohort developed invasive carcinoma [31]. Nevertheless, the group suggested that due to the high percentage of patients with cancer after the diagnosis of LN, an EBB is warranted [31]. Supporting this recommendation, other studies performed using CNB also found that LN lesions had a higher risk for developing breast cancer and an underestimation of 8–19% if CNB alone was performed without a completion EBB [32, 33]. To further stratify the exact criteria of ALH or LCIS (LN lesions) that warranted surgical excision, histologic findings of these lesions with more than 1 lobule per core involvement were considered to be diffuse lobular neoplasia while those with 1 or less lobules affected in each core (focal lobular neoplasia) did not require full excision [34]. In summary, ADH and ALH are radiologically difficult to diagnose as they have features similar to DCIS and LCIS respectively and thus are best diagnosed and managed by excisional breast biopsy (EBB).

2.2. Carcinoma in situ of the breast (DCIS and LCIS)

2.2.1. Ductal carcinoma in situ (DCIS)

Ductal carcinoma in situ (DCIS) are pre-malignant breast lesions that can present both symptomatically and asymptomatically as an incidental finding on breast imaging. It accounts for up to 30% of breast cancer lesions detected on mammography [35]. These numbers have risen significantly following the introduction of screening mammography as compared to previous diagnosis of DCIS, which comprised of only 0.8–5% of all breast cancers primarily diagnosed clinically due to symptomatic DCIS [6, 35]. It represents a premalignant proliferation of malignant epithelial cells in the lumen of the breast ducts that have not invaded the basement membrane and retains its myoepithelium layer [36]. DCIS may present with symptoms of a palpable breast lump, nipple changes and discharge or asymptomatically for smaller sized lesions seen on mammography, which has been associated with a higher risk for the development of invasive carcinoma and treatment failure [6, 37]. The risk of invasive cancer in patients diagnosed with DCIS on CNB is 11-fold and vary from 17 to 50% depending on the type of DCIS lesion as the invasive cancers tends to occur in the same location as the DCIS lesion [38, 39]. DCIS is associated with similar risk factors to that of invasive breast cancer such as increasing age (peak at postmenopausal age), family history of breast cancer, nulliparity or late first pregnancy after the age of 30 and the use of hormone replacement therapy [40].

Radiologic findings account for the majority of DCIS detection. The majority of DCIS lesions appear as microcalcifications on mammography [41]. However, they can also present as circumscribed masses or focal nodular patterns [41]. Screening mammography has led to the early diagnosis and investigation of breast cancer lesions. The early implementation of the appropriate management of breast cancer has reduced mortality rates by 30% [42]. This is relevant in the case of DCIS lesions as a large percentage of the higher grade lesions have potential to become invasive and early diagnosis and management is key to reduce this risk [42]. A focused ultrasound can also be carried out once a lesion is detected on mammography to further evaluate the characteristics of the lesion and can aid in the CNB of the lesion [43]. Typical findings representing DCIS on ultrasound include features of a microlobulated irregular mass with no acoustic shadowing [43].

As mentioned previously, DCIS and ADH have similar morphology [15]. However, DCIS lesions are more proliferative and can be diagnosed based on CNB [44]. DCIS are localised lesions that usually present in one quadrant of the breast and can be as larger as 5 cm in size [44]. It can be classified based on its size, nuclear grade, architectural subtype and the presence of necrosis following the 2009 College of American Pathologists/American Society of Clinical Oncology protocol [45]. The nuclear grades are subdivided into low (Grade I), intermediate (Grade II) or high grade (Grade III) [45]. High grade DCIS is comprised of proliferative large pleomorphic cells with abundant normal and abnormal mitoses [36]. Intermediate grade DCIS have similar characteristics of both high and low grade DCIS with an intermediate degree of pleomorphism [36]. They tend to present more commonly as a solid cribiform pattern [36]. Low grade DCIS has small cells that are in a uniform pattern [36]. Architectural subtypes include comedo, Paget's disease of the nipple, cribriform, micropapillary, papillary and solid patterns (listed in increasing order towards a higher grade subtype of DCIS) [45]. DCIS lesions was also found to have varying risk of developing invasive breast cancer based on genetic alterations and receptor status of the lesion with a majority of lesions exhibiting ER positivity on immunohistochemistry staining [37, 44]. Palpable DCIS lesions were more commonly associated with negative ER and PR status, which confirms its association to a higher grade DCIS and leading to more aggressive phenotype compared to DCIS found incidentally on screening [37].

As with other pre-malignant disease of the breast, the diagnosis of DCIS warrants further management with either surgery and/or other adjuvant treatments due to its nature to progress to invasive malignancy [46]. Multiple trials have been carried out to determine the effectiveness of these treatments in the prevention of recurrence after DCIS diagnosis [46]. The options for the surgical management of DCIS consist of mastectomy of the affected breast or breast conserving surgery such as wide local excision (WLE) [46]. Suitability for either type of surgery is based on the grade of the lesion and presence of microinvasion, the patient's age at diagnosis and pre-existing co-morbidities (life expectancy) as these may influence the decision to perform a more definitive surgery like mastectomy instead of WLE due to the risk of having to re-excise the margins and the chance of local recurrence [46]. Rutter et al. reported on the increasing use of mastectomy as a treatment of DCIS especially in patients with higher grade DCIS and younger age [47]. This was due to the increased risk of recurrence and development of invasive breast cancer. Other authors have reported the effectiveness of nipple-sparing mastectomy in comparison with mastectomy whereby the probability of local recurrence was similar and low in the case of DCIS treatment [48]. However, these results were not similarly replicated favourably when the breast conserving treatment of DCIS was used as a solitary treatment modality. The RTOG 9804 trial was conducted to evaluate the effectiveness of breast conserving surgery (BCS) with or without adjuvant radiotherapy in patients diagnosed with low or intermediate risk DCIS on CNB [49]. Results showed a low risk for recurrence with BCS alone at 6.7%; however, this was significantly lower in the adjuvant radiotherapy arm at 0.9% recurrence risk [49]. This opened up the possibility of DCIS subtype with good prognosis to be considered for BCS treatment alone without further adjuvant therapy; however, the authors concluded that a longer follow-up time of more than 7 years was required to give more reproducible results as the BCS and adjuvant radiotherapy cohort had much better response [49]. In contrary to this, other studies have not yielded promising results as patients treated with BCS alone had recurrence rates of approximately 14–16%, despite the stratification of patients into the low risk DCIS category [50, 51]. Conflicting evidence has been reported regarding the need for sentinel lymph node biopsy (SLNB) in the treatment of DCIS. Some studies suggest that SLNB should not be part of the standard surgical treatment of all subtypes of DCIS as the percentage of positive SLNB range from 1 to 22% with majority of the studies reporting a lower percentage of positive findings, hence rendering it unnecessary [52]. Furthermore, some authors argue that performing a SLNB in these patients could disrupt the diagnosis of future lymphatic spread in the case where invasive carcinoma occurs [53]. The general consensus surrounding the addition of SLNB as part of the surgical treatment of DCIS is to be only reserved for those lesions with high grade of DCIS exhibiting microinvasion, large lesions of more than 5 cm in size, lesions treated with mastectomy and DCIS subtypes with high risk of developing invasive cancer [52, 53].

2.2.2. Lobular carcinoma in situ (LCIS)

Lobular carcinoma in situ (LCIS) is similar in histology to ALH; however, it is more extensive and proliferative compared to ALH [27]. It is on the higher spectrum of lobular neoplasia (LN) [27]. LCIS lesions are usually diagnosed incidentally via breast imaging such as through mammographic screening or are detected incidentally as part of a CNB or an EBB for another breast lesion diagnosis [54]. LCIS is a pre-malignant lesion that has a 15% risk of developing subsequent invasive carcinoma (IDC and ILC) on the ipsilateral breast, as well as a 9% risk of developing invasive carcinoma on the contralateral breast (mostly ILC) [27, 55, 56]. Its estimated incidence is varied between 0.5 and 3.8% as it is most often overlapped with other premalignant or invasive lesions in the breast [57–59]. The risk of DCIS or invasive carcinoma after the diagnosis of LCIS is 17% at 15 years post diagnosis of LCIS with a relative risk of 8–10 [59]. Similarly to ALH, LCIS may be affected by menopausal status. Its incidence was observed to be higher in premenopausal women with only 10% incidence in postmenopausal women, suggesting it may be affected by reproductive history such as age at the birth of first child and ovarian function status [8, 60].

Due to the majority of LCIS being detected incidentally on CNB, it is difficult to characterise its possible findings on breast imaging. A retrospective study evaluated the appearance of LCIS on breast imaging after the diagnosis was confirmed on CNB in an attempt to define the characteristics of LCIS [61]. They described the mammographic findings of LCIS as micro calcifications [61]. Choi et al. used ultrasound imaging to characterise the feature of LCIS and described it as ill-defined, asymmetrical, elongated or round lesions with hypoechogenicity [62].

Histological findings of LCIS are well defined on CNB. LCIS morphology consists of type A and B cells [27]. The type A cells have a smaller sized nuclei compared to the larger and more pleomorphic type B cells that are usually polygonal, cuboidal or round shaped [27]. These cells fill and expand more than half of the acini in the lobular unit with loss of central lumina, which differentiates it from the features of ALH [27, 61]. There has been an ongoing debate whether CNB is sufficient to diagnose LCIS without further EBB. Murray et al. performed a prospective study that investigated the underdiagnoses rate of LN (LCIS and ALH) in samples obtained from their institution over 5 years [63]. When there was radiologic and histologic disconcordance, 50% of samples diagnosed as LCIS by CNB turned out to be DCIS on EBB [63]. However, when there is radiologic and histologic concordance, there were no underdiagnosed LCIS lesions by CNB [63]. They compared their results with previous studies and discovered that the underdiagnoses risk of DCIS or invasive carcinoma in samples that had radiologic and histologic disconcordance is significant in ~38–67% of CNB samples diagnosed as LCIS [63].

The management of LCIS is another controversial issue due to its low incidence and lack of distinguishing mammographic findings, as well as its incidental co-diagnosis with other breast lesions such as DCIS and IDC [58, 59]. Conflicting opinions have risen with some indicating that surgical excision is unnecessary, while others disagree and recommend the excision of LCIS is crucial to prevent future development of invasive carcinoma. Nagi et al. agreed with the recommendation that type A cell LCIS lesions should be treated conservatively. The reasoning is that the cohort of patients with this type of lesion, who did not have surgical excision, did not develop progressive disease up to 8 years of follow-up [26]. The authors rationale was that as long as strict criteria were followed histologically and close monitoring were performed radiologically, surgical excision did not provide further benefit in these type A lesions [26]. The type B cell LCIS lesions have poorer prognosis compared to type A, hence will require surgical excision [26]. Similar to the management of ALH, lesions diagnosed, as LCIS also did not require surgical excision unless associated or is adjacent to other co-existing more aggressive premalignant or malignant breast lesions or in the case where there is discordance between radiologic and histologic diagnosis [28]. In more aggressive forms of LCIS that can present in the contralateral breast, some studies have recommended the option to manage LCIS by bilateral prophylactic mastectomies as part of a risk reduction surgery [64]. However, the decision to follow through with these surgeries required meticulous discussion with a multidisciplinary team (MDT) to assess the patient's risk of future carcinoma and the best management plan for the patient [64].

2.3. Columnar cell pre-malignant lesions of the breast

Types of columnar cell pre-malignant lesions of the breast include columnar alteration with prominent apical snouts and secretions (CAPSS; also known as columnar cell lesions: CCL) and flat epithelial atypia (FEA; also known as CCL with atypia) [65]. Fraser et al. described a type of breast lesion that had similar features on imaging to ADH and DCIS [66]. Although the lesion on imaging did not appear benign, it could not be classified specifically as either ADH or DCIS on histology as it lacked some features that can confirm these diagnoses [66]. These spectra of lesions were described as architecturally complex lesions that exhibited columnar epithelial cells with prominent apical cytoplasmic snouts and intraluminal secretions, which may or may not have nuclear atypia lining the terminal duct lobular unit (TDLU) [66]. This group of lesions were therefore named as columnar alteration with prominent apical snouts and secretions (CAPSS) [66]. CAPSS lesions lie on a spectrum depending on the atypia of the cells and were routinely diagnosed on ultrasound-guided CNB [67]. Studies have shown that CAPSS lesions with atypia closely resembled DCIS and had a higher risk of association with invasive cancer when compared to CAPSS lesions without atypia [67]. CAPSS and FEA lesions are described as clustered microcalcifications that may have amorphous or fine pleomorphic features located in the TDLU on mammography [68]. Again, these features are similar to other pre-malignant disease such as ADH and DCIS, hence it is difficult to diagnose without a CNB [68]. FEAs are observed histologically as dilated basophilic acini, which consists of layers of cuboidal to columnar epithelial cells with low-grade atypia on cytology and distended TDLUs [65, 69].

The presence of CAPSS in the breast was found to increase the risk of breast cancer due to its co-occurrence with other proliferative breast lesions such as DCIS [70]. However, these lesions independently did not confer a high risk of developing breast cancer [71]. FEAs have also been associated with an approximately 20% risk of developing breast cancer and a high underestimation rate for malignancy when diagnosed on CNB due to its similar co-existence with other pre-malignant lesions such as ADH and DCIS [72].

The suggested clinical recommendation for the management of columnar cell pre-malignant lesions of the breast is EBB for both CAPSS and FEA based on radiographic and histologic correlations [67, 72, 73].

2.4. Papillary lesions of the breast

Papillary lesions of the breast are composed of benign and malignant types. The papillomatosis of the breast and atypical papilloma lesions may be considered premalignant due to its association to the development of breast cancer [74]. Pre-malignant papilloma lesions can be associated with calcifications on mammogram and appear as a homogeneous solid or intra-cystic lesion that is complex on ultrasound [74]. Clinically, patients with this disease may present with symptomatic findings such as a breast mass or nipple discharge [74]. Histologically, breast papilloma is described as clusters of epithelium in the ducts that develop into branching papillae, which protrude into the lumen [75]. Due to the varying spectrum of pathological findings seen in the papilloma disease of the breast, it is difficult to distinguish between true benign and malignant or premalignant lesions. Multiple studies have shown that the diagnostic technique using either FNA or CNB may be inaccurate as benign findings were often either co-existing with premalignant lesions or were underestimated [75, 76]. The suggested management of breast papillomas diagnosed on FNA or CNB is for active surveillance if there is no atypia and no discordance between imaging and histologic findings [74]. When there is doubt on biopsy or the presence of high-risk papilloma lesions then an EBB is warranted [74].

2.5. Radial scar/complex sclerosing lesion

A radial scar or complex sclerosing lesions of the breast are considered to be pre-malignant breast lesions due to its common association with other more proliferative lesions leading to its increase in breast cancer risk [77]. On mammography, a radial scar/complex sclerosing lesion is described as the presence of radiolucency in the centre of the lesion with spicules that are longer compared to malignant lesions. There is also the presence of radiating radiolucent linear structures and the absence of macrocalcifications [77]. Histologically, radial scars have a fibroelastic core with entrapped ducts and variable surrounding benign epithelial features; however, it can also be associated with atypia usually at the edges of the lesion [78]. The term radial scars was given to lesions smaller than or equal to 1 cm while the term complex sclerosing lesions is larger than 1 cm [78]. There have been various opinions among pathologists and surgeons regarding the most appropriate management of radial scars. Some suggest that a large gauge CNB was adequate to sample radial scars and there was no need for EBB as long as there is no atypia and the radiology and histology correlate [79]. However, other authors still classify radial lesions as high-risk lesions and EBB is the recommend management [79].

3. Adjuvant therapies for the treatment of high-risk breast disease

Adjuvant therapies have been considered in an attempt to reduce the risk of breast cancer following the diagnosis of a pre-malignant breast lesion via CNB or EBB. Several trials have been conducted to determine if adjuvant radiotherapy and/or endocrine therapy may be useful as a measure to reduce this risk [80].

Trials involving the use of adjuvant radiotherapy were performed on pre-malignant carcinoma in situ lesions, predominantly, DCIS. Adjuvant radiotherapy used in a study involving patients with BCS following a DCIS diagnosis, yielded promising results as there was a significant risk reduction compared to the control group especially in the postmenopausal patient cohort [81]. A meta-analysis carried out by the Early Breast Cancer Trialists' Collaborative Group (EBCTCG) evaluating the results from four randomised clinical trials involving adjuvant radiotherapy in the management of DCIS showed that radiotherapy after BCS was successful in reducing the absolute risk of developing ipsilateral DCIS recurrence and invasive breast cancer development by 15% in the 10 year follow-up duration [80]. As similarly seen in the previous study, a greater risk reduction was seen in postmenopausal women and that radiotherapy did not have a significant effect on the contralateral breast or on distant metastatic occurrence [80]. This led to the suggestion that the patients receiving adjuvant radiotherapy as part of the BCS treatment of DCIS should be further stratified to avoid unnecessary exposure to radiotherapy, which carries its own risks [80]. The EORTC 10853 Randomised Phase III Trial further confirmed the benefit of adjuvant radiotherapy as it reduced the risk of any local recurrences after an EBB of DCIS by almost half (48%) after a 15 year follow-up [82]. The treatment of LCIS with adjuvant radiotherapy has not been explored to the same extent as DCIS lesions. A small study carried out with 25 patients treated for LCIS lesions with lumpectomy and radiotherapy reported promising findings as only 1 patient had a local recurrence after a median follow-up of 153 months [83].

Apart from radiotherapy, multiple studies have been performed to explore the effects of oral selective oestrogen receptor modulators (SERMs) and aromatase inhibitors (AIs) as part of a preventative measure to reduce the risk of developing breast carcinoma as well as an adjuvant treatment following EBB or BCS of DCIS lesions [84–86]. The randomised International Breast Cancer Intervention Study (IBIS-I) trial was not aimed specifically at women with a known diagnosis of DCIS but was targeted for women with an increased risk for the development of DCIS and invasive breast cancer [85]. The trial reported the benefit of prophylactic tamoxifen in high-risk women leading to a 34% reduced risk of developing invasive cancer [85]. The benefit of tamoxifen was also found to outweigh the risk in this subset of high-risk patients [85]. Although this study was not investigating the adjuvant treatment of DCIS, however, the rationale of this study can still apply to the management of this disease. Most patients have a high risk of developing invasive cancer after a DCIS diagnosis and may benefit from adjuvant treatment with selective oestrogen receptor modulators because of the ER positive nature of DCIS. The National Surgical Adjuvant Breast and Bowel Project (NSABP) B-17 and B-24 randomised clinical trials were performed to determine the effectiveness of lumpectomy alone as a surgical treatment of DCIS compared to lumpectomy with adjuvant radiotherapy or tamoxifen therapy [86]. The trial focussed on the long-term prognosis of DCIS with these various treatment combinations and the risk of ipsilateral invasive breast cancer recurrence [86]. The trial reported that the cumulative incidence of ipsilateral invasive breast cancer recurrence (15 year follow-up) was 19.4% for lumpectomy only compared to 8.9% for lumpectomy plus adjuvant radiotherapy while the incidence was 10.0% in the lumpectomy plus radiotherapy combination treatment group compared to 8.5% for the combination treatment of lumpectomy plus adjuvant radiotherapy and tamoxifen [86]. Radiotherapy and tamoxifen therapy were concluded to be effective as adjuvant treatments to lumpectomy to reduce the risk of tumour recurrence [86]. Another prospective cohort study carried out by Thompson et al. over a follow-up period of 62 months reported similar findings to Wapnir et al. with a reduction of risk in developing DCIS recurrence or ipsilateral breast cancer in patients given adjuvant therapy combination with radiotherapy and tamoxifen after BCS [87].

4. Conclusion

High-risk breast lesions vary in the degree of risk of developing either in situ carcinoma or invasive carcinoma. Multi-observer disparities in histology reporting had previously been a concern; however, standardised criteria have been developed to overcome this issue. There is a general consensus that radiologic and histologic concordance is important to formulate an accurate diagnosis to help direct the appropriate treatment regime. The management of high-risk breast lesions is rather confusing and needs to be determined by the risk of developing invasive breast cancer. Risk reduction strategies for these high-risk breast lesions described in this chapter vary from active surveillance to surgical excision in form of an excisional biopsy or a mastectomy with or without adjuvant therapies. These strategies are largely influenced by the patient and the clinicians' decisions.

Acknowledgements

The authors would like to acknowledge the Beaumont Hospital Cancer Research and Development Trust for the grant received for this book chapter.

Author details

Azlena Ali Beegan and Gozie Offiah*

*Address all correspondence to: gozieoffiah@rcsi.ie

Royal College of Surgeons in Ireland, Education and Research Centre, Beaumont Hospital, Dublin, Ireland

References

[1] Ferlay JSI, Ervik M, Dikshit R, Eser S, Mathers C, Rebelo M, Parkin DM, Forman D, Bray F. GLOBOCAN 2012 v1.0, Cancer Incidence and Mortality Worldwide: IARC CancerBase No. 11. 2013. Available from: http://globocan.iarc.fr/Pages/fact_sheets_cancer.aspx [Accessed: June 1, 2017]

[2] Sharma GN et al. Various types and management of breast cancer: An overview. Journal of Advanced Pharmaceutical Technology & Research. 2010;1(2):109-126

[3] Guray M, Sahin AA. Benign breast diseases: Classification, diagnosis, and management. The Oncologist. 2006;11(5):435-449

[4] Chapa J, An G, Kulkarni SA. Examining the relationship between pre-malignant breast lesions, carcinogenesis and tumor evolution in the mammary epithelium using an agent-based model. PloS One. 2016;11(3):e0152298

[5] Lebeau A. Precancerous lesions of the breast. Breast Care. 2010;**5**(4):204-206

[6] Schnitt SJ et al. Ductal carcinoma in situ (intraductal carcinoma) of the breast. The New England Journal of Medicine. 1988;**318**(14):898-903

[7] Flegg KM, Jeffrey JF, Anne MB, Sanjiv J. Surgical outcomes of borderline breast lesions detected by needle biopsy in a breast screening program. World Journal of Surgical Oncology. 2010;**8**:78-78

[8] Page DL et al. Atypical hyperplastic lesions of the female breast. A long-term follow-up study. Cancer. 1985;**55**(11):2698-2708

[9] Degnim AC et al. Stratification of breast cancer risk in women with Atypia: A Mayo cohort study. Journal of Clinical Oncology. 2007;**25**(19):2671-2677

[10] Boughey JC et al. Evaluation of the Tyrer-Cuzick (International Breast Cancer Intervention Study) model for breast cancer risk prediction in women with atypical hyperplasia. Journal of Clinical Oncology. 2010;**28**(22):3591-3596

[11] Hartmann LC et al. Understanding the premalignant potential of atypical hyperplasia through its natural history: A longitudinal cohort study. Cancer Prevention Research. 2014;**7**(2):211-217

[12] London SJ et al. A prospective study of benign breast disease and the risk of breast cancer. Journal of the American Medical Association. 1992;**267**(7):941-944

[13] Marshall LM et al. Risk of breast cancer associated with atypical hyperplasia of lobular and ductal types. Cancer Epidemiology Biomarkers & Prevention. 1997;**6**(5):297-301

[14] Menes TS et al. Subsequent breast cancer risk following diagnosis of atypical ductal hyperplasia on needle biopsy. JAMA Oncology. 2017;**3**(1):36-41

[15] Kohr JR et al. Risk of upgrade of atypical ductal hyperplasia after stereotactic breast biopsy: Effects of number of foci and complete removal of calcifications. Radiology. 2010;**255**(3):723-730

[16] Hartmann LC et al. Atypical hyperplasia of the breast—Risk assessment and management options. New England Journal of Medicine. 2015;**372**(1):78-89

[17] Simpson JF. Update on atypical epithelial hyperplasia and ductal carcinoma in situ. Pathology. 2009;**41**(1):36-39

[18] Moon WK et al. US of ductal carcinoma in situ. Radiographics. 2002;**22**(2):269-280 discussion 280-1

[19] Mesurolle B et al. Atypical ductal hyperplasia diagnosed at sonographically guided core needle biopsy: Frequency, final surgical outcome, and factors associated with underestimation. AJR. American Journal of Roentgenology. 2014;**202**(6):1389-1394

[20] Page DL. Cancer risk assessment in benign breast biopsies. Human Pathology. 1986; **17**(9):871-874

[21] Schnitt SJ et al. Interobserver reproducibility in the diagnosis of ductal proliferative breast lesions using standardized criteria. The American Journal of Surgical Pathology. 1992;**16**(12):1133-1143

[22] Moore MM et al. Association of breast cancer with the finding of atypical ductal hyperplasia at core breast biopsy. Annals of Surgery. 1997;**225**(6):726-731 discussion 731-3

[23] Gadzala DE et al. Appropriate management of atypical ductal hyperplasia diagnosed by stereotactic core needle breast biopsy. Annals of Surgical Oncology. 1997;**4**(4):283-286

[24] Forgeard C et al. Is surgical biopsy mandatory in case of atypical ductal hyperplasia on 11-gauge core needle biopsy? A retrospective study of 300 patients. American Journal of Surgery. 2008;**196**(3):339-345

[25] Page DL, Dupont WD, Rogers LW. Ductal involvement by cells of atypical lobular hyperplasia in the breast: A long-term follow-up study of cancer risk. Human Pathology. 1988;**19**(2):201-207

[26] Nagi CS et al. Lobular neoplasia on core needle biopsy does not require excision. Cancer. 2008;**112**(10):2152-2158

[27] Simpson PT et al. The diagnosis and management of pre-invasive breast disease: Pathology of atypical lobular hyperplasia and lobular carcinoma in situ. Breast Cancer Research : BCR. 2003;**5**(5):258-262

[28] Bauer VP et al. The management of lobular neoplasia identified on percutaneous core breast biopsy. The Breast Journal. 2003;**9**(1):4-9

[29] Renshaw AA et al. Lobular neoplasia in breast core needle biopsy specimens is associated with a low risk of ductal carcinoma in situ or invasive carcinoma on subsequent excision. American Journal of Clinical Pathology. 2006;**126**(2):310-313

[30] Atkins KA et al. Atypical lobular hyperplasia and lobular carcinoma in situ at core breast biopsy: Use of careful radiologic-pathologic correlation to recommend excision or observation. Radiology. 2013;**269**(2):340-347

[31] Foster MC et al. Lobular carcinoma in situ or atypical lobular hyperplasia at core-needle biopsy: Is excisional biopsy necessary? Radiology. 2004;**231**(3):813-819

[32] Karabakhtsian RG et al. The clinical significance of lobular neoplasia on breast core biopsy. The American Journal of Surgical Pathology. 2007;**31**(5):717-723

[33] Cangiarella J et al. Is surgical excision necessary for the management of atypical lobular hyperplasia and lobular carcinoma in situ diagnosed on core needle biopsy?: A report of 38 cases and review of the literature. Archives of Pathology & Laboratory Medicine. 2008;**132**(6):979-983

[34] Esserman LE et al. Should the extent of lobular neoplasia on core biopsy influence the decision for excision? The Breast Journal. 2007;**13**(1):55-61

[35] Yamada T et al. Radiologic-pathologic correlation of ductal carcinoma in situ. Radiographics. 2010;**30**(5):1183-1198

[36] Pinder SE, Ellis IO. The diagnosis and management of pre-invasive breast disease: Ductal carcinoma in situ (DCIS) and atypical ductal hyperplasia (ADH)—Current definitions and classification. Breast Cancer Research. 2003;**5**(5):254

[37] Sundara Rajan S et al. Palpable ductal carcinoma in situ: Analysis of radiological and histological features of a large series with 5-year follow-up. Clinical Breast Cancer. 2013;**13**(6):486-491

[38] Kurniawan ED et al. Risk factors for invasive breast cancer when core needle biopsy shows ductal carcinoma in situ. Archives of Surgery. 2010;**145**(11):1098-1104

[39] Page DL et al. Continued local recurrence of carcinoma 15-25 years after a diagnosis of low grade ductal carcinoma in situ of the breast treated only by biopsy. Cancer. 1995;**76**(7):1197-1200

[40] Virnig BA et al. Ductal carcinoma in situ: Risk factors and impact of screening. Journal of the National Cancer Institute. Monographs. 2010;**2010**(41):113-116

[41] Ikeda DM, Andersson I. Ductal carcinoma in situ: Atypical mammographic appearances. Radiology. 1989;**172**(3):661-666

[42] D'Orsi CJ. Imaging for the diagnosis and management of ductal carcinoma in situ. Journal of the National Cancer Institute. Monographs. 2010;**2010**(41):214-217

[43] Shin HJ et al. Screening-detected and symptomatic ductal carcinoma in situ: Differences in the sonographic and pathologic features. AJR. American Journal of Roentgenology. 2008;**190**(2):516-525

[44] Lopez-Garcia MA et al. Breast cancer precursors revisited: Molecular features and progression pathways. Histopathology. 2010;**57**(2):171-192

[45] Lester SC et al. Protocol for the examination of specimens from patients with ductal carcinoma in situ of the breast. Archives of Pathology & Laboratory Medicine. 2009;**133**(1):15-25

[46] Park TS, Hwang ES. Current trends in the Management of Ductal Carcinoma in Situ. Oncology (Williston Park). 2016;**30**(9):823-831

[47] Rutter CE et al. Growing use of mastectomy for ductal carcinoma-in situ of the breast among young women in the United States. Annals of Surgical Oncology. 2015;**22**(7):2378-2386

[48] Sakurai T et al. Long-term follow-up of nipple-sparing mastectomy without radiotherapy: A single center study at a Japanese institution. Medical Oncology. 2013;**30**(1):481

[49] McCormick B et al. RTOG 9804: A prospective randomized trial for good-risk ductal carcinoma in situ comparing radiotherapy with observation. Journal of Clinical Oncology. 2015;**33**(7):709-715

[50] Wong JS et al. Eight-year update of a prospective study of wide excision alone for small low- or intermediate-grade ductal carcinoma in situ (DCIS). Breast Cancer Research and Treatment. 2014;**143**(2):343-350

[51] Solin LJ et al. Surgical excision without radiation for ductal carcinoma in situ of the breast: 12-year results from the ECOG-ACRIN E5194 study. Journal of Clinical Oncology. 2015;**33**(33):3938-3944

[52] Francis AM et al. Is sentinel lymph node dissection warranted in patients with a diagnosis of ductal carcinoma in situ? Annals of Surgical Oncology. 2015;**22**(13):4270-4279

[53] Farkas EA et al. An argument against routine sentinel node mapping for DCIS. The American Surgeon. 2004;**70**(1):13-17 discussion 17-8

[54] Frykberg ER. Lobular carcinoma in situ of the breast. The Breast Journal. 1999;**5**(5):296-303

[55] Sullivan ME et al. Lobular carcinoma in situ variants in breast cores: Potential for misdiagnosis, upgrade rates at surgical excision, and practical implications. Archives of Pathology & Laboratory Medicine. 2010;**134**(7):1024-1028

[56] Chuba PJ et al. Bilateral risk for subsequent breast cancer after lobular carcinoma-in-situ: Analysis of surveillance, epidemiology, and end results data. Journal of Clinical Oncology. 2005;**23**(24):5534-5541

[57] Haagensen CD et al. Lobular neoplasia (so-called lobular carcinoma in situ) of the breast. Cancer. 1978;**42**(2):737-769

[58] Liberman L et al. Lobular carcinoma in situ at percutaneous breast biopsy: Surgical biopsy findings. American Journal of Roentgenology. 1999;**173**(2):291-299

[59] Page DL et al. Lobular neoplasia of the breast: Higher risk for subsequent invasive cancer predicted by more extensive disease. Human Pathology. 1991;**22**(12):1232-1239

[60] Wohlfahrt J et al. A comparison of reproductive risk factors for CIS lesions and invasive breast cancer. International Journal of Cancer. 2004;**108**(5):750-753

[61] Cutuli B et al. Lobular carcinoma in situ (LCIS) of the breast: Is long-term outcome similar to ductal carcinoma in situ (DCIS)? Analysis of 200 cases. Radiation Oncology. 2015;**10**(1):110

[62] Choi BB et al. Radiologic findings of lobular carcinoma in situ: Mammography and ultrasonography. Journal of Clinical Ultrasound. 2011;**39**(2):59-63

[63] Murray MP et al. Classic lobular carcinoma in situ and atypical lobular hyperplasia at percutaneous breast core biopsy: Outcomes of prospective excision. Cancer. 2013;**119**(5):1073-1079

[64] Oppong BA, King TA. Recommendations for women with lobular carcinoma in situ (LCIS). Oncology (Williston Park). 2011;**25**(11):1051-1056 1058

[65] Pandey S et al. Columnar cell lesions of the breast: Mammographic findings with histopathologic correlation. Radiographics. 2007;**27**(suppl_1):S79-S89

[66] Fraser JL et al. Columnar alteration with prominent apical snouts and secretions: A spectrum of changes frequently present in breast biopsies performed for microcalcifications. The American Journal of Surgical Pathology. 1998;**22**(12):1521-1527

[67] Guerra-Wallace MM, Christensen WN, White RL. A retrospective study of columnar alteration with prominent apical snouts and secretions and the association with cancer. The American Journal of Surgery. 2004;**188**(4):395-398

[68] Kim MJ et al. Columnar cell lesions of the breast: Mammographic and US features. European Journal of Radiology. 2006;**60**(2):264-269

[69] Lerwill MF. Flat epithelial atypia of the breast. Archives of Pathology & Laboratory Medicine. 2008;**132**(4):615-621

[70] Abdel-Fatah TM et al. High frequency of coexistence of columnar cell lesions, lobular neoplasia, and low grade ductal carcinoma in situ with invasive tubular carcinoma and invasive lobular carcinoma. The American Journal of Surgical Pathology. 2007;**31**(3):417-426

[71] Aroner SA et al. Columnar cell lesions and subsequent breast cancer risk: A nested case-control study. Breast Cancer Research. 2010;**12**(4):R61

[72] Ingegnoli A et al. Flat epithelial atypia and atypical ductal hyperplasia: Carcinoma underestimation rate. The Breast Journal. 2010;**16**(1):55-59

[73] Calhoun BC et al. Management of flat epithelial atypia on breast core biopsy may be individualized based on correlation with imaging studies. Modern Pathology. 2015;**28**(5):670-676

[74] Lam WWM et al. Role of radiologic features in the management of papillary lesions of the breast. American Journal of Roentgenology. 2006;**186**(5):1322-1327

[75] Mercado CL et al. Papillary lesions of the breast at percutaneous core-needle biopsy. Radiology. 2006;**238**(3):801-808

[76] Mercado CL et al. Papillary lesions of the breast: Evaluation with stereotactic directional vacuum-assisted biopsy. Radiology. 2001;**221**(3):650-655

[77] Kennedy M et al. Pathology and clinical relevance of radial scars: A review. Journal of Clinical Pathology. 2003;**56**(10):721-724

[78] King TA et al. A better understanding of the term radial scar. The American Journal of Surgery. 2000;**180**(6):428-433

[79] Rakha EA et al. Outcome of breast lesions diagnosed as lesion of uncertain malignant potential (B3) or suspicious of malignancy (B4) on needle core biopsy, including detailed review of epithelial atypia. Histopathology. 2011;**58**(4):626-632

[80] Early Breast Cancer Trialists' Collaborative, G. Overview of the randomized trials of radiotherapy in ductal carcinoma in situ of the breast. Journal of the National Cancer Institute. Monographs. 2010;**2010**(41):162-177

[81] Holmberg L et al. Absolute risk reductions for local recurrence after postoperative radiotherapy after sector resection for ductal carcinoma in situ of the breast. Journal of Clinical Oncology. 2008;**26**(8):1247-1252

[82] Donker M et al. Breast-conserving treatment with or without radiotherapy in ductal carcinoma in situ: 15-year recurrence rates and outcome after a recurrence, from the EORTC
10853 randomized phase III trial. Journal of Clinical Oncology. 2013;**31**(32):4054-4059

[83] Cutuli B et al. Breast conserving surgery and radiotherapy a possible treatment for lobular carcinoma in situ ? European Journal of Cancer. 2005;**41**

[84] Cuzick J et al. Anastrozole for prevention of breast cancer in high-risk postmenopausal
women (IBIS-II): An international, double-blind, randomised placebo-controlled trial.
Lancet. 2014;**383**(9922):1041-1048

[85] Cuzick J et al. Long-term results of tamoxifen prophylaxis for breast cancer—96-month
follow-up of the randomized IBIS-I trial. Journal of the National Cancer Institute.
2007;**99**(4):272-282

[86] Wapnir IL et al. Long-term outcomes of invasive ipsilateral breast tumor recurrences
after lumpectomy in NSABP B-17 and B-24 randomized clinical trials for DCIS. Journal
of the National Cancer Institute. 2011;**103**(6):478-488

[87] Thompson AM et al. Treatment and outcomes from a large, prospective, national longitudinal cohort study of screen detected ductal carcinoma in situ (DCIS). Journal of
Clinical Oncology. 2016;**34**(15_suppl):1570-1570

9

Initial Clinical Evaluation of Observer Performance Using a Tablet Computer with a 4K High-Resolution Display for Detection of Breast Cancer by Digital Mammography

Ryusuke Murakami, Nachiko Uchiyama,
Hitomi Tani and Shinichiro Kumita

Abstract

Purpose: To compare observer performance using medical-purpose 5-megapixel liquid crystal display monitors (5-MP LCDs) and a tablet PC with a 4K high-resolution display for detection of breast cancer by digital mammography. **Materials and methods:** Mammograms from 40 patients with primary breast cancer (18 mass, 16 microcalcifications, 3 artificial distortions, and 3 focal asymmetries) and 60 control patients were consecutively collected. Four experienced radiologists assessed 100 mammograms to rate using the BI-RADS lexicon. The BI-RADS assessments were subjected to receiver operating characteristic (ROC) curve analysis. Also, the observers assessed the image quality in terms of brightness, contrast, sharpness, and noise using 5-step Likert scale. **Results:** The average under the curve (AUC) values for use of the 5-MP LCDs and 4K monitors were 0.921 and 0.936; the difference between them was small and not significant. In terms of image quality, the 4K was rated better for brightness, contrast, and sharpness. **Conclusion:** Observer performance for detecting breast cancer on a 4K tablet PC with a high-resolution display is similar to that using a 5-MP LCD. This appears adequate for displaying mammograms of diagnostic quality and could be useful for patient consultations, clinical demonstrations, or educational and teaching purposes.

Keywords: breast cancer, mammography, soft-copy, tablet PC, 4K

1. Introduction

Since the introduction of the Apple iPad in April 2010, the use of the mobile tablet PC has increased rapidly and such devices now comprise a major portion of the PC market.

With new developments in technology, opportunities for the use of tablet PCs in hospitals for management or diagnosis have increased because of the great advantages they have in terms of portability and applications for teleradiology [1–4]. An increasing number of reports have compared the use of mobile device screens with liquid-crystal displays (LCDs) for diagnosis, and the accuracy of the former is now considered to be almost equal to that of the latter, or at least acceptable, for MRI diagnosis of spinal injury, radiography and CT diagnosis of intracranial hemorrhage and orthopedic injury, and CT diagnosis of pulmonary embolism [5–8].

The viewing of digital mammograms using a soft-copy reading device has many advantages in terms of image display, better handling, postprocessing capability, computer-assisted diagnosis, archiving of image information, and image data transmission [9]. High-grade (so-called medical purpose) LCDs, such as the 5-megapixel (MP) LCD, are recommended for soft-copy reading in digital mammography [10–12].

Recently, a high-resolution 4K color display has also been developed and is commercially available. 4K resolution refers to a display device or content having a horizontal resolution in the order of 4000 pixels. Several examples of 4K resolution exist in the fields of digital television and digital cinematography. To our knowledge, however, there is no definite consensus as to whether a 4K high-resolution display monitor would be acceptable for reading of mammograms. In terms of access, portability and cost effectiveness, it would be useful to clarify whether 4K images actually afford better diagnostic accuracy.

The purpose of this study was to assess the observer performance of 4K tablet PCs with a high-resolution calibrated grayscale display monitor for detection of breast cancers on digital mammograms, in comparison with 5-MP LCDs.

2. Methods and materials

2.1. Mammogram selection

The study cohort included 40 cases surgically verified and pathologically proven breast cancers (mean age, 51.2 years; age range, 29–83 years). Histologic analysis demonstrated invasive ductal carcinoma in 25 cases, ductal carcinoma *in situ* in 10, and special type in 5. The median size of the lesions revealed by pathologic examination was 18.3 mm (range 3–45 mm). In addition, 60 cases (mean age, 48.4 years; age range, 28–82 years) including 48 with normal breast findings and 12 with benign conditions (mastopathy in 6; cyst in 3; fibroadenoma in 2; papilloma in 1) were selected. Mention this in abstract as well. Finally, 100 cases (48 normal, 40 with cancer, and 12 with benign lesions) were examined. ACR BI-RADS for density, a predetermined breast density distribution was followed when selecting the cases: 10 were for cases with extremely dense breasts, 55 with heterogeneously dense breasts, 30 with scattered fibroglandular tissue, and 5 with entirely fatty breasts.

2.2. Image acquisition and display

Mammograms were acquired using a flat-panel digital mammography system (Senographe DS LaVerite; GE Healthcare). The spatial resolution was 100 μm per pixel (pixel dimension: 1800 × 2304) and the contrast resolution was 14 bits.

The images were displayed on two types of display: (i) two monochrome 5-MP LCDs (MFGD5621HD, 2048 × 2560 pixels, 21.3 inch; BARCO); and (ii) two commercially available 4K tablet PCs with high-resolution color monitors (4K UT-MA6, 2560 × 3840 pixels, 20.8 inch; Panasonic) (**Figures 1** and **2**).

The physical properties of the two types of monitors are shown in **Table 1**.

The displays run with the PACS software (We VIEW Z; HITACHI) and viewing software specialized for MGs (Plissimo MG, Panasonic). The luminance of both monitors was calibrated as recommended by the suppliers and at the start of the reading test.

2.3. Image interpretation

Four board-certified radiologists assessed the mammograms in a dark environment (<10 lux). Each of the observers independently assessed 200 images (100 patients × 2 sides; MLO and CC views). The observers were asked to rate the images on the level of confidence using the BI-RADS lexicon: 1, negative; 2, benign; 3, probably benign; 4, suspicious; and 5, highly suggestive of malignancy.

In addition, on another occasion, the observers assessed the image quality in terms of brightness, contrast, sharpness, and noise, side-by-side for the 5-MP LCDs versus the 4K tablet PCs (5-step Likert scale, −2 = 5-MP definitely better and +2 = 4K definitely better).

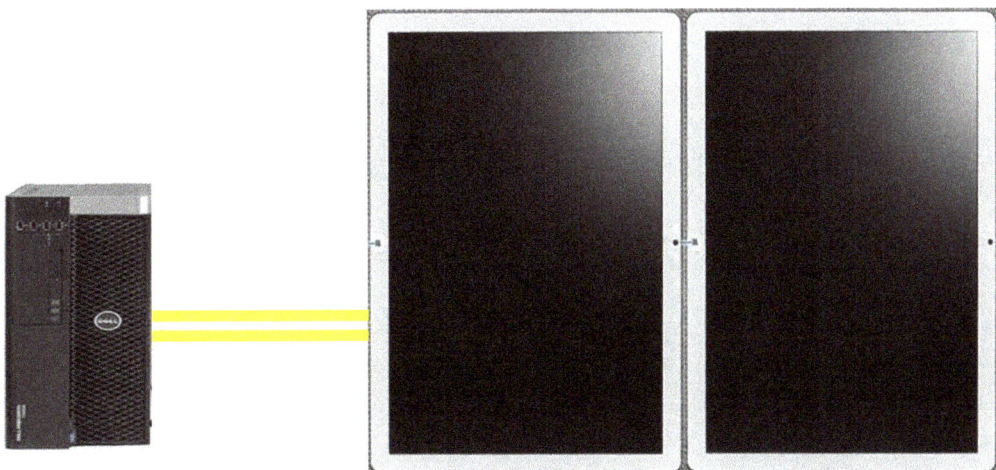

Figure 1. 4k UT-MA6 (TOUGHPAD) 20.8 inches; Panasonic.

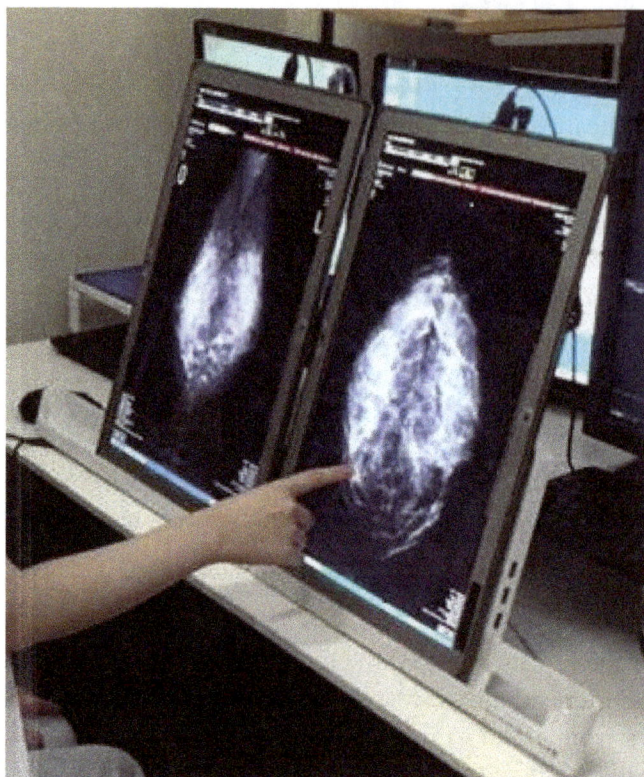

Figure 2. Two sets of 4K tablet PCs with high-resolution color monitors (4K UT-MA6, 2560 × 3840 pixels, 20.8 inch; Panasonic).

	Screen size	Matrix size	Color	Maximum luminance (cd/m²)	Contrast ratio	Product name (manufacturer)
4K tablet PC	20.8 (inches)	2560 × 3840	Color	300	850:1	UT-MA6 (Panasonic)
5-MP LCD	21.3 (inches)	2048 × 2560	Monochrome	450	800:1	MFGD5621HD (Barco)

Table 1. The physical properties of the 5-MP LCDs and 4K display monitors used in comparison with observer performance.

2.4. Data and statistical analysis

The observers' detection performance was evaluated using receiver operating characteristic (ROC) curve analysis. The confidence level results were used to construct ROC curves. This allowed to obtain the sensitivity, specificity, positive predictive value (PPV), negative predictive value (NPV), and accuracy of each monitor. Image quality ratings were tabulated for each reader and summarized across all readers. The confidence interval (CI) for the proportion of 4K ratings as similar (0), slightly better (±1), or better (±2) was obtained, considering the side-by-side comparison to be a single test condition. In the statistical analysis, differences at $P < 0.05$ were considered to be statistically significant.

3. Results

Table 2 and **Figure 3** show the average under the curve (AUC) values and ROC curves for detection of breast cancers using the 5-MP LCDs and the 4K tablet PCs, respectively. The mean AUC values for use of the 5-MP LCDs and the 4K tablet PCs were 0.921 and 0.936, respectively. The difference was not statistically significant ($P = 0.27$). Sensitivity, specificity, positive and negative predictive values, and accuracy were comparable (**Table 3**).

	BI-LADS	
	5-MP LCD	4K
Reader 1	0.858	0.903
Reader 2	0.932	0.954
Reader 3	0.945	0.945
Reader 4	0.949	0.958
Mean	0.921	0.936

Table 2. The area under the ROC curve for the 5-MP and 4K in BI-RADS scores.

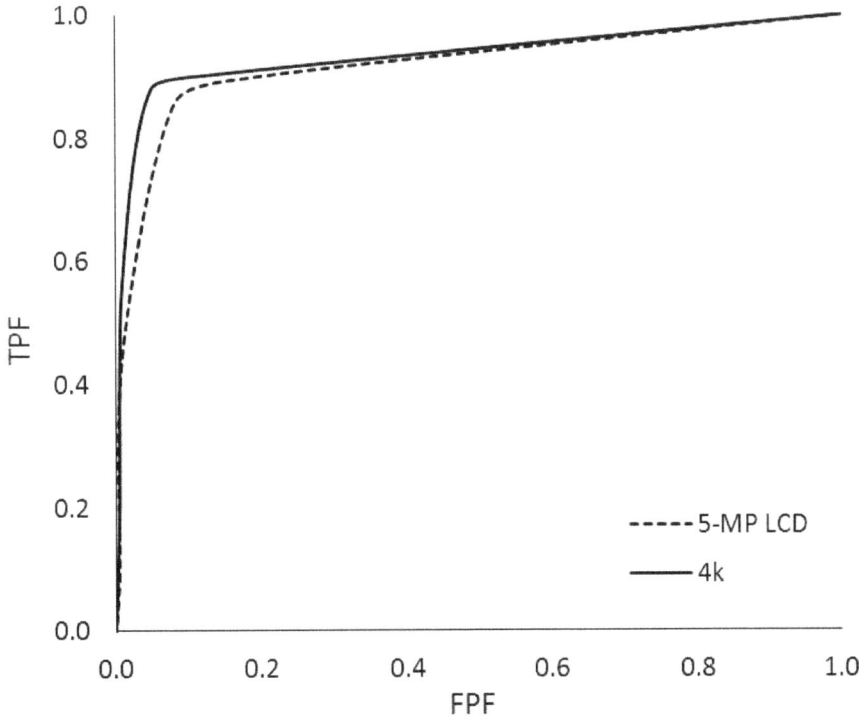

Figure 3. ROC curves for the detection of breast cancers. FPF, false positive fraction; TPF, true positive fraction. The thick line shows the ROC curve for a set of 4K tablet PC with high-resolution color monitors and the dashed line shows the ROC curve for a set of 5-MP LCDs. There was no significant difference between the two types of display modes ($P = 0.27$).

	5-MP LCD	4K
Sensitivity	0.857 (0.863/0.956)	0.881 (0.788/0.937)
Specificity	0.918 (0.889/0.936)	0.963 (0.939/0.978)
PPV	0.735 (0.643/0.794)	0.860 (0.769/0.915)
NPV	0.960 (0.931/0.980)	0.969 (0.945/0.984)
Accuracy	0.905 (0.860/0.934)	0.946 (0.908/0.969)

Table 3. Sensitivity, specificity, positive and negative predictive values and accuracy with the 5-MP and 4K.

With regard to image quality, brightness for the 4K tablet PC was rated as similar to that of the 5-MP LCD in 12% of the study readings, slightly better in 54%, and better in 27%. Contrast for the 4K tablet PC was rated as similar to that of the 5-MP LCD in 26% of the study readings, slightly better in 40%, and better in 15%. Sharpness for the 4K tablet PC was rated as similar to that of the 5-MP LCD in 38% of the study readings, slightly better in 26%, and better in 12%. Noise for the 4K tablet PC was rated as similar to that of the 5-MP LCD in 85% of the study readings, and slightly better in 5% (**Table 4** and **Figure 4**). **Figures 5–8** demonstrated breast cancers displayed on 5-MP and 4K monitors.

	4K better (+2)	4K slightly better (+1)	Similar (0)	5-MP slightly better (−1)	5-MP better (−2)	Mean	Lower 95% CL	Upper 95% CL
Brightness	27	54	12	7	0	1.00	0.84	1.16
Contrast	15	40	26	19	0	0.51	0.32	0.70
Sharpness	12	26	38	24	0	0.26	0.07	0.45
Noise	0	5	85	10	0	−0.05	−0.13	0.03

Table 4. Image quality on the basis of brightness, contrast, sharpness and noise, for side-by-side feature visibility rating with 5-MP versus 4K. Values are presented as numbers (also percentages). Mean is average preference by percentage. Positive numbers indicate a preference for 4K and negative numbers indicate a preference for 5-MP. CL; confidence limits.

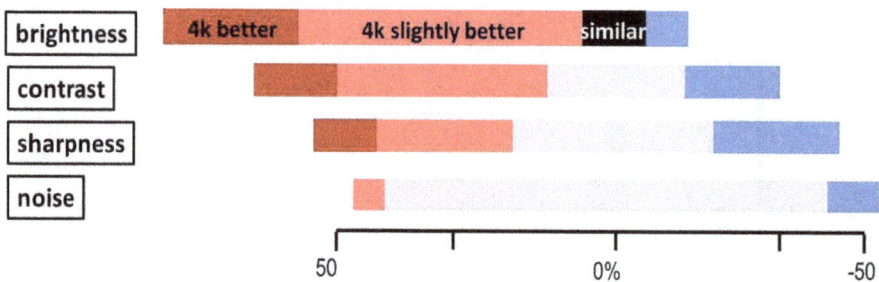

Figure 4. Likert scale scores (*n* = 100 eligible patients). Image quality on the basis of brightness, contrast, sharpness, and noise, for side-by-side feature visibility rating with 4K and 5-MP LCD. Values are presented as percentages.

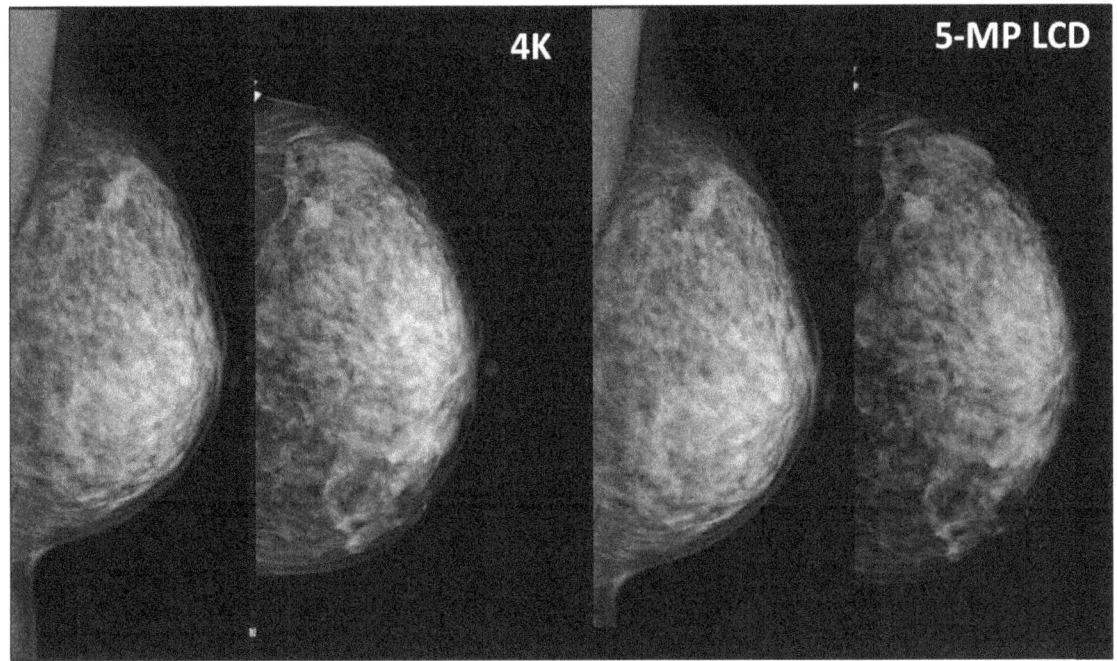

Figure 5. Microlobulated mass in the left upper area *captured images.

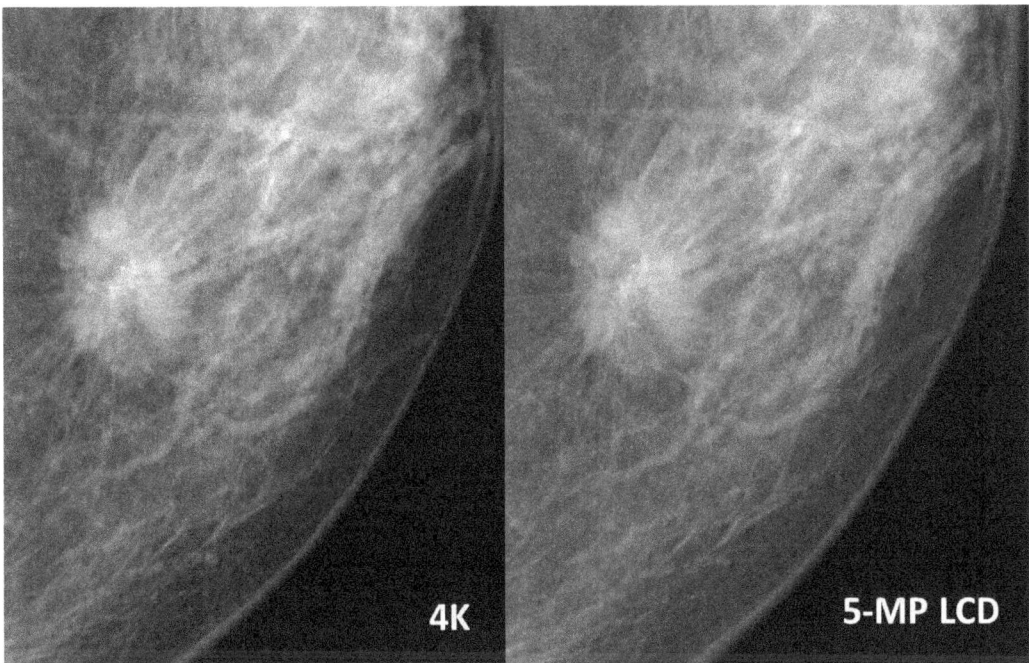

Figure 6. Spiculated mass *captured images.

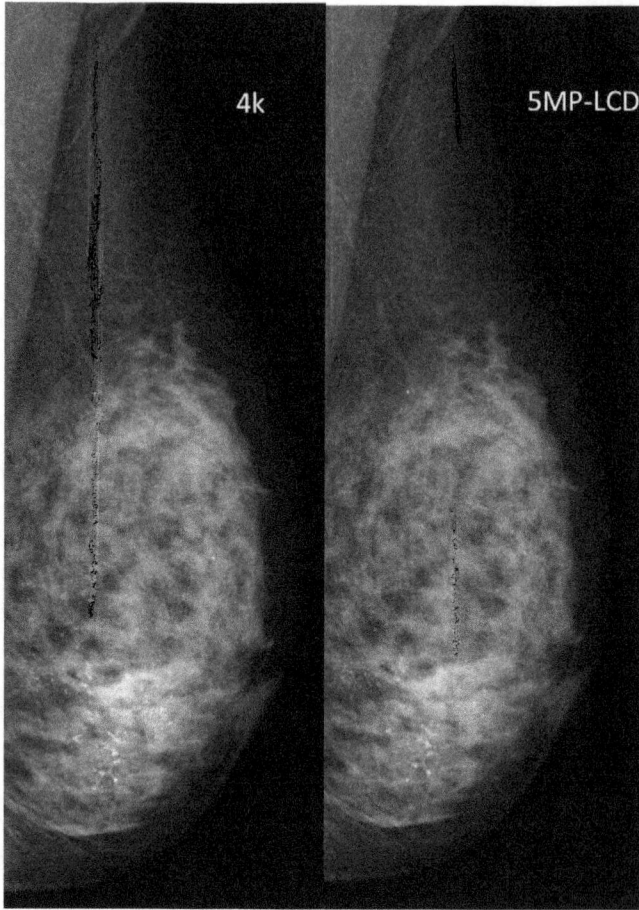

Figure 7. Finelinear branching calcifications in the left lower area *captured images.

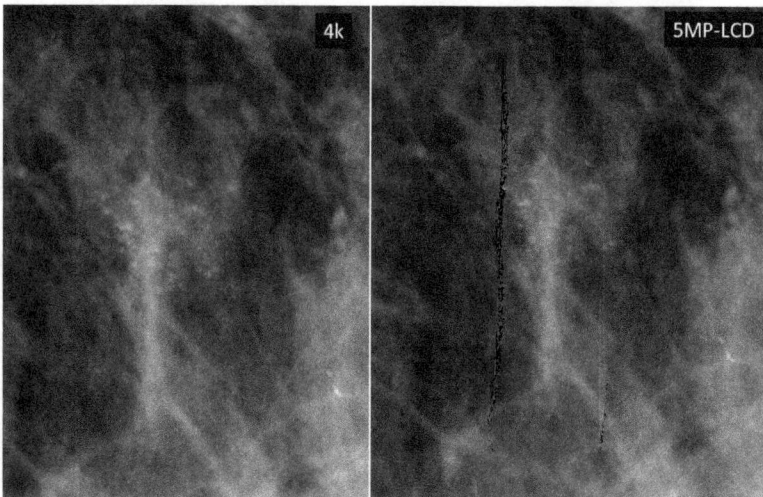

Figure 8. Amorphous grouped calcifications *captured images.

4. Discussion

The purpose of the present study using images from actual patients was to obtain initial data to indicate whether or not the newer tablet PCs with a 4K high-resolution color display monitor could be deployed for mammographic imaging. Only one previous study has evaluated the display quality of tablet PCs [13]. This study represented the first attempt to evaluate the display quality of tablet PCs (iPad 2 and 3) with a dedicated 10-MP LCD using a standardized CDMAM phantom. It was concluded that the evaluated iPads, especially version 3, would likely be adequate for display of diagnostic-quality mammograms [13].

Our present study found no significant difference between the performances of the 5-MP LCDs and the 4K tablet PCs for detecting breast cancers on mammograms. Moreover, in terms of the image quality, 4K tablet PCs were rated as having better brightness, contrast, and sharpness. This is the first confirmation that observer performance for detection of breast cancers using soft-copy readings on digital mammograms is comparable between the current standard 5-MP LCDs and 4K tablet PCs with a high-resolution display monitor. The 4K tablet PC seems suitable for displaying mammograms in a variety of tasks such as patient consultation, clinical demonstrations, or educational and teaching purposes, and its large high-resolution screen seems to meet the legal requirements. As many patients are interested in taking a look at their images, one of the most promising applications of tablet PC-based mammographic display would be patient consultation. This would give patients a clearer idea of their disease and might have a positive impact on patient compliance.

The greatest benefits of the 4K tablet PC with a high-resolution display monitor are its low cost and possible application for multiple purposes, such as reporting systems and referencing of color images including endoscopic, PET/CT, and SPECT/CT images. In addition, the performance of 4K high-resolution color display monitors has recently improved, and they now have high-resolution (5-MP or more) capability, as is the case for medical LCDs. However, the development of tablet PCs is progressing rapidly; the 4K display used in the present study might now be considered a relatively old model. If the 4K display is suitable for medical display purposes, the cost would increase.

5. Conclusion

Our findings suggest that observer performance for detection of breast cancers on digital mammograms using 4K tablet PCs with a high-resolution display monitor is comparable to that obtained using 5-MP LCDs. Therefore, 4K tablet PCs, as a result of the advanced technology, might be adequate for diagnostic-quality mammogram display and could be useful for patient consultation, clinical demonstration, or educational and teaching purposes. Because of the promising potential advantages of tablet PCs, such as their portability, further assessments of their potential clinical use are warranted.

Author details

Ryusuke Murakami[1]*, Nachiko Uchiyama[2], Hitomi Tani[1] and Shinichiro Kumita[1]

*Address all correspondence to: rywakana@nms.ac.jp

1 Department of Radiology, Nippon Medical School, Tokyo, Japan

2 Department of Radiology, National Cancer Center, Tokyo, Japan

References

[1] Volonté F, Robert JH, Ratib O, Triponez F. A lung segmentectomy performed with 3D recon-struction images available on the operating table with an iPad. Interactive CardioVascular and Thoracic Surgery. 2011;**12**:1066-1068

[2] Mc Laughlin P, Neill SO, Fanning N, Mc Garrigle AM, Connor OJ, Wyse G, Maher MM. Emergency CT brain: Preliminary interpretation with a tablet device—Image quality and diagnostic performance of the Apple iPad. Emergency Radiology. 2012;**19**:127-133

[3] Takao H, Murayama Y, Ishibashi T, Karagiozov KL, Abe T. A new support system using a mobile device (smartphone) for diagnostic image display and treatment of stroke. Stroke. 2012;**43**:236-239

[4] Yoshimura K, Nihashi T, Ikeda M, Ando Y, Kawai H, Kawakami K, Kimura R, Okada Y, Okochi Y, Ota N, Tsuchiya K, Naganawa S. Comparison of liquid crystal dis-play monitors calibrated with gray-scale standard display function and with γ 2.2 and iPad: Observer performance in detection of cerebral infarction on brain CT. American Journal of Roentgenology. 2013;**200**:1304-1309

[5] John S, Poh AC, Lim TC, Chan EH, Chong LR. The iPad tablet computer for mobile on-call radiology diagnosis? Auditing discrepancy in CT and MRI reporting. Journal of Digital Imaging. 2012;**25**:628-634

[6] McNulty JP, Ryan JT, Evanoff MG, Rainford LA. Flexible image evaluation: iPad versus secondary-class monitors for review of MR spinal emergency cases—A comparative study. Academic Radiology. 2012;**19**:1023-1028

[7] Toomey RJ, Ryan JT, McEntee MF, Evanoff MG, Chakraborty DP, McNulty JP, Manning DJ, Thomas EM, Brennan PC. Diagnostic efficacy of handheld devices for emergency radiology consultation. American Journal of Roentgenology. 2010;**194**:469-474

[8] Johnson PT1, Zimmerman SL, Heath D, Eng J, Horton KM, Scott WW, Fishman EK. The iPad as a mobile device for CT display and interpretation: Diagnostic accuracy for iden-tification of pulmonary embolism. Emergency Radiology. 2012;**19**:323-327

[9] Kamitani T, Yabuuchi H, Matsuo Y, Setoguchi T, Sakai S, Okafuji T, Sunami S, Hatakenaka M, Ishii N, Kubo M, Tokunaga E, Yamamoto H, Honda H. Diagnostic performance in

differentiation of breast lesion on digital mammograms: Comparison among hard-copy film, 3-megapixel LCD monitor, and 5-megapixel LCD monitor. Clinical Imaging. 2011;**35**:341-345

[10] Yamada T, Suzuki A, Uchiyama N, Ohuchi N, Takahashi S. Diagnostic performance of detecting breast cancer on computed radiology (CR) mammograms: Comparison of hard copy film, 3-megapixel liquid-crystal-display (LCD) monitor and 5-megapixel LCD monitor. European Radiology. 2008;**18**:2363-2369

[11] Schueller G, Schueller-Weidekamm C, Pinker K, Memarsadeghi M, Weber M, Helbich TH. Comparison of 5-megapixel cathode ray tube monitors and 5-megapixel liquid crystal monitors for soft-copy reading in full-field digital mammography. European Journal of Radiology. 2010;**76**:68-72

[12] Yabuuchi H, Kawanami S, Kamitani T, Matsumura T, Yamasaki Y, Morishita J, Honda H. Detectability of BI-RADS category 3 or higher breast lesions and reading time on mammography: Comparison between 5-MP and 8-MP LCD monitors. Acta Radiologica. 2017;**58**:403-407

[13] Hammon M, Schlechtweg PM, Schulz-Wendtland R, Uder M, Schwab SA. iPads in breast imaging—A phantom study. Geburtshilfe Frauenheilkd. 2014;**74**:152-156

10

Breast Ultrasound Past, Present, and Future

Jocelyn A. Rapelyea and Christina G. Marks

Abstract

This chapter will review the utilization of breast ultrasound for screening and diagnostic purposes. Currently, ultrasound is primarily used to investigate palpable lesions in women less than 30 years old, to provide further characterization of abnormal mammographic findings, and to guide invasive breast interventions. Innovations in ultrasound technology have improved the detection and diagnosis of breast cancer. Computer-aided detection (CAD), elastography, quantitative breast ultrasound technology, and ultrasound contrast agents (microbubbles) were developed to improve diagnostic accuracy. These advancements have the potential to impact overall survival by detecting cancers that are smaller and less aggressive.

Keywords: screening ultrasound, elastography, CAD, quantitative ultrasound, breast cancer, breast ultrasound, targeted breast ultrasound, automated whole breast ultrasound, breast density, ultrasound guided biopsy

1. Introduction

Breast ultrasound is an integral component of the diagnostic evaluation of breast lesions. It is the primary modality used to examine palpable abnormalities in young women (<30 years old), is routinely employed to further characterize mammographic abnormalities as solid or cystic, and provides direction for image-guided breast interventions [1].

For many years, the primary utility of breast ultrasound was differentiating cysts from solid masses. Cysts can occur at any age, but are most commonly found in pre- and perimenopausal women. To classify a lesion as a simple cyst, it must meet a strict set of criteria; it must be entirely anechoic, sharply marginated, round or oval in shape, and demonstrate posterior acoustic enhancement [2]. Lesions containing low-level echoes, which otherwise meet the criteria for simple cysts, are referred to as complicated cysts. Complicated cysts may also have fluid-fluid or fluid-debris levels that may shift with changes in a patient's position. Complex cystic masses with discrete solid components are suspicious for malignancy and require further evaluation with biopsy [2].

Today, there is a paradigm shift in the application of breast ultrasound. Its new role as a primary screening tool in women with dense breast tissue is growing. The limitation of mammography in women with dense breast tissue has opened the door to supplemental screening with ultrasound and magnetic resonance imaging (MRI). Ultrasound has become the supplemental screening tool of choice for breast cancer detection in this select group of women given that it is low in cost, is widely available and has no ionizing radiation. Whether breast ultrasound is used for diagnosis or screening, evidence of its utilization over the last 50 years has deemed it an invaluable tool.

2. Background/historical perspective

In the mid to late 1960s, there was a significant amount of research involving breast ultrasound. Issues such as transducer design and manipulation of the ultrasonic beam became the focus of many researchers. Improvement in resolution and the advent of grayscale imaging segued to modern day imaging and an effort to shift from evaluating pathological breast findings toward screening healthy women.

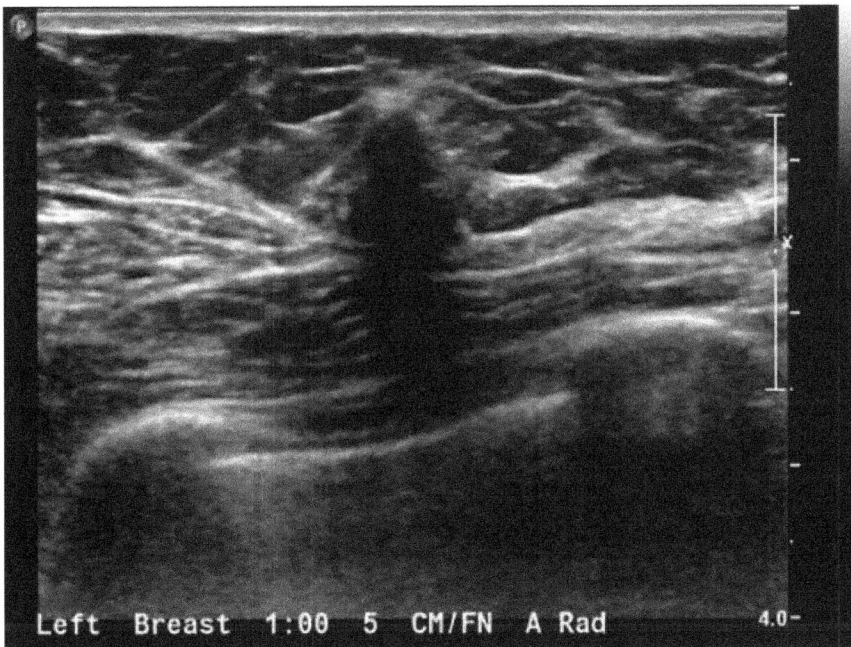

Figure 1. Transverse ultrasound of the left breast demonstrates an irregular, antiparallel mass with posterior acoustic shadowing.

It was not until 1970 that there was regular clinical use of breast ultrasound, mainly in the United States and Asia. During this time, Japanese authors Kobayashi et al. published several papers [3, 4] discussing the various characteristics that could differentiate benign and malignant breast disease. Published work from these authors linked the characteristic descriptor of acoustic shadowing with breast malignancy [5]. Further development in the late 1980s and early 1990s of Doppler ultrasound helped complement B-mode grayscale images, augmenting the ability to differentiate cancerous masses from benign findings (**Figure 1**). In 1995, Stavros and colleagues described a set of criteria to improve specificity in determining benign and malignant features of breast masses [6]. By the late 1990s and early 2000, advancement and application of tissue harmonics and spatial compounding further refined ultrasound images; helping to improve image resolution and reduce noise [7, 8].

Optimization of the ultrasound image is essential, but not the only component needed to properly classify masses as benign vs. malignant. The knowledge of normal breast anatomy, breast scanning technique (artifactual tissue shadowing will resolve with increase in transducer pressure), along with the understanding of common artifacts encountered can improve the overall effectiveness of the examination. Recent publication of the American College of Radiology's (ACR's) Breast Ultrasound Lexicon (++) has helped to standardize the descriptive language of breast lesions, thus improving the positive predictive value (PPV) and confidence in determining the likelihood of malignancy.

3. Basics of breast ultrasound

3.1. Anatomy

The female breast is made up of glandular tissue and fat, held together by a framework of fibers called Cooper's ligaments. The female breast, representing a modified sweat gland, spans the distances between the second and sixth anterior ribs, sternum, and midaxillary line. Normal anatomical structures imaged during breast ultrasound include the skin, nipple, fat, Cooper's ligaments, ducts, breast parenchyma, pectoralis muscles, pleura, and ribs (**Figure 2**). These appear as six distinct layers on ultrasound images as follows (from anterior to posterior): skin, subcutaneous fat, breast parenchyma (including ducts and lobules), retroglandular (retromammary) fat, pectoralis muscles, and chest wall (**Figure 3**). It is the sonographic appearance of the breast fat which gives reference for comparing other structures within the breast [9]. Breast fat appears dark gray on ultrasound images. Ducts and cysts are anechoic. The nipple and blood vessels appear hypoechoic, while breast parenchyma, Cooper's ligaments, and skin appear hyperechoic.

Ultrasound imaging of the skin and nipple can best be imaged using a stand off pad, which can help eliminate the acoustic shadowing commonly seen posterior to the nipple [1]. The skin is usually less than or equal to 2 mm in thickness, except over the areola where the skin is often thicker.

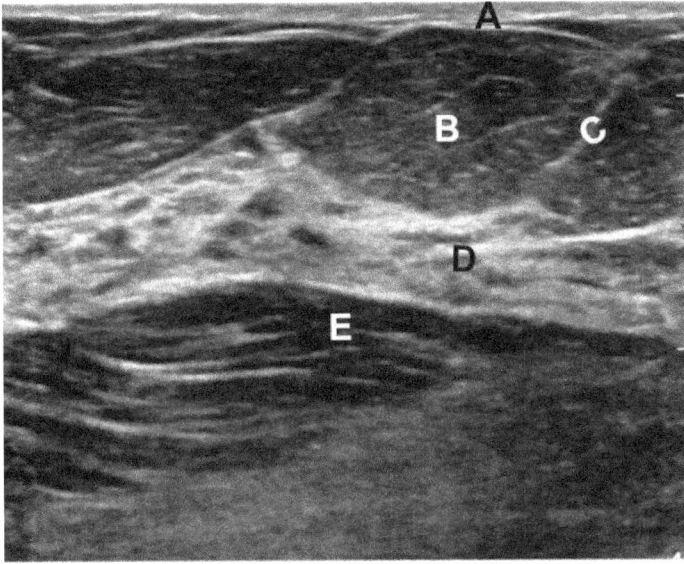

Figure 2. Breast anatomy. Transverse ultrasound shows normal breast anatomy. (A) Skin, (B) fat lobule, (C) Cooper ligament, (D) fibroglandular zone, and (E) muscle.

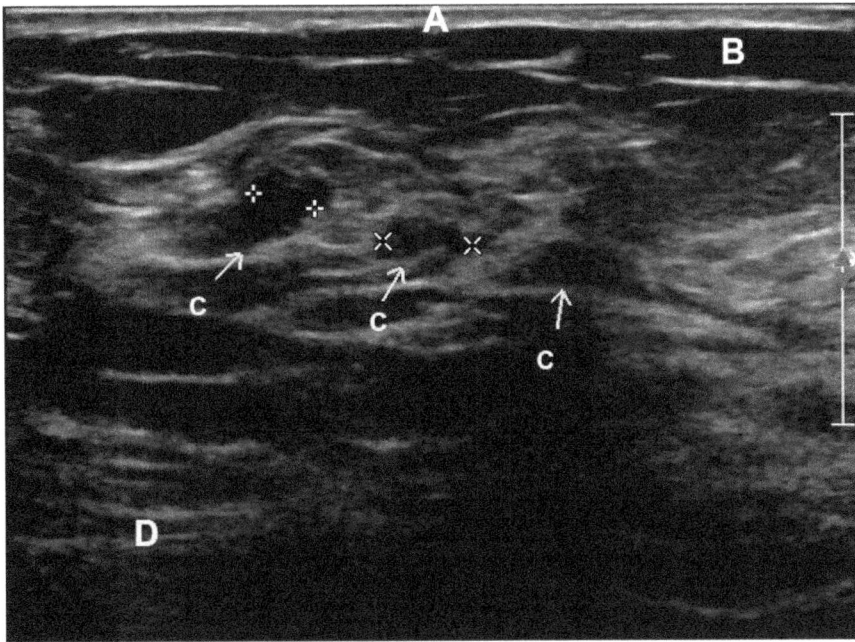

Figure 3. Breast anatomy. Transverse ultrasound shows normal breast anatomy. (A) Skin, (B) subcutaneous fat, (C) terminal duct lobular unit, and (D) muscle.

3.1.1. Male vs. female

In contrast to the female breast in which ducts, stroma, and glandular tissue are found, the male breast contains mostly fatty tissue with a few ducts and stroma. The sparse ductal and stromal elements within the male breast give rise to the most common disease seen within the male breast, gynecomastia. Gynecomastia is typically bilateral and appears on ultrasound images as subareolar glandular tissue, which may be hypoechoic to hyperechoic. There are no standard protocols for imaging the male breast with many institutions performing a mammogram prior to ultrasound. Male breast cancer is very rare, representing only about 1% of all breast cancers [10].

3.1.2. Maturation phases

Mastogenesis begins around the sixth week of development and by the eighth week, a mammary gland is formed from the thickening located at the epidermic "milk line" [11]. During puberty, both estrogen and progesterone stimulate breast development.

3.1.3. Lactation changes

During pregnancy and lactation, the breast undergoes many hormonal changes resulting in glandular proliferation, ductal distention, and stromal involution. Ultrasound is the modality of choice for evaluating palpable masses, bloody nipple discharge, and focal pain in the lactating breast. Masses unique to the lactating breast include lactating adenomas and galactoceles [12].

3.1.4. The postoperative breast

Patients who have undergone lumpectomy surgery often present with postoperative fluid collections such as seromas, hematomas, and lymphoceles with spontaneous resorption of these fluid collections occurring over time. It is important not to confuse scar formation for recurrent cancer in this patient population, as areas of scarring can appear as areas of acoustic shadowing [1]. In patients who have undergone radiation therapy, skin thickening, and breast edema are frequently identified and eventually decrease over time.

3.1.5. The postimplant breast

Breast implants include both silicone and saline implants which are surgically placed for either breast augmentation or reconstruction. While MRI is the imaging modality of choice to evaluate for silicone implant integrity, there are characteristic sonographic appearances associated with silicone implant rupture. The appearance of an intact breast implant on ultrasound is similar to a large cyst, with presence of an anechoic implant lumen surrounded by a hyperechoic linear shell [13]. The "stepladder sign," which appears as horizontal, hyperechoic, straight, or curvilinear lines across the implant lumen, is characteristic of intracapsular silicone implant rupture (**Figure 4**) [13]. The "snowstorm sign" is reportedly the most significant sonographic finding for extracapsular rupture and appears as hyperechoic nodules with defined anterior margin and posterior acoustic shadowing within the breast parenchyma or axillary lymph nodes [13]. The ability to diagnose extracapsular rupture on sonography approaches accuracy of MRI, with one study finding 100% diagnostic accuracy for extracapsular rupture with ultrasound (**Figure 5**) [13].

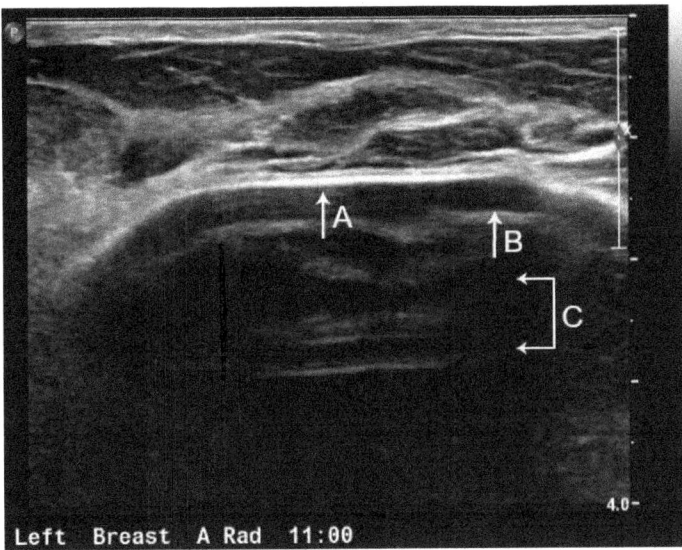

Figure 4. "**Stepladder sign.**" Transverse ultrasound demonstrates an intracapsular silicone implant rupture. (A) Outer capsule, (B) shell of collapsed implant, and (C) "Linguine sign".

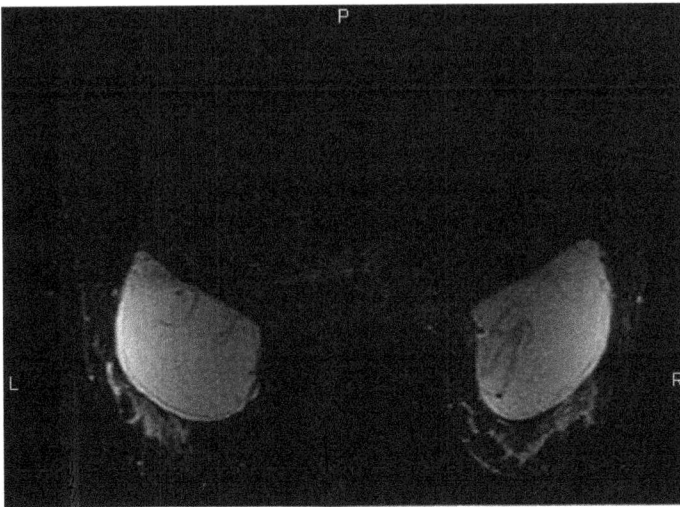

Figure 5. Axial T2W MRI demonstrates bilateral intracapsular silicone implant ruptures.

3.2. B-mode and Doppler

B-mode or brightness mode, ultrasound images are the standard two-dimensional grayscale images routinely obtained during breast ultrasound. The higher the probe frequency, the better the axial resolution, which is the ability to resolve objects within the imaging plane located at different depths [14]. For this reason, high frequency probes (12–18 mHz) are often utilized for breast ultrasound, which requires relatively steep time gain curve to compensate for rapid beam attenuation (**Figure 6**). If a large breast is being imaged, a lower frequency probe may be preferable to image deep lesions close to the pectoralis muscle given that high frequency

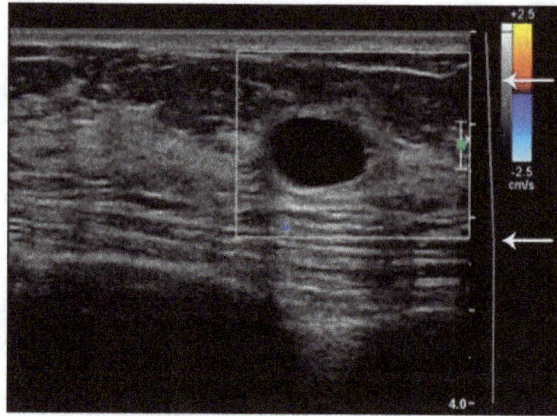

Figure 6. Gain. Transverse ultrasound illustrates gain. Ultrasound waves are absorbed by tissue. The deeper the tissue, the greater the absorption. A gradual increase in the gain with deeper tissues is recommended.

probes often do not penetrate as deeply as lower frequency probes. Alternatively, adjusting the patient's position or compressing the breast can help bring the lesion into the focal zone [1]. Ensuring the focal zone is centered at the depth of interest within the breast is also essential to ensure optimization of lateral resolution (**Figure 7**). Lateral resolution is the ability to resolve objects located side by side at the same depth and is best at the focal zone, where the ultrasound beam is at its narrowest [14]. Doppler ultrasound utilizes the Doppler Effect to analyze the frequency of the returning echo allowing for color Doppler images to be obtained demonstrating both tissue morphologies in grayscale as well as blood flow in color [14]. While the use of color Doppler can help differentiate solid masses from complicated cysts [9], some propose that Doppler ultrasound will further improve ultrasound performance by aiding in the assessment of tumor vascularity and tumor blood flow [15].

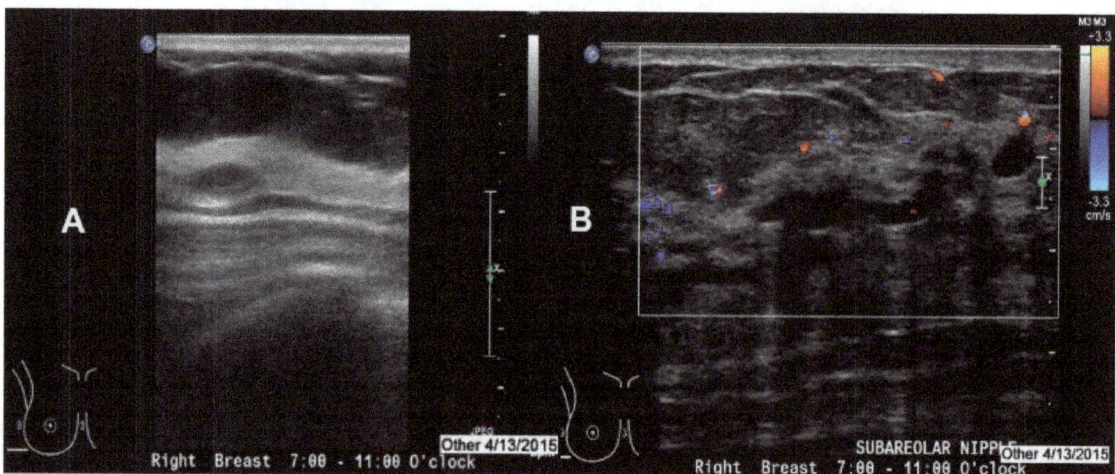

Figure 7. Focal zone. Transverse ultrasound of the right breast illustrating focal zone settings. The focal zone should be set at the anterior to middle third of the region of interest. (A) Partial volume averaging—loss of detail and (B) image with appropriate focal zone setting.

3.3. Artifacts

Ultrasound is a modality with many artifacts. Some artifacts most commonly encountered in breast ultrasound include acoustic shadowing, posterior acoustic enhancement, refraction, speckle, and reverberation. While some artifacts make detection or differentiation of lesions more difficult, other artifacts help identify and characterize lesions in the breast. Acoustic shadowing and posterior acoustic enhancement are both artifacts that routinely aid in characterization of breast lesions. Acoustic shadowing is secondary to a decrease in the energy of transmitted sound either secondary to reflection and/or absorption and appears on ultrasound images as a dark or hypoechoic band beneath an object of high attenuation [14, 16]. Sound is gradually attenuated as it passes through solid structures. Alternatively, sound is less attenuated as it passes through fluid-filled structures, giving the appearance of a brighter signal deep to cystic structures [14, 16]. The presence of posterior acoustic enhancement helps distinguish cystic versus solid breast lesions, although it is important to note that some solid lesions also demonstrate posterior acoustic enhancement. Refraction is often encountered in breast ultrasound when the sound beam is refracted at a curved interface between the higher velocity soft tissues and a lower velocity cyst resulting in narrow refractive bands along the margins [17]. Refractive artifacts should not be confused with acoustic shadowing. Speckle refers to a granular appearance of an otherwise fat homogeneous region of breast tissue. It can affect image contrast and reduce visibility of lesions by masking small differences in the level of gray (**Figure 8**). Reverberation artifact occurs when sound is reflected off strong acoustic interfaces creating a ping-pong of echoes resulting in an image of parallel, linear bright bands or diffuse low-level echoes in the superficial most aspect of a cyst [14, 16, 17]. Decreasing the gain can help reduce reverberation artifact [14].

3.4. Spatial compound imaging

Compound imaging refers to the technique by which images are acquired from multiple angles of isonation and then added together while maintaining a static transducer position. Each image has its own artifact profile and when multiple images are averaged together, the artifacts become less apparent and true structures are better visualized [18]. One benefit of spatial compound imaging is reduced speckle artifact (**Figure 9**). Reduced image speckle has been shown to improve the conspicuity of low contrast lesions, enhance the delineation of tumor margins, and improve the depiction of the internal architecture of solid lesions and microcalcifications. One limitation of spatial compound imaging is the reduced visibility of the posterior echo pattern (acoustic shadowing or enhancement), artifacts often used to aid in characterization of lesions as cystic or solid [19]. Additionally, spatial compound imaging requires frame averaging during compounding, producing motion blurring if the ultrasound probe is moved too quickly [15].

3.5. Clutter

Clutter is a noise artifact caused by either aberration or reverberation of echoes, which causes filling in and loss of contrast [20, 21]. On ultrasound images, clutter appears as a diffuse haze thereby reducing image contrast and is most easily visualized in anechoic or hypoechoic

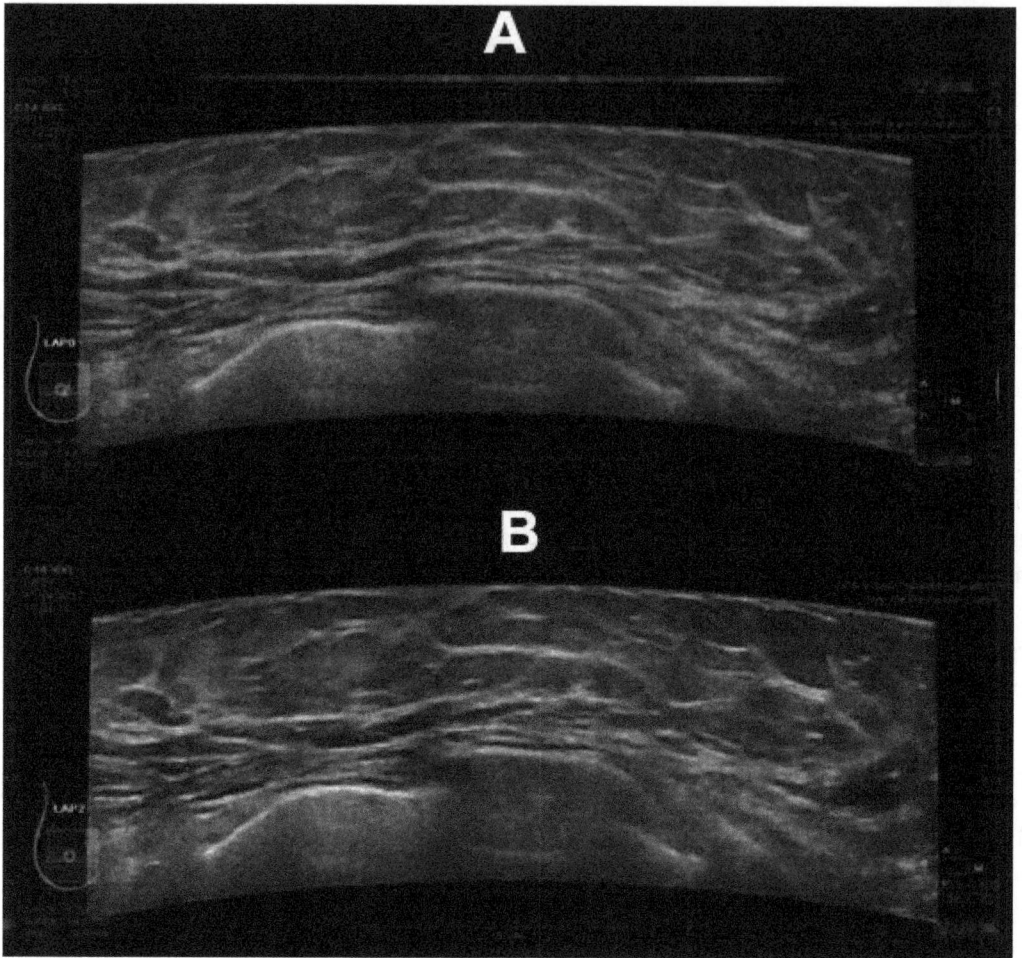

Figure 8. (A) Long axis view of transverse ultrasound demonstrating speckle artifact. Increased noise noted throughout the image and (B) long axis view of transverse ultrasound demonstrating speckle reduction.

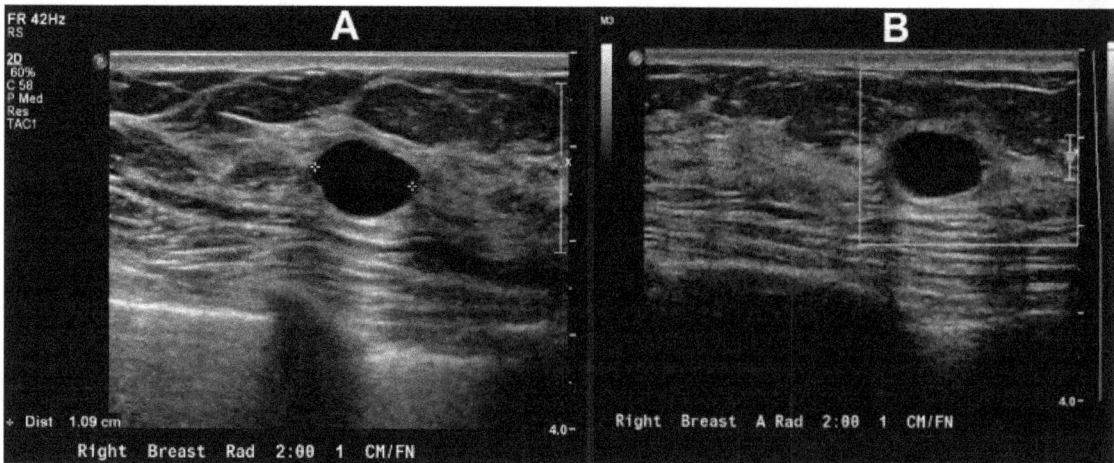

Figure 9. Compound imaging. Transverse ultrasound of the right breast illustrates compound imaging. (A) Utilization of compound imaging and (B) without compound imaging.

structures [21]. Clutter is of particular concern when imaging small, low-contrast lesions [21]. Methods to reduce clutter include second-order ultrasound field imaging, short-lag spatial coherence imaging, filtering techniques, and tissue harmonic imaging [20].

3.6. Tissue harmonic imaging

Tissue harmonic imaging is an ultrasonographic technique that can potentially provide images of higher quality than those obtained with conventional ultrasound techniques. Tissue harmonic imaging involves the use of harmonic frequencies that originate within the tissue

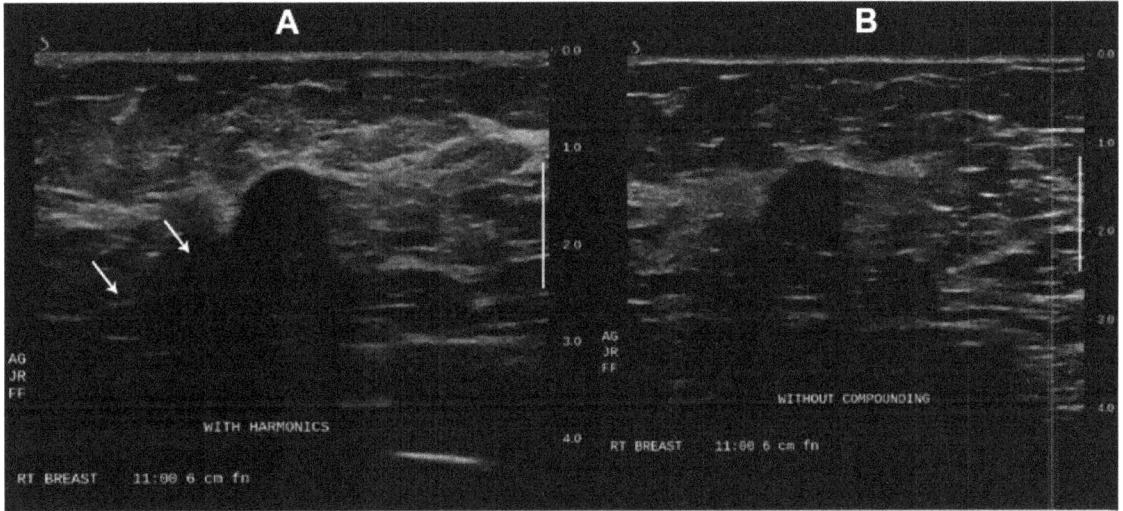

Figure 10. Harmonics increase real echoes. Transverse ultrasound of the right breast shows harmonics increasing real echoes. (A) With harmonics and (B) without harmonics.

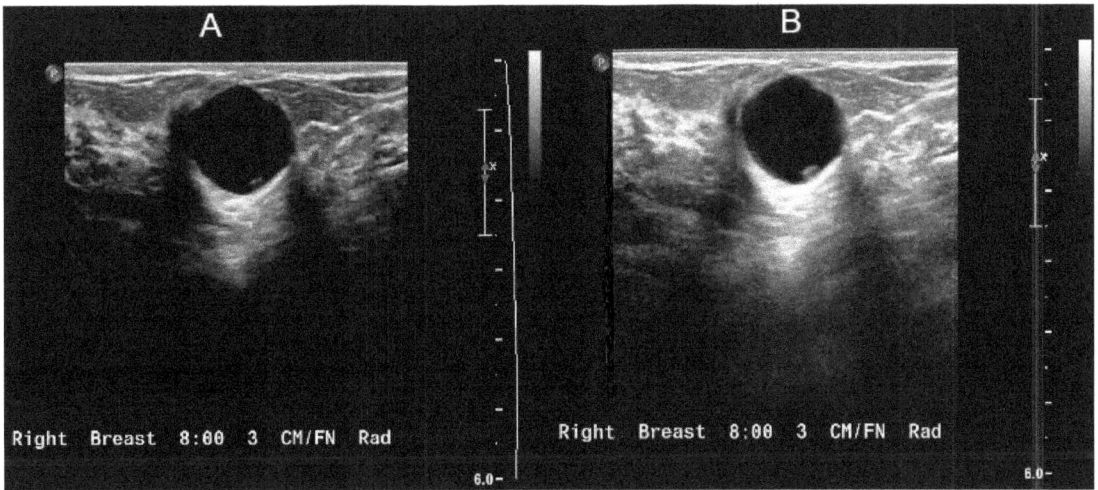

Figure 11. Harmonics reduce artefactual echoes. Transverse ultrasound of the right breast shows harmonics reducing artefactual echoes. (A) With harmonics and (B) without harmonics.

as a result of nonlinear wave front propagation and are not present in the incident beam (**Figure 10**). These harmonic signals are generated differently at anatomic sites with similar impedances and thus lead to a higher contrast resolution. In addition, use of tissue harmonic imaging helps reduce many of the artifacts that occur with conventional ultrasound, such as side-lobe, near-field, reverberation, and clutter artifacts, and improves the signal to noise ratio (**Figure 11**) [22, 23, 20].

4. Lesion characterization with BI-RADS Lexicon

4.1. Correlative BI-RADS classifications and positive predictive value (PPV)

Similar to the BI-RADS system used to standardize the language of mammography reporting, the American College of Radiology (ACR) also developed a BI-RADS lexicon for breast sonography for the characterization of the sonographic lesions. This lexicon includes descriptors of masses such as shape, orientation, margin, echo pattern, and posterior features as well as associated features such as architectural distortion, duct changes, breast edema, skin changes, vascularity, and elastography. Special cases delineated by BI-RADS lexicon include simple cyst, clustered microcysts, complicated cyst, skin masses, foreign bodies (including implants), intramammary and axillary lymph nodes, vascular abnormalities, and postsurgical fluid collections. BI-RADS lexicon defines a simple cyst as oval or round in shape, anechoic, circumscribed margin, and with posterior acoustic enhancement (BI-RADS) (**Figures 12–14**). BI-RADS descriptors showing a high predictive value for malignancy include spiculated margin, irregular shape, and nonparallel orientation (**Figure 15**). Circumscribed margin, oval shape, and parallel orientation are characteristics predictive of a benign lesion [24, 25].

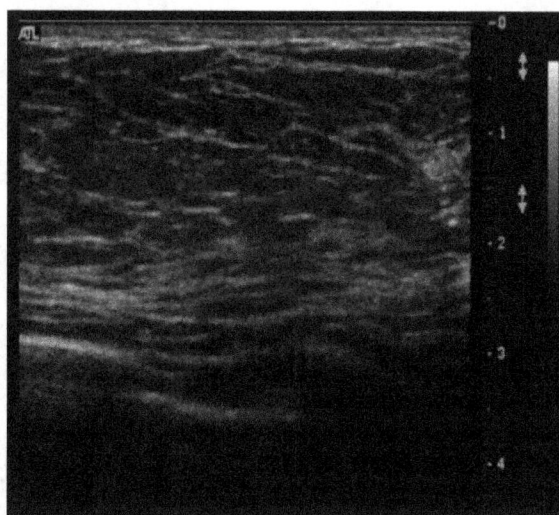

Figure 12. Homogenous background echotexture — fat. Transverse ultrasound demonstrates fat lobules, with uniform echogenic bands of supporting structures making up the bulk of the breast tissue.

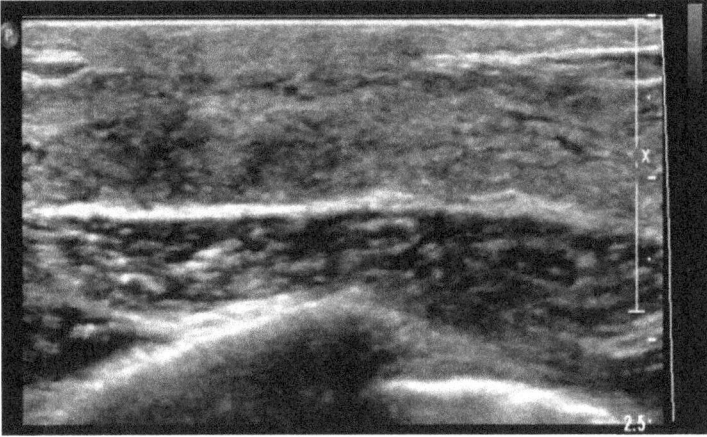

Figure 13. Homogenous background echotexture—fibroglandular. Transverse ultrasound shows a thick zone of homogenously echogenic fibroglandular tissue present beneath a thin hypoechoic layer of fat lobules.

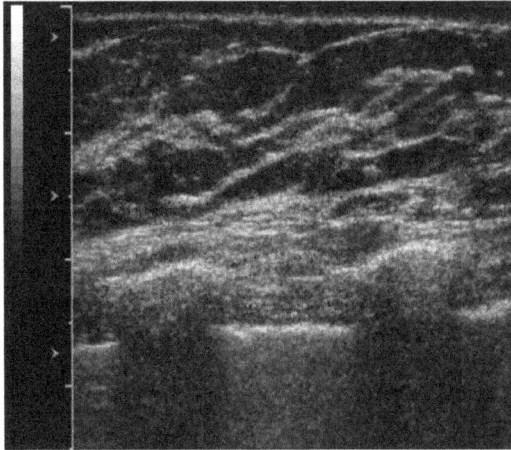

Figure 14. Heterogeneous background echotexture. Transverse ultrasound depicts multiple areas of increased and decreased echogenicity. Heterogeneity can be either focal or diffuse.

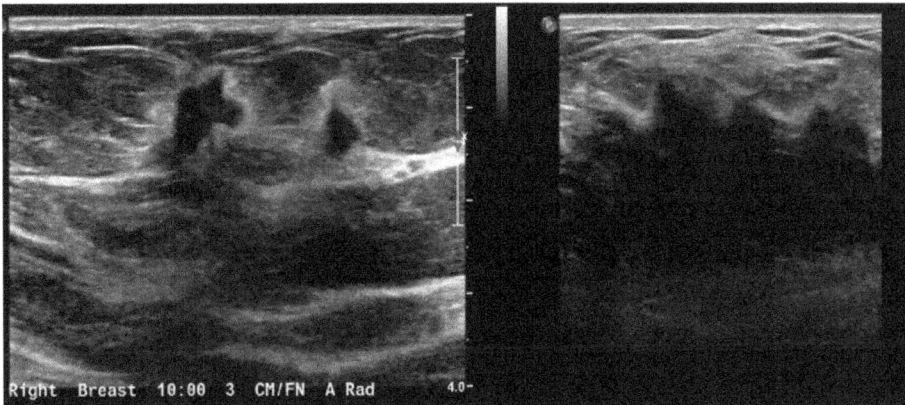

Figure 15. Margin assessment. Transverse ultrasound of the right breast demonstrates an irregular mass with angular margins. Some or all of the margins has sharp corners, often forming acute angles.

5. Indications for targeted breast ultrasound

5.1. Characterization of a mammographic mass

Ultrasound is an adjunct to mammography for mass characterization and is the next examination to perform for characterization of a mammographic mass, per ACR appropriateness
criteria [26]. It is critical to establish the location and depth of the mass identified on mammography to ensure that the same area is imaged during breast ultrasound. If a mass is
identified on breast ultrasound and is thought to correlate with the mammographic mass,
the size, shape, location, and surrounding tissue composition should correlate between the
two modalities [27]. If no sonographic correlate is found for a mass identified on mammogram, then revaluation of the mammogram should be performed. If mammographic findings
remain suspicious for a sonographically occult mass, then further evaluation with a different
imaging modality and/or biopsy can be pursued (**Figure 16**).

5.2. Evaluation of a palpable mass in a patient with negative mammogram

Fifty years ago, women who presented with a palpable mass eventually underwent surgical
excision to exclude malignancy [28]. With advances in ultrasound imaging, many women
now who present with a palpable mass and no mammographic correlate undergo diagnostic targeted ultrasound, often on the same day as diagnostic mammogram, to evaluate
the region of palpable concern. If no mammographic or sonographic abnormality is identified, women can be safely reassured that there is no abnormality instead of undergoing

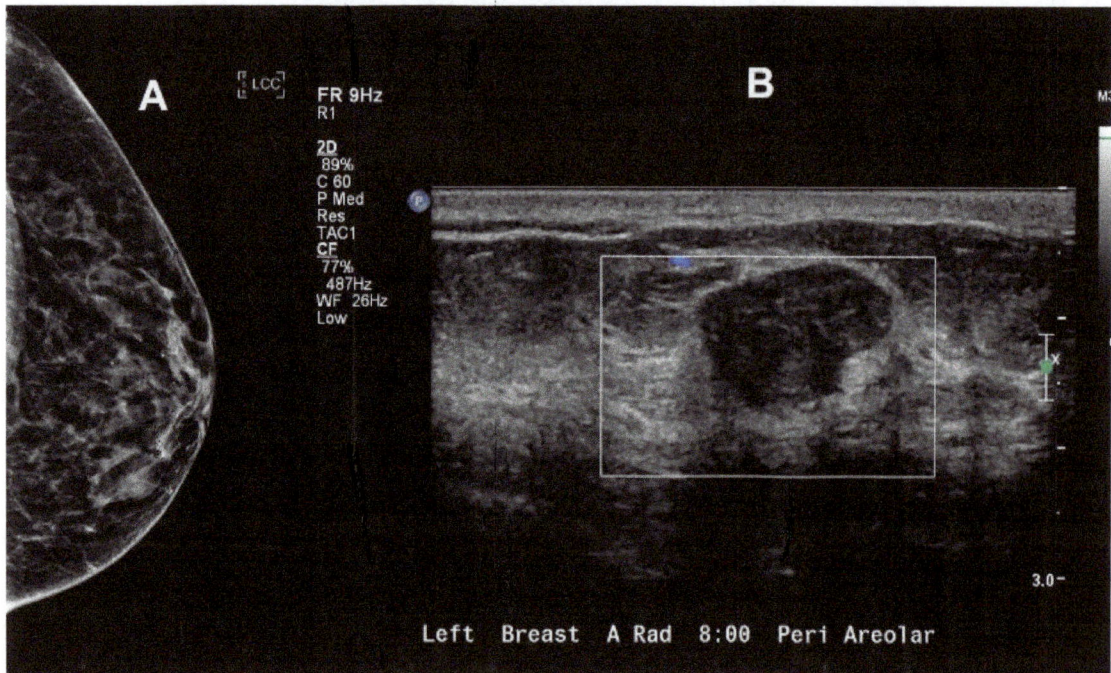

Figure 16. Lesion visibility. (A) CC mammogram of the left breast and (B) transverse ultrasound of the left breast.

unnecessary surgery or biopsy [29]. However, if a patient presents with a palpable mass with negative mammogram, ultrasound has been shown to be effective in identifying an abnormality in about 50% of cases, with the majority of these abnormalities characterized as benign (mostly cysts) or likely benign [30]. Recent studies also question whether a repeat mammogram is even necessary when a woman presents with a new palpable mass within 12 months of prior negative mammogram, given that ultrasound has been shown to yield the most diagnostic information [30].

5.3. Evaluation of a palpable mass in young patients (<30 years old)

Ultrasound is the initial imaging modality used to evaluate a palpable mass in a patient less than 30 years old [26]. After an abnormality is detected with ultrasound, it is debatable as to whether the next examination to perform is a unilateral mammogram imaging the breast with the sonographic abnormality, a bilateral mammogram, or an ultrasound guided biopsy of the abnormality. Per ACR appropriateness criteria, either mammography or a biopsy is appropriate and the determination of the next examination is likely patient dependent [26]. Masses often found in this patient population include cysts, fibroadenomas, and very infrequently breast cancer.

5.4. Ultrasound guided interventional breast procedures

Historically, the most important role of breast ultrasound was differentiating a solid from a cystic mass [1], for which ultrasound has a reported accuracy of 96–100% [27]. However, as ultrasound imaging has improved, the indications for utilization of ultrasound have expanded from lesion characterization to real-time sampling of the lesion using ultrasound guidance. Some are now also using ultrasound guidance for treatment of breast lesions with percutaneous ablation. The real-time nature of ultrasound imaging, lack of radiation, cost effectiveness, and relative patient comfort make ultrasound an ideal modality with which to perform biopsies and treat breast lesions.

Ultrasound guided interventional breast procedures include fine needle aspiration, ultrasound guided core biopsy, ultrasound guided vacuum assisted biopsy, and ultrasound guided pre-surgical localization. Indications for ultrasound guided fine needle aspiration include symptomatic relief of a painful cyst and confirmation of cystic nature of an indeterminate mass [1]. Varying needle sizes are used for ultrasound guided fine needle aspirations ranging from 25 up to 18 gauge. Percutaneous image guided core-needle biopsies have almost completely replaced surgical needle-localization biopsy of breast lesions as they are faster, less invasive, less expensive, safe, and accurate, with specificity and positive predictive value for detection of malignancy nearing 100% [31]. Not only does a negative core needle biopsy prevent a patient from undergoing unnecessary surgery, but ultrasound guided core needle biopsy for malignancy reduces the incidence of positive margins after local excision and decreases the number of surgeries for definitive breast cancer treatment [31]. Ultrasound guided 14-gauge automated core biopsy was described almost 25 years ago with 100% concordance between ultrasound guided core biopsy results and surgery [32]. While many practices still perform ultrasound guided core biopsies with an automated 14-gauge biopsy needle, there are now a wide array of gauges and needles available for breast biopsy. Automated biopsy needles range from 20 to 14 gauge and vacuum assisted biopsy needles range from 13 to 9 gauge. The needle chosen to perform an ultrasound guided core biopsy is physician and patient dependent. While the risks of severe complications from ultrasound guided breast biopsy are very rare, occurring in less than 1% of procedures, there has been slightly more severe bleeding events associated with vacuum-assisted biopsies than with automated gun biopsies [33]. Perhaps this can be attributed in part to the needle size as most vacuum-assisted biopsy needles are larger in size than automated biopsy guns and other studies also support increased risk of hematoma formation after biopsy with a larger gauge needle (9-gauge) compared to a smaller gauge needle (12- or 14-gauge) [34]. Historically, percutaneous breast biopsies performed on patients on antithrombotic therapies, including clopidogrel, daily non-steroidal anti-inflammatory drugs, aspirin, and warfarin, have been performed with caution given concern for increased risk of bleeding and hematoma formation with many breast imagers requiring patients to cease antithrombotic therapy prior to biopsy. Recent data suggest that patients may be able to safely undergo percutaneous breast biopsy without stopping antithrombotic therapy, with one prospective studying showing no clinically significant hematomas in women taking antithrombotics [34].

Ultrasound-guided percutaneous ablation procedures, including cryoablation, irreversible electroporation, laser therapy, microwave ablation, radiofrequency ablation, and high-intensity focused ultrasound, of benign and malignant breast lesions that are 2 cm or less in size are also being performed [35]. These ultrasound-guided ablation techniques are particularly appealing for patients who are not surgical candidates; however, identifying the group of patients best suited for percutaneous ablation procedures is evolving [35]. While many of these percutaneous ablation techniques can be performed with local anesthesia alone, both radiofrequency ablation and high-intensity focused ultrasound must be performed with sedation and may be performed with MRI guidance instead of ultrasound guidance [35].

5.5. Targeted breast ultrasound secondary to abnormal MRI or molecular breast imaging

The use of breast magnetic resonance imaging (MRI) and molecular breast imaging (MBI) has increased over the past several years, with breast MRI offering the highest sensitivity of all modalities. A "second-look ultrasound" is a targeted reevaluation of the breast with ultrasound after an abnormality, which is not characteristically benign, is identified on either MRI or MBI [36]. Similar to mammographic-sonographic correlation of masses, it is critical to establish the location and depth of the abnormality identified on MRI or MBI to ensure that the same area is imaged during breast ultrasound. Studies suggest identification of MRI-detected abnormalities on ultrasound imaging range between 23 and 89%, with lesion type being the most important predictor [37]. If a sonographic correlate for the MRI or MBI detected abnormality is discovered, then most breast imagers will proceed with an ultrasound guided biopsy of the abnormality. This is advantageous to the patient who can undergo biopsy without breast compression in a relatively comfortable reclined position and the ability to often use a smaller gauge needle for biopsy. In contrast, MRI guided biopsies are performed with the breast in compression with the patient in a prone position and utilize large gauge vacuum assisted needles. Additionally, ultrasound guided biopsies are less expensive and less time consuming. However, if there is concern that the abnormality biopsied under ultrasound did not correspond to the MRI detected abnormality, then confirmatory MRI images could be obtained with attention to susceptibility artifact from the metallic clip placed at the time of ultrasound guided core biopsy [38]. Some recommend a T1-weighted, axial, noncontrast, gradient-echo sequence MRI to verify metallic marker placement [36]. If no ultrasound correlate is identified for the MRI or MBI abnormality, revaluation of the MRI or MBI is required with possible recommendations for MRI or MBI guided biopsy of the abnormality.

6. Screening breast ultrasound

Although mammography is the only screening modality proven to reduce mortality [39, 40], its performance is diminished in women with dense breast tissue. Dense tissue refers to the mammographic appearance and the amount of stromal, epithelial, and connective tissue elements of the breast – all of which are radiodense on the mammographic image [41]. All of which are radiodense on the mammographic image. Breast density can change based on hormonal activity, BMI, and age. Mammographic sensitivity may be as low as 30–48% in women with dense breasts [42]. The association of breast density identified on mammography, using the American College of Radiology BI-RADS classification [43], C and D (heterogeneous or extremely dense) is coupled with a reduction in the effectiveness of the examination. This is in large part due to the masking effect observed when dense fibroglandular tissue is superimposed over breast cancer, limiting visualization of the known cancer. In a recent study, 78% of tumors were found to be mammographically occult secondary to overlapping tissue [44]. Furthermore, the inherent four- to sixfold increased risk of developing breast cancer in women with dense tissue compared to women with predominantly fatty breast composition [45] is associated with a higher occurrence rate of interval breast cancers [5, 46–48]. For these reasons, supplemental screening with other modalities is considered.

Breast ultrasound is not limited by breast density, and its use as an adjunct screening tool can improve the diagnostic accuracy of the screening examination. The use of ultrasound can detect early, node negative invasive cancers and interval breast cancers, thus improving the prognosis and morbidity in women diagnosed with the disease [48]. Based on earlier studies published by Kolb et al. 42% more invasive cancers were identified using adjunct screening with ultrasound [49]. Results from other single institutional studies validate these findings, demonstrating a range between 0.4 and 5.7 additional cancers detected per 1000 women screened (see tables). The ACRIN 6666 trial, a multi-center observational study, confirmed that cancer detection could improve with the addition of ultrasound, by approximately 4.2 additional cancers per 1,000 women screened [42]. In both Kolb's analysis and the ACRIN study, nearly 1/3 to 1/2 of all women undergoing supplemental screening with breast ultrasound were considered at increased risk for developing breast cancer.

Thus, the incremental increase in cancer detection may in part be due to the higher prevalence of disease detected in the cohort of women [49]. Subsequent studies focusing on evaluating women at average risk with mammographically dense breast tissue, demonstrate an additional 3.2 cancers detected per 1000 women screened with breast ultrasound [50, 51]. The advantage of supplemental screening ultrasound, regardless of the population screened or the variation in study design, demonstrates an incremental increase in cancer detection. Whether this translates to a decrease in breast cancer mortality is unknown, as there are no randomized control trials assessing this outcome.

While optimizing breast cancer screening is of utmost importance, establishing a balance between improving sensitivity while maintaining specificity proves to be difficult. Of main concern, is the possibility of increasing the number of false positive findings which can lead to unnecessary tests and biopsies. Many studies have demonstrated that screening breast ultrasound does have a higher false positive rate than mammography alone [52]. This includes the Japan Strategic Anti-cancer randomized Trial (J-START), where the sensitivity was significantly higher in the intervention group (mammography plus ultrasound screening) than in the control group but the specificity was significantly lower (87.7% decreased from 91.4%) [53]. Alternatively, in another multiinstitutional trial including 12,519 Chinese women, the authors found comparable PPVs between mammography and ultrasound screening (72.7 vs. 70.0%), which did not reach statistical significance [54]. The lack of decline in the PPV from one modality to the next in this study may be secondary to emphasis on consistency. Radiologists participating in the study had to undergo additional training in interpretation in order to keep consistency among all study centers.

Another major concern is the time needed to perform the screening ultrasound examination. Depending on the number of pathological findings and the patient's breast size, the time to perform screening with handheld ultrasound can range from 3 minutes and 59 seconds [55] to 4 minutes and 39 seconds [49]. In both studies, the screening ultrasound was performed by an experienced radiologist, alleviating operator variability. Ultrasound, which relies on the examiner's experience and acquisition and interpretation of the exam, is operator dependent. In the ACRIN 6666 trial, in order to keep consistency among all study centers, ultrasound scans were performed by the physician per strict protocol. The time it took to perform a bilateral handheld screening ultrasound was on average 19 minutes. Given the long acquisition times and the limited number of trained personnel, real world implementation would be impractical. Thus in recent years, there have been a number of manufacturers that have developed automated whole breast ultrasound systems that may minimizing the aforementioned time constraints and improving the through-put of the patient.

Automated whole breast ultrasound systems were approved on the premise that they could improve efficiency in the diagnostic and screening setting. Some manufacturers have attached a computer-guided articulating arm to the existing 4 cm transducer, while others have distinguished themselves with a larger 15 cm transducer (Invenia, GE healthcare; Acuson S2000, Siemens healthcare) that can methodically map and image the breast in a reproducible way. The use of automation allows for images to be obtained of the entire breast in under 5 minutes. Images obtained with the larger transducer can be reconstructed in multiple planes with the potential to decrease false positive findings and improve diagnostic accuracy. All systems have software to generate a cine loop of the images to be reviewed by the radiologist which can be read at time of completion or at a later time and date. Authors of the Somo-Insight multicenter study, assessed outcome measures using automated whole breast ultrasound and found an overall improvement in cancer detection rate of 1.9 per 1000 women screened, similar to prior single institution studies yet PPV was significantly reduced [56] (**Figure 17**, **Tables 1** and **2**).

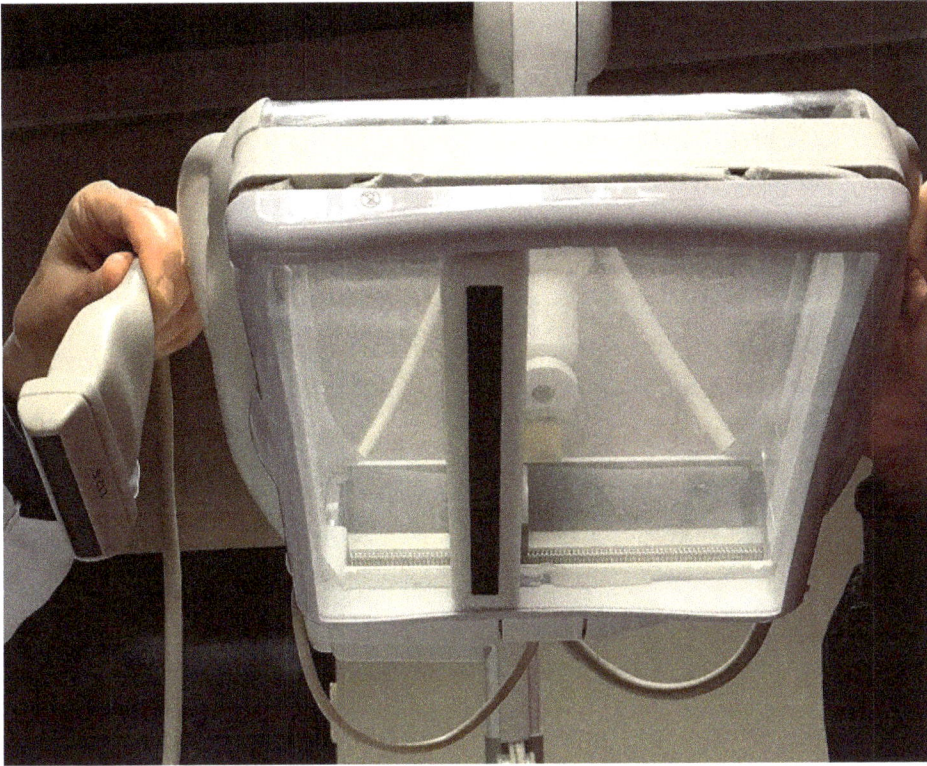

Figure 17. Handheld (left) vs. automated whole breast ultrasound (right).

Study	No. of Cancers	No. of Women	Incremental Cancer Detection Rate (per 1000)	PPV$_3$ (%)	Comments	Country and Year
Single Institution						
Girardi et al [70]	41	22131	1.9	–	Women were at average risk. CDR for dense breasts – 2.2, nondense breasts – 1.6, AVG RISK	Italy, 2013
Parris et al [71]	10	5519	1.8	5.5	Women were at average risk.	US, 2013
Hooley et al [50]	3	935	3.2	6.5	Women were at average risk.	US, 2012
Leong et al [72]	2	141	1.4%	14.3	Reported CDR. Included women at increased risk.	Singapore, 2012
De Felice et al [73]	12	1754	6.8	6.4	Women were at average risk.	Italy, 2007
Brancato et al [74]	2	5227	0.4	3.2	Women were at average risk.	Italy, 2007
Leconte et al [75]	16	4236	3.8	–	Included nondense breasts, palpable lesions, diagnostic exams, and women at increased risk.	Belgium, 2003

Study	No. of Cancers	No. of Women	Incremental Cancer Detection Rate (per 1000)	PPV$_3$ (%)	Comments	Country and Year
Crystal et al [76]	7	1517	4.6	18.4	Included women at increased risk.	Israel, 2003
Kolb et al [49]	33	4897; 12193 exams	2.7	10.3	CDR based on patients with normal mammogram and dense breasts. Included scattered fibroglandular tissue and women at increased risk.	US, 2002
Kaplan [77]	6	1862	3.2	11.8	Included women with focal abnormal mammographic findings or palpable lesions	US, 2001
Buchberger et al [78]	32	8103	3.9	8.8	Included scattered fibroglandular tissue, CDR based on patients with normal mammogram and nonpalpable lesions	Austria, 2000
Maestro et al [79]	2	350	5.7	13.3	Included women at increased risk. Solid mass incidentally detected in 14% of patients.	France, 1999
Multi-Institution						
Ohuchi et al [53]	67	36752	1.8	–	Women were at average risk.	Japan, 2016
Weigert and Steenbergen [51]	28	8647	3.2	6.7	Women were at average risk.	US, 2012
Berg et al [42]	32	7473	4.3	5.9	1st year US screen – 2659 women, 2nd year US screen – 2493 women, 3rd year US screen – 2321 women, 612 women had MR screen after 3rd US screen. Included women at increased risk.	US, 2012
Corsetti et al [48]	21	8865; 19728 exams	1.1	–	CDR based on negative screening exams. Women were at average risk.	Italy, 2011
	37	9157	4.0	5.9	Women were at average risk. 13/50 cancers found were excluded due to symptoms/ palpable lesion	Italy, 2008
Schaefer et al [80]	116	59514; 62006 exams	1.9	5.2	Included nondense breasts and women at increased risk.	Germany, 2010

Table 1. Incremental cancer detection rate of handheld ultrasound.

Study	No. of Cancers	No. of Women	Incremental Cancer Detection Rate (per 1000)	PPV$_3$ (%)	Comments	Country and Year
Single Institution						
Wilczek et al [81]	4	1668	2.4	33.3	Decreased PPV3 for mammography + ultrasound. Included women at increased risk.	Sweden, 2016
Giuliano et al [82]	42	3418	12.3 (Mammography + ABUS)	–	CDR for mammography alone – 4.6. Women were at average risk in the test group.	US, 2012
Multi-Institution						
Brem et al [56]	30	15318	1.9	–	SomoInsight Study – Increased sensitivity and recall rate associated with a decreased specificity and PPV3. Included women at increased risk.	US, 2015
Kelly et al [83]	23	4419; 6425 exams	3.6	38.4	Included women at increased risk	US, 2010

Table 2. Incremental cancer detection rate of automated breast ultrasound.

7. Future directions in breast ultrasound

Innovations in ultrasound technology have improved our ability to detect and diagnose breast cancer. Computer-aided detection (CAD), elastography, quantitative breast ultrasound technology, and ultrasound contrast agents (microbubbles) were developed to improve diagnostic accuracy. These advancements have the potential to impact overall survival by detecting cancers that are smaller and less aggressive.

7.1. Computer-aided detection

To date, there are a limited number of computer-aided detection (CAD) systems approved by the Food and Drug Administration (FDA) for ultrasound. CAD for ultrasound is analogous to CAD for mammography in that it can improve the overall diagnostic performance of the interpreting radiologist. The software will interpret regions of interests marked by the radiologist for further characterization—providing anatomical shape and potential for malignancy based on the ACR BI-RADS Lexicon. Similar to other modalities, the radiologist can accept or reject the analysis based on his or her interpretation. Interpreting automated whole breast ultrasound images has also demonstrated an improvement in overall specificity and differentiation of true and false positive findings with the use of computer-aided detection [57].

7.2. Elastography

Elastography can help differentiate normal tissue from adjacent tumors improving specificity and diagnostic performance, and is routinely incorporated into the ultrasound equipment. The two most frequently used elastography techniques in the breast are strain elastography and shear-wave elastography [58]. Shear-wave technology is reported to be highly reproducible [59] unlike strain elastography which can have a significant amount of interobserver variability [60]. Both techniques are used in conjunction with B-mode ultrasound, but differ in how they measure tissue stiffness. Shear-wave technology uses an impulse produced by a focused ultrasound beam to measure propagation of speed within the tumor and surrounding tissue, quantifying the stiffness in kilopascals. The quantitative estimates in stiffness are independent of the morphologic features of a mass. In contrast, strain elastography determines the underlying elasticity of the lesion by repeated manual compression of the transducer (strain) over a lesion. Both techniques can improve specificity of ultrasonography (US) breast masses without a reduction in sensitivity. However, the sensitivity and specificity of strain and shear-wave elastography can differ based on the underlying pathology and grade of a tumor [58, 61].

7.3. Quantitative breast ultrasound

Quantitative breast ultrasound measures the transmission and speed of sound through the breast. Images are obtained using a ring transducer that emits acoustic transmissions through the breast, receiving information on the attenuation and transmission of sound through the breast. In addition, the reflective (analogous to b-mode images) properties of the fibrous stroma of the breast is evaluated. The transmission data that is acquired is used to construct a cross-sectional tomographic image. Dense tissue tends to have high transmission and attenuation of sound (characterized as white on the tomographic image), while fatty tissue demonstrates low-sound speed and low attenuation (appears as dark on the tomographic image). Given these parameters some authors have suggested that it can provide a surrogate measure of breast density [62]. Others suggest that it can improve specificity by determining solid masses from complicated cysts [63].

7.4. Contrast enhanced ultrasound of the breast

Early published work documents the improved visibility and visual intensity of Doppler signals with the use of ultrasound contrast agents (microbubbles) at the size of 100 um or less [64]. This work has led to more recent developments that can quantify tumor neovascularity using contrast agents (microbubbles) at the size of 1–8 um. Contrast-enhanced ultrasound imaging is based on the principle of acoustic excitation of the microbubbles which produces nonlinear frequency components that can be received at the transducer. The differences in the received signal relative to the transmitted signal produces what is called harmonic imaging. Signals identified below transmission are called subharmonic emissions which can be differentiated from the inherent tissue signals allowing for improved visualization of tumor angiogenesis [65]. Additional studies have investigated the use of certain algorithms using ultrasound contrast agents to quantify breast vasculature, density, and perfusion patterns [66–68]. This novel approaches to differentiating between benign and malignant lesions and promises to improve overall diagnostic accuracy.

8. Summary

The role of breast ultrasound has evolved over the last 50 years, progressively gaining recognition as a diagnostic tool. Current and future applications of this modality can assist the radiologist in improving sensitivity, specificity, and differentiation between benign and malignant findings. The prospect of ultrasound-guided minimally invasive therapy to target breast cancer tumor angiogenesis with therapy-bound microbubbles is an exciting prospect, and one that may be on the horizon for future clinical implementation [69]. Ultrasound provides a significant contribution in the management of breast cancer and will continue to be considered as an indispensable diagnostic and screening tool.

Author details

Jocelyn A. Rapelyea[1,2]* and Christina G. Marks[3]

*Address all correspondence to: jrapelyea@mfa.gwu.edu

1 Breast Imaging & Intervention, George Washington University Medical Faculty Associates, Washington, DC, USA

2 Department of Radiology, George Washington University School of Medicine & Health Sciences, Washington, DC, USA

3 University of Mississippi Medical Center, Jackson, MS, USA

References

[1] Venta LA, Dudiak CM, Salomon CG, Flisak ME. Sonographic evaluation of the breast. Radiographics. 1994;**14**(1):29-50

[2] Berg WA, Campassi CI, Ioffe OB. Cystic lesions of the breast: Sonographic-pathologic correlation. Radiology. 2003;**227**(1):183-191

[3] Kobayashi T, Takatani O, Hattori N, Kimura K. Differential diagnosis of breast tumors. The sensitivity graded method of ultrasonotomography and clinical evaluation of its diagnostic accuracy. Cancer. 1974;**33**(4):940-951

[4] Kobayashi T. Diagnostic ultrasound in breast cancer: Analysis of retrotumorous echo patterns correlated with sonic attenuation by cancerous connective tissue. Journal of Clinical Ultrasound. 1979;**7**(6):471-479

[5] Dempsey P. The history of breast ultrasound. Journal of Ultrasound. Medicine. 2004;**23**: 887-894

[6]   Stavros AT, Thickman D, Rapp CL, Dennis MA, Parker SH, Sisney GA. Solid breast nod-
      ules: Use of sonography to distinguish between benign and malignant lesions. Radiology.
      1995;**196**(1):123-134

[7]   Haerten R, Lowery C, Becker G, Gebel M, Rosenthal S, Sauerbrei E. ""Ensemble" Tissue
      Harmonic Imaging": The technology and clinical utility. Electromedica-Erlangen. 1999;**67**:
      50-56

[8]   Kwak JY, Kim EK, You JK, Oh KK. Variable breast conditions. Journal of Ultrasound in
      Medicine. 2004;**23**(1):85-96

[9]   Mundinger A. Ultrasound of the breast, including interventions: An update. Diseases of
      the Heart and Chest, Including Breast. 2011;**2011-2016**:259-266

[10] Iuanow E, Kettler M, Slanetz PJ. Spectrum of disease in the male breast. American
      Journal of Roentgenology. 2011;**196**(3):W247-W259

[11] Zucca-Matthes G, Urban C, Vallejo A. Anatomy of the nipple and breast ducts. Gland
      Surgery. 2016;**5**(1):32

[12] Robbins J, Jeffries D, Roubidoux M, Helvie M. Accuracy of diagnostic mammography and
      breast ultrasound during pregnancy and lactation. American Journal of Roentgenology.
      2011;**196**(3):716-722

[13] Telegrafo M, Moschetta M. Role of US in evaluating breast implant integrity. Journal of
      Ultrasound. 2015;**18**(4):329-333

[14] Middleton WD, Kurtz AB, Hertzberg BS. Ultrasound: The Requisites. 2nd ed. St. Louis,
      Mo: Mosby; 2004. p. 5-19

[15] Sehgal CM, Weinstein SP, Arger PH, Conant EF. A review of breast ultrasound. Journal
      of Mammary Gland Biology and Neoplasia. 2006;**11**(2):113-123

[16] Feldman MK, Katyal S, Blackwood MS. US artifacts 1. Radiographics. 2009;**29**:1179-1189

[17] Scanlan KA. Sonographic artifacts and their origins. American Journal of Roentgenology.
      1991;**156**(6):1267-1272

[18] Weinstein SP, Conant EF, Sehgal C. Technical advances in breast ultrasound imaging.
      Seminars in Ultrasound, CT and MRI. 2006;**27**(4):273-283

[19] Cha JH, Moon WK, Cho N, Chung SY, Park SH, Park JM, Han BK, Choe YH, Cho G, Im
      JG. Differentiation of benign from malignant solid breast masses: Conventional US versus
      spatial compound imaging 1. Radiology. 2005;**237**(3):841-846

[20] Dahl JJ, Sheth NM. Reverberation clutter from subcutaneous tissue layers: Simulation
      and in vivo demonstrations. Ultrasound in Medicine & Biology. 2014;**40**(4):714-726

[21] Lediju MA, Pihl MJ, Dahl JJ, Trahey GE. Quantitative assessment of the magnitude,
      impact and spatial extent of ultrasonic clutter. Ultrasonic Imaging. 2008;**30**(3):151-168

[22] Cha JH, Moon WK, Cho N, Kim SM, Park SH, Han BK, Choe YH, Park JM, Im JG. Characterization of benign and malignant solid breast masses: Comparison of conventional US and tissue harmonic imaging 1. Radiology. 2007;**242**(1):63-69

[23] Strobel K, Zanetti M, Nagy L, Hodler J. Suspected rotator cuff lesions: Tissue harmonic imaging versus conventional US of the shoulder 1. Radiology. 2004;**230**(1):243-249

[24] Hong AS, Rosen EL, Soo MS, Baker JA. BI-RADS for sonography: Positive and negative predictive values of sonographic features. American Journal of Roentgenology. 2005;**184**(4): 1260-1265

[25] Rahbar G, Sie AC, Hansen GC, Prince JS, Melany ML, Reynolds HE, Jackson VP, Sayre JW, Bassett LW. Benign versus malignant solid breast masses: US differentiation 1. Radiology. 1999;**213**(3):889-894

[26] Harvey JA, Mahoney MC, Newell MS, Bailey L, Barke LD, D'Orsi C, Hayes MK, Jokich PM, Lee SJ, Lehman CD, Mainiero MB. ACR appropriateness criteria palpable breast masses. Journal of the American College of Radiology. 2013;**10**(10):742-748

[27] Whitman GJ, Arribas E, Uppendahl L. Mammographic-sonographic correlation. Seminars in Roentgenology. 2011;**46**(4):252-259

[28] Joe BN, Sickles EA. The evolution of breast imaging: Past to present. Radiology. 2014; **273**(2S):S23-S44

[29] Dennis MA, Parker SH, Klaus AJ, Stavros AT, Kaske TI, Clark SB. Breast biopsy avoidance: The value of normal mammograms and normal sonograms in the setting of a palpable lump 1. Radiology. 2001;**219**(1):186-191

[30] Leung SE, Ben-Nachum I, Kornecki A. New palpable breast lump with recent negative mammogram: Is repeat mammography necessary? American Journal of Roentgenology. 2016;**207**(1):200-204

[31] White RR, Halperin TJ, Olson Jr JA, Soo MS, Bentley RC, Seigler HF. Impact of core-needle breast biopsy on the surgical management of mammographic abnormalities. Annals of Surgery. 2001;**233**(6):769-777

[32] Parker SH, Jobe WE, Dennis MA, Stavros AT, Johnson KK, Yakes WF, Truell JE, Price JG, Kortz AB, Clark DG. US-guided automated large-core breast biopsy. Radiology. 1993;**187**(2):507-511

[33] Bruening W, Fontanarosa J, Tipton K, Treadwell JR, Launders J, Schoelles K. Systematic review: Comparative effectiveness of core-needle and open surgical biopsy to diagnose breast lesions. Annals of Internal Medicine. 2010;**152**(4):238-246

[34] Chetlen AL, Kasales C, Mack J, Schetter S, Zhu J. Hematoma formation during breast core needle biopsy in women taking antithrombotic therapy. American Journal of Roentgenology. 2013;**201**(1):215-222

[35] Fleming MM, Holbrook AI, Newell MS. Update on image-guided percutaneous ablation of breast cancer. American Journal of Roentgenology. 2017;**208**:267-264

[36] Trop I, Labelle M, David J, Mayrand MH, Lalonde L. Second-look targeted studies after breast magnetic resonance imaging: Practical tips to improve lesion identification. Current Problems in Diagnostic Radiology. 2010;**39**(5):200-211

[37] Leung JW. Utility of second-look ultrasound in the evaluation of MRI-detected breast lesions. Seminars in Roentgenology. 2011;**46**(4):260-274

[38] Leung JW. Second-look ultrasound: Only for biopsy or more? European Journal of Radiology. 2012;**81**:s87-s89

[39] Tabár L, Yen AMF, WYY W, Chen SLS, Chiu SYH, Fann JCY, MMS K, Smith RA, Duffy SW, Chen THH. Insights from the breast cancer screening trials: How screening affects the natural history of breast cancer and implications for evaluating service screening programs. The Breast Journal. 2015;**21**(1):13-20

[40] Smith RA, Duffy SW, Gabe R, Tabar L, Yen AM, Chen TH. The randomized trials of breast cancer screening: What have we learned? Radiologic Clinics of North America. 2004;**42**(5):793-806

[41] Boyd NF, Dite GS, Stone J, Gunasekara A, English DR, McCredie MR, Giles GG, Tritchler D, Chiarelli A, Yaffe MJ, Hopper JL. Heritability of mammographic density, a risk factor for breast cancer. New England Journal of Medicine. 2002;**347**(12):886-894

[42] Berg WA, Blume JD, Cormack JB, Mendelson EB, Lehrer D, Böhm-Vélez M, Pisano ED, Jong RA, Evans WP, Morton MJ, Mahoney MC. Combined screening with ultrasound and mammography vs mammography alone in women at elevated risk of breast cancer. Journal of the American Medical Association. 2008;**299**(18):2151-2163

[43] D'orsi CJ, Mendelson EB, Ikeda DM. Breast Imaging Reporting and Data System: ACR BI-RADS—Breast Imaging Atlas. American College of Radiology: Reston, VA; 2003

[44] Bae MS, Moon WK, Chang JM, Koo HR, Kim WH, Cho N, Yi A, La Yun B, Lee SH, Kim MY, Ryu EB. Breast cancer detected with screening US: Reasons for nondetection at mammography. Radiology. 2014;**270**(2):369-377

[45] Harvey JA, Bovbjerg VE. Quantitative assessment of mammographic breast density: Relationship with breast cancer risk 1. Radiology. 2004;**230**(1):29-41

[46] Mandelson MT, Oestreicher N, Porter PL, White D, Finder CA, Taplin SH, White E. Breast density as a predictor of mammographic detection: Comparison of interval-and screen-detected cancers. Journal of the National Cancer Institute. 2000;**92**(13):1081-1087

[47] Boyd NF, Guo H, Martin LJ, Sun L, Stone J, Fishell E, Jong RA, Hislop G, Chiarelli A, Minkin S, Yaffe MJ. Mammographic density and the risk and detection of breast cancer. New England Journal of Medicine. 2007;**356**(3):227-236

[48] Corsetti V, Houssami N, Ghirardi M, Ferrari A, Speziani M, Bellarosa S, Remida G, Gasparotti C, Galligioni E, Ciatto S. Evidence of the effect of adjunct ultrasound screening in women with mammography-negative dense breasts: Interval breast cancers at 1year follow-up. European Journal of Cancer. 2011;**47**(7):1021-1026

[49] Kolb TM, Lichy J, Newhouse JH. Comparison of the performance of screening mammography, physical examination, and breast us and evaluation of factors that influence them: An analysis of 27,825 patient evaluations 1. Radiology. 2002;**225**(1):165-175

[50] Hooley RJ, Greenberg KL, Stackhouse RM, Geisel JL, Butler RS, Philpotts LE, Screening US. in patients with mammographically dense breasts: Initial experience with Connecticut Public Act 09-41. Radiology. 2012;**265**(1):59-59

[51] Weigert J, Steenbergen S. The Connecticut experiment: The role of ultrasound in the screening of women with dense breasts. The Breast Journal. 2012;**18**(6):517-522

[52] Chae EY, Kim HH, Cha JH, Shin HJ, Kim H. Evaluation of screening whole-breast sonography as a supplemental tool in conjunction with mammography in women with dense breasts. Journal of Ultrasound in Medicine. 2013;**32**(9):1573-1578

[53] Ohuchi N, Suzuki A, Sobue T, Kawai M, Yamamoto S, Zheng Y, Shiono Y, Saito H, Kuriyama S, Tohno E, Endo T, Fukao A, Tsuji I, Yamaguchi T, Ohashi Y, Fukuda M, Ishida T. Sensitivity and specificity of mammography and adjunctive ultrasonography to screen for breast cancer in the Japan Strategic Anti-cancer Randomized Trial (J-START): A randomised controlled trial. Lancet. 2016;**387**:341-348

[54] Shen S, Zhou Y, Xu Y, Zhang B, Duan X, Huang R, Li B, Shi Y, Shao Z, Liao H, Jiang J, Shen N, Zhang J, Yu C, Jiang H, Li S, Han S, Ma J, Sun QA. multi-centre randomised trial comparing ultrasound vs. mammography for screening breast cancer in high- risk Chinese women. British Journal of Cancer. 2015;**112**:998-1004

[55] Kolb TM, Lichy J, Newhouse JH. Occult cancer in women with dense breasts: Detection with screening US—diagnostic yield and tumor characteristics. Radiology. 1998;**207**:191-219

[56] Brem RF, Tabar DSW, Inciardi MF, Guingrich JA, Hashimoto BE, Lander MR, Lapidus RL, Peterson MD, Rapelyea JA, Roux S, Schilling KJ, Shah BA, Torrente J, Wynn RT, Miller DP. Assessing improvement in detection of breast cancer with three-dimensional automated breast US in women with dense breast tissue: The SomoInsight study. Radiology. 2015;**3**:663-672

[57] QV Medical Inc. QV Medical, INC [Internet]. 2015. Available from: http://www.qview-medical.com/home [Accessed: February 17, 2017]

[58] Chang JM, Won JK, Lee KB, Park IA, Yi A, Moon WK. Comparison of shear-wave and strain ultrasound elastography in the differentiation of benign and malignant breast lesions. American Journal of Roentgenology. 2013;**201**(2):W347-W356

[59] Cosgrove DO, Berg WA, Doré CJ, Skyba DM, Henry JP, Gay J, Cohen-Bacrie C, BE1 Study Group. Shear wave elastography for breast masses is highly reproducible. European Radiology. 2012;**22**(5):1023-1032

[60] Chang JM, Moon WK, Cho N, Kim SJ. Breast mass evalution: Factors influencing the quality of US elastography. Radiology. 2011;**259**:59-64

[61] Berg WA, Cosgrove DO, Dore CJ, Schafer FK, Hooley RJ, Ohlinger R, Mendelson EB, Balu-Maestro C, Locatelli M, Tourasse C, Cavanaugh BC, Juhan V, Stavros AT, Tardivon A, Gay J, Henry J, Cohen-Bacrie C, for the BE! Investigators. Shear-wave elastography improves the specificity of breast US: The BE1 multinational study of 939 masses. Radiology. 2012;**262**(2):435-449

[62] O'flynn EA, Fromageau J, Ledger AE, Messa A, D'aquino A, Schoemaker MJ, Schmidt M, Duric N, Swerdlow AJ, Bamber JC. Ultrasound tomography evaluation of breast density. Investigative Radiology. 2017;**52**:343-348

[63] Duric N, Li C, Littrup P, Glide-Hurst C, Huang L, Lupinacci J, Schmidt S, Rama O, Bey-Knight L, Xu Y. Multi-modal breast imaging with ultrasound tomography. International Society for Optics and Photonics. 2008;**6920**:69200O

[64] Kedar RP, Cosgrove D, McCready VR, Bamber JC, Carter ER. Microbubble contrast agent for color Doppler US: Effect on breast masses-work in progress. Radiology. 1996;**198**:679-686

[65] Sridharan A, Eisenbrey JR, Dave JK, Forsberg F. Quantitative nonlinear contrast-enhanced ultrasound of the breast. American Journal of Roentgenology. 2016;**207**(2):274-281

[66] Eisenbrey JR, Dave JK, Merton DA, Palazzo JP, Hall AL, Forsberg F. Parametric imaging using subharmonic signals from ultrasound contrast agents in patients with breast lesions. Journal of Ultrasound in Medicine. 2011;**30**(1):85-92

[67] Eisenbrey JR, Joshi N, Dave JK, Forsberg F. Assessing algorithms for defining vascular architecture in subharmonic images of breast lesions. Physics in Medicine and Biology. 2011;**56**(4):919

[68] Lam L, Lee SW, Suen CY. Thinning methodologies-a comprehensive survey. IEEE Transactions on Pattern Analysis and Machine Intelligence. 1992;**14**(9):869-885

[69] Javitt MC. Section editor's notebook: The future of breast imaging—find it and fix it. American Journal of Roentgenology. 2017;**208**:245-247

[70] Girardi V, Tonegutti M, Ciatto S, Bonetti F. Breast ultrasound in 22,131 asymptomatic women with negative mammography. The Breast. 2013;**22**(5):806-809

[71] Parris T, Wakefield D, Frimmer H. Real world performance of screening breast ultrasound following enactment of Connecticut Bill 458. The Breast Journal. 2013;**19**(1):64-70

[72] Leong LC, Gogna A, Pant R, Ng FC, Sim LS. Supplementary breast ultrasound screening in Asian women with negative but dense mammograms—A pilot study. Annals of the Academy of Medicine-Singapore. 2012;**41**(10):432

[73] De Felice C, Savelli S, Angeletti M, Ballesio L, Manganaro L, Meggiorini ML, Porfiri LM. Diagnostic utility of combined ultrasonography and mammography in the evaluation of women with mammographically dense breasts. Journal of Ultrasound. 2007;**10**(3):143-151

[74] Brancato B, Bonardi R, Catarzi S, Iacconi C, Risso G, Taschini R, Ciatto S. Negligible advantages and excess costs of routine addition of breast ultrasonography to mammography in dense breasts. Tumori. 2007;**93**(6):562

[75] Leconte I, Feger C, Galant C, et al. Mammography and subsequent whole-breast sonography of nonpalpable breast cancers: The importance of radiologic breast density. AJR American Journal of Roentgenology. 2003;**180**(6):1675-1679

[76] Crystal P, Strano SD, Shcharynski S, Koretz MJ. Using sonography to screen women with mammographically dense breasts. AJR American Journal of Roentgenology. 2003;**181**(1): 177-182

[77] Kaplan SS. Clinical utility of bilateral whole-breast US in the evaluation of women with dense breast tissue. Radiology. 2001;**221**(3):641-649

[78] Buchberger W, Niehoff A, Obrist P, DeKoekkoek-Doll P, Dünser M. Clinically and mammographically occult breast lesions: Detection and classification with high-resolution sonography. Seminars in Ultrasound, CT and MRI. 2000;**21**(4):325-336

[79] Maestro C, Cazenave F, Marcy PY, Bruneton JN, Chauvel C, Bleuse A. Systematic ultrasonography in asymptomatic dense breasts. European Journal of Radiology. 1998;**26**(3):254-256

[80] Schaefer F, Waldmann A, Katalinic A, et al. Influence of additional breast ultrasound on cancer detection in a cohort study for quality assurance in breast diagnosis: Analysis of 102,577 diagnostic procedures. European Radiology. 2010;**20**:1085-1092

[81] Wilczek B, Wilczek H, Rasouliyan L, et al. Adding 3D automated breast ultrasound to mammography screening in women with heterogeneously and extremely dense breasts: Report from a hospital-based, high-volume, single-center breast cancer screening program. European Journal of Radiology. 2016;**85**:1554-1563

[82] Giuliano V, Giulian C. Improved breast cancer detection in asymptomatic women using 3D-automated breast ultrasound in mammographically dense breasts. Clinical Imaging. 2013;**37**:480-486

[83] Kelly K, Dean J, Comulada W, et al. Breast cancer detection using automated whole breast ultrasound and mammography in radiographically dense breasts. European Journal of Radiology. 2010;**20**:734-742

11

An Innovative Concept of 3D X-Ray Imaging Systems for Painless Breast Cancer Detection

Mohammed Ali Alnafea

Abstract

Breast cancer is a life-threatening disease and considered one of the most common forms of cancer among women worldwide. Early and accurate detection with mass screening programmes helps improve a woman's chances for successful treatment. The current and the most effective technique used for screening and diagnosis of breast cancer is the X-ray mammography. The photon transport detection of such technique is mostly based on a forward scattering mechanism as well as makes use of attenuation and penetration coefficients. The painful compression and the double X-ray exposure of both patients' breasts carried out during the imaging process remain unavoidable. In addition, the conventional 2D mammography has two major limitations: sensitivity in detecting breast cancers (~ <80%) and the high recall rate (~10%). It suffers from certain limitations, most important of which is tissue overlap and false diagnoses arising thereof. To overcome this and as an alternative, a new 3D imaging method for breast cancer screening and diagnosis, namely, tomosynthesis, has recently been used. In such method, a limited number of low-dose 2D projection images of a patient are used to reconstruct the 3D tissue information. Tomosynthesis systems incorporate an X-ray source that moves over a certain angle to acquire images. This tube motion is a major limitation because it degrades image quality, increases the scan time and causes prolonged patient discomfort. Therefore, the goal of this work was to overcome all of the above limitations by developing an innovative proof of concept for painless 3D X-ray mammography to be hopefully used as a screening and as diagnostic methods for breast cancer detection by utilizing the scattered X-ray photon information. Most imaging modalities required a wide spectrum of capabilities, which span biomedical sciences, physical sciences and clinical medicine; thus, the ongoing methodology aims to establish a collaborative cross-disciplinary research engaging together with scientists in universities and clinicians in hospitals. Consequently, we hope that this work provides the potential to score some successes in clinical imaging science. In order to do this and since it is generally not possible or feasible to use real components to build and optimize a system repeatedly, a Monte Carlo simulation was used. The first phase focused on realistic computer simulation of the proposed imaging system to find the optimum setup as well as to aid in the analysis of the effect of various factors on the system performance. Thus, the main focus was on 3D mammography imaging simulation setup. Five main steps have been carefully checked and successfully produced: (a) the production of X-ray radiation or source after careful and detailed physics check. This includes the interaction between the X-ray photons and the object (the 3D breast phantom) that is used on scan as well as the detector system and its associated electronics modelled. (b) Next is the realistic modelling of anthropomorphic breast phantoms to check if the effectiveness of prediction of the simulation is successfully achieved. A computer simulation model is developed to estimate the radiation dose to the breast that would be incurred using mammography. Mono-energetic normalized glandular dose coefficients, DgN(E), were computed for energies 11–120 keV using breast phantoms of various sizes and compositions.

Keywords: mammography, breast cancer detection, 3D imaging

1. Introduction

Breast cancer is one of the most common cancers in Saudi Arabia [1] and, thus, is an important health problem [2]. In the Western world, it is the second most frequent cause of cancer death in women (after lung cancer) [3]. Statistics show that a large number of women in Europe, North America, Australia and many Latin-American countries suffer from this life-threatening disease [4]. Worldwide, in the year 2005, the number of new cases exceeded 1.2 million [3]. Breast cancer is rare in women below the age of 20 years and less common below the age of 30 years, but it is more aggressive and thus has a lower survival rate. The incidence rate, however, rises dramatically over the age of 50 years. This could be due to several risk factors such as family history, genetics, early menstruation, late menopause and other factors that have not yet been identified. Breast cancer can also occur in males and often fatal, but it is extremely rare. The above problems have prompted global governments to put constant efforts to increase patient's recovery level against this disease. Early and accurate detection with mass screening programmes helps improve a woman's chances for successful treatment. It also minimizes pain, suffering and anxiety that surround patients and their families.

The current and the most cost-effective technique used for screening and diagnosis of breast cancer is X-ray mammography. It is the state of the art for earlier detection to improve both prognosis and survival rate [5]. This may be due to its good availability, high sensitivity and relatively low cost/patient. Despite the above efforts, the mortality rate of breast cancer still remains high and in the UK, for example, accounts for ~17% of all female deaths [6, 7]. This is due to some limitations of the current mammographic procedures. As a result, a large number of cases with positive mammography results undergo invasive surgical breast biopsies. Breast biopsy is still widely used and thus is the only fail-safe method to determine whether a lesion is malignant. Of all biopsy cases, only about 25% prove to be malignant. Moreover, a majority of the diagnosed women below the age of 50 have a dense breast tissue. This is a problem as it obscures lesions and results in false-negative mammography.

In addition, the size, shape and appearance of the female breast are not constant but undergo a number of changes during the lifetime of women. For instance, changes occur during the menstrual cycle and more pre-/postmenopause. In addition, the age of the subject not only influences the shape but also parenchymal density of the breast. Thus younger women tend to have denser breasts (more fibro-glandular tissue), whilst postmenopausal women have breasts containing a larger adipose component. This makes the X-ray mammogram far more effective in older women as the fat content is more radio-translucent (appears darker) than glandular tissue (appears underexposed) in younger women [8].

The above discussion suggests that both the shape and parenchymal density of the breast impose particular constraints on the choice of imaging modality. The imaging technique should be powerful for initial detection and subsequent follow-up of the diseases. At present, no single technique can be used for all cases of breast cancer detection without showing certain clinical or technical limitations. This implies necessity to address the specific needs that can help for breast tumour imaging to overcome these limitations. For instance, breast compression is often needed as it holds the breast still and enhances the spatial resolution. It also evens out the breast thickness and reduces scatter in X-ray or gamma-ray imaging in case of scintimammography (SM) [9], thus increasing image sharpness. Moreover, it spreads out the tissue so that small abnormalities will not be obscured by the overlying breast tissue. Since the breast is an external organ and extends to the chest wall, it requires appropriate views to be taken. For instance, in X-ray mammography a lateral (from the side) view of the breast allows separation of the chest wall from lesions deep within the breast.

Furthermore, mammography involves the radiological examination of the breast using equipment specifically designed for, and dedicated to, imaging breast tissue. This equipment is primarily used for the detection of breast cancer at an early stage. It is widely used in screening programme involving healthy populations of women. Early detection of breast cancer in a healthy population places particular demands on radiological equipment as high-quality images are required at a low dose. Symptomatic patients may also benefit from the development of mammography equipment that produces high-quality images for breast screening. Perhaps because of the exacting demands of mammography, acceptability criteria and suspension levels are well developed [10, 11]. It has been an accepted practice that mammography should be performed on X-ray equipment designed and dedicated specifically for imaging breast tissue, due to the clinical imaging requirements for high-quality image. In practice, either film/screen or digital detectors may be used. Both qualitative and quantitative acceptability criteria have been published for X-ray mammography by considering the image quality needed clinically in screening programmed.

2. Literature review

Cancer is a disease that starts in a localized organ or tissue and then grows out of control. Breast cancer is an important health problem as in the western world; it is the second most frequent cause of cancer death in women (after lung cancer) [6, 7]. Statistics show that a large number of women in Europe, North America, Australia and many Latin-American countries suffer from this life-threatening disease [8]. Worldwide, in the year 2005, the number of new cases exceeded 1.2 million [7]. Breast cancer is a heterogeneous disease as it has different cell types and different behavioural characteristics and appearances. Understanding the types of breast cancer and their growth pattern is important for imaging purposes. Breast cancer is usually categorized into two main types: invasive (infiltrating) and non-invasive (in situ) cancer. In situ means that the cancer cells are at early stage, i.e. remains localized to ducts (milk passages) or lobule (milk producing glands) with no micro-invasion to the surrounding fatty tissue. Once the basement membrane is penetrated, the cancer cells break into the surrounding tissue and are referred to as invasive breast carcinoma. Breast cancer is rare in women below the age of 20 years and less common below the age of 30 years, but it is more aggressive and thus has a lower survival rate. The incidence rate, however, rises dramatically over the age of 50 years. This is may be due to several risk factors such as family history, genetics, early menstruation, late menopause and other factors that have not yet been identified. Breast cancer can also occur in males and often fatal, but it is extremely rare. The above problems have prompted global governments to put constant efforts to increase patient's recovery level against this disease. Early and accurate detection with mass screening programmes helps improve a woman's chances for successful treatment. It also minimizes pain, suffering and anxiety that surround patients and their families. The current and the most cost-effective technique used for screening and diagnosis of breast cancer is X-ray mammography. It is the state of the art for earlier detection to improve both prognosis and survival rate [9].

Mammography is a low-energy (25–32 keV) X-ray examination of the soft tissues of the breast. It uses the variation in density between normal mammary features and abnormal tissue structures (lesion) to produce the image. The current widely used technique is based on screen-film technology. It is considered the gold standard in breast imaging as it is fast and available and has a lower cost than the scintimammography. It has two main applications: as a screening method in asymptomatic patients and as a diagnostic method in symptomatic populations. The former application is extremely important, and its introduction has significantly reduced the mortality rate of breast cancer in many countries [10, 11]. The American Cancer Society (ACS), the Department of Health and Human Services (HHS), the American Medical Association (AMA) and the American College of Radiology (ACR) recommend screening mammography every year for women, beginning at age 40. This is because the screening services accurately detect micro-calcifications and non-palpable soft tissue masses which until now have been beyond other imaging methods thanks to the high spatial resolution (50100 μm). Research has shown that annual mammograms lead to early detection of breast cancers, when they are most curable and breast-conservation therapies are available. The National Cancer Institute (NCI) adds that women who have had breast cancer and those who are at increased risk due to a genetic history of breast cancer should seek expert medical advice about whether they should begin screening before age 40 and about the frequency of screening. A recent review [12] estimated that screening leads to a reduction in breast cancer mortality of 15 and to 30% overdiagnosis and overtreatment. This means that for every 2000 women invited for screening throughout 10 years, one will have her life prolonged. In addition, 10 healthy women, who would not have been diagnosed if there had not been screening, will be diagnosed as breast cancer patients and will be treated unnecessarily. Furthermore, more than 200 women will experience important psychological distress for many months because of false-positive findings. Normally, screening is achieved by exposing the breast to X-rays after being gently compressed between two plates and then taking two views for each breast. A craniocaudal (imaging from above to below) and lateral views are generally taken. A lead grid is used to reduce scattering photons that reach the film. Diagnostic mammography is used for assessing the size of the lesion, for pre-surgical localization of suspicious areas of breast and in the guidance of needle biopsies.

The reported sensitivity (the fraction of patients actually having the disease and correctly diagnosed as positive) in lesion detection varies between 69 and 90% [13] depending on the breast density. The specificity (the fraction of patients without the disease, correctly diagnosed as negative) is the major drawbacks of conventional mammography. A variation in specificity between 87 and 97% and a low positive predictive value as low as 15% have also been reported in Ref. [14]. This 'less than perfect' performance may be due to several confounding factors, e.g. poor mammographic technique, observer error, the lesions are non-palpable or at a cellular level and/or the lesions are obscured by the normal breast tissues. In addition, the presence of scars or tissue distortion may hide true small tumours on the mammogram. Moreover, in mammography the ultimate challenge with regard to X-ray image quality and, thus, improving the reliability of screening and early diagnosis, requires better epidemiological understanding of breast tissues, improved diagnostic tools, enhanced quality control, continuous training and efficient management of data and records. Nevertheless, conventional mammography remains the most valuable and cost-effective technique for breast tumour diagnosis.

Over the last two decades, considerable efforts have been carried out to improve the current screen-film mammographic technique. These improvements include image quality, acquisition techniques and interpretation protocol in order to reduce some of the mammographic limitations [15]. Furthermore, a new research effort started 5 years ago focusing on 'digital mammography' (DM) as a possible future direction in breast imaging. Digital mammography, also called full-field digital mammography (FFDM), is a mammography system in which the X-ray film is replaced by solid-state detectors that convert X-rays into electrical signals. These detectors are similar to those found in digital cameras. The electrical signals are used to produce images of the breast that can be seen on a computer screen or printed on special film similar to conventional mammograms. This technique offers many advantages compared to the conventional screen-film-based method [16, 17]. For instance, processing with digital systems increases dynamic range (two to four times the dynamic range of typical film screen) and improved quantum efficiency and storage and display mechanisms. In addition, the use of computer-assisted image interpretation is claimed to be helpful for the physician. This may enhance different features such as computer-aided diagnosis which may further improve the visibility of lesions and improve mammographic sensitivity [18]. Therefore, repeated exposures (which are sometimes needed when using conventional mammography) are not required, and this may reduce the radiation dose. Moreover, it does not need either cassettes or dark rooms or processors and thus allegedly saves space and time in archiving and retrieving DM images. However, DM requires large disk space for saving image data.

Despite several advantages, DM does not yet replace screen-film mammography in many centres. However, with continuous technical improvements of the digital system, it is gradually taking over the conventional systems. Both conventional and DM systems suffer from substantial technical and clinical limitations. For instance, these systems are unreliable in imaging patients with dense parenchyma tissue especially in the younger female population due to more glandular tissue. Breast implants can also impede accurate mammogram readings because both silicone and saline implants are not transparent on X-rays. Thus, it blocks a clear view of the tissues behind them. This is true especially if the implant has been placed in front of, rather than beneath, the chest muscles. This issue requires an experienced technologists and radiologists to carefully compress the breasts to improve the view without rupturing the implant. All the above limitations and problems of imaging need to be dealt with to enhance detection efficiency and overcome the drawback. One of the methods that recently employed is the computer-aided detection (CAD) systems. Such systems use a digitized mammographic image that can be obtained from either a conventional film mammogram or a digitally acquired mammogram. The computer software then searches for abnormal areas of density, mass or calcification that may indicate the presence of cancer. The CAD system highlights these areas on the images, alerting the radiologist to the need for further analysis. Despite that mammographic findings are non-specific (cannot always differentiate benign from malignant disease) and often underestimate the size of the detected lesion, X-ray–based imaging is also not useful for breast diagnosis following surgery or radiotherapy as the patient's breasts in these cases have architectural distortion. Mammography is not recommended for women with breast implants and is also not useful following hormonal replacement therapy due to the increase of breast density. It is worth mentioning that X-ray mammography is not always useful for non-palpable tumours. Another group of women— close carrying a mutation in BRCA1 (human gene called breast cancer 1, early onset) or BRCA2 (breast cancer 2) genes—are at high genetic risk of cancer, some even having opted for preventative bilateral mastectomy. It is preferred not to repeat scan this group due to X-ray dose, and thus, a more sensitive diagnostic test would be advisable.

Moreover, the size, shape and appearance of the female breast are not constant but undergo a number of changes during the lifetime of women. For instance, changes occur with pregnancy, breast feeding and during the menstrual cycle. In addition, the age of the subject not only influences the shape but also parenchymal density of the breast. That is why young women tend to have dense breasts (more fibro-glandular tissue), creating a rounded appearance. On the other hand, postmenopausal women have breasts containing a large amount of fat. This makes the X-ray mammogram far more effective in older women as the fat content is more radio-translucent (appears darker) than glandular tissue (appears underexposed) in younger women [19]. The above discussion suggests that both the shape and parenchymal density of the breast imposes particular constraints on the choice of imaging modality. The imaging technique should be powerful for initial detection and subsequent follow-up of the diseases. At present, no single technique can be used for all cases of breast cancer detection without showing certain clinical or technical limitations. This implies necessity to address the specific needs that can help for breast tumour imaging to overcome these limitations. For instance, breast compression is often needed as it holds the breast still and enhances the spatial resolution. It also evens out the breast thickness and reduces scatter in X-ray or gamma-ray imaging [20], thus increasing image sharpness. Moreover, it spreads out the tissue so that small abnormalities will not be obscured by the overlying breast tissue. Since the breast is an external organ and extends to the chest wall, it requires appropriate views to be taken. For instance, in X-ray mammography a lateral (from the side) view of the breast allows separation of the chest wall from lesions deep within the breast. On the other hand, in single photon-ray emission imaging, one needs to separate the breast from the heart by employing an appropriate prone (face down) position. However, it has been claimed that with prone imaging view, there is a possibility of missing a small low-intensity medial lesion because of attenuation. This implies that another image is needed but with the camera positioned in the lateral view. In addition, shielding the camera from the background cardiac flux is very useful in tumour detection in terms of contrast and resolution [21, 22].

Having discussed the golden diagnostic technique for breast tumour imaging, the following section will describe the complementary imaging techniques of the breast. The image reconstruction techniques will be then discussed. Section 3 will be closed by presenting some preliminary results and a description of the design details.

3. Complementary diagnostic techniques

From the previous discussion, it is clear that there are some clinical situations where there are significant limitations to use mammography in isolation. In such cases, there is a great need to use sensitive tests to achieve a high confidence and accurate diagnostic decision. The use of breast biopsies is necessary if breast cancer is indicated or suspected in such cases. Of the performed breast biopsies, about 60–80% [23] are negative breast cancer or have benign lesions. In these cases, breast biopsies are considered unnecessary. This has led many breast cancer experts to propose complementary imaging modalities to provide additional diagnostic information and reduce unnecessary breast biopsies.

Ultrasonography (US) uses high-frequency acoustic waves that reflect at boundaries with different acoustic properties. It is a non-invasive technique, easily available and relatively cheap. Breast US provides unique information in assessing both palpable and non-palpable breast abnormalities. For instance, it clearly differentiates between solid masses and cystic lesions [24]. It is also considered to be useful in cancer staging, measuring tumour sizes, easy accessing lesions located in peripheries and reducing the number of unnecessary biopsies. It allows accurate needle placement during biopsy and is very useful for aspiration of cysts. The members of the European group for breast cancer screening recommended using US as a complementary method to X-ray mammography. In addition, the use of high-frequency transducers has improved spatial resolution and thus claimed to be useful in axillary node evaluation. However, breast US technique is time-consuming and operator/observer dependent. It has also a number of other limitations that may be due to overlapping in sonographic characteristics. For instance, it cannot detect calcifications (micro-calcifications or macro-calcifications) in DCIS. It could also miss solid lesions especially in a fatty breast and if detected cannot determine whether a solid lump is benign or malignant. For these reasons, US is not used as a screening technique for asymptomatic breast cancer as it is difficult to ensure that the entire breast has been scanned.

Magnetic resonance imaging (MRI) images are created by the recording of signals generated after radio-frequency excitation of nuclear particles exposed to strong magnetic field. Breast MRI is a non-ionizing tomographic functional technique that may be used when the diagnosis is uncertain with mammography [25]. The technique is valuable for specific clinical indications such as patients with (1) axillary adenopathy (enlargement or inflammation of the lymph gland), (2) possible tumour recurrence after surgery or radiotherapy, (3) lesions overlying implants or (4) those requiring staging of multifocal carcinoma (two or more discrete lesions in one breast) [26]. Breast MRI with dedicated breast coil has excellent soft tissue resolution that enhances the ability to both identify the location and in some cases determine the full extent of the lesion. The use of intravenous contrast agent, gadolinium, which accumulates in tissues with a dense blood vessel network, has also increased the sensitivity of breast MRI [13]. However, the reported specificity (ability to determine if lesion is benign or malignant) is 56–72% [27]. This technique has a limited application in patients with implanted metal devices or other metallic materials inside the body. MRI cannot also differentiate between inflammatory breast cancer and abscesses. In addition, several clinical limitations have been reported in the literature suggested not to use MRI in premenopausal women. For example, changes that do occur in the T1 value of the breast tissue during the menstrual cycle [13] mean that patients should be scanned between the 6th and 16th days of the cycle. In summary, researchers have concluded that breast MRI is limited by lack of availability and inconsistent quality, and the technique is too expensive for routine use in breast cancer screening.

The need to improve the breast cancer detection and to reduce the unnecessary invasive breast biopsies has stimulated researchers to investigate functional imaging modalities. These techniques produce a range of different imaging approaches such as positron emission tomography (PET), single-photon emission computed tomography (SPECT), planar imaging and dedicated imaging instrumentation with and without breast compression. These imaging techniques of the breast potentially over additional information in breast cancer diagnosis. This is because these imaging methods rely on the physiological and biochemical characteristics of a lesion. Thus, they are considered as the best hope to differentiate between benign/normal and malignant diseases. These functional techniques have also been used to assess and monitor the effect of cancer prevention drugs. The current radionuclide imaging techniques used for breast tumour imaging are briefly discussed.

In PET a small amount of positron emitter radio-tracer, 18fluorodeoxyglucose (FDG), is administered intravenously to the patient [27]. It is then distributed in the body, and as it decays, the radionuclide emits a positron in any random direction. If the positron whilst travelling interacts with an electron within the body, the two particles then annihilate and produce two rays of 511 keV each. Either a whole-body scanner or a breast-specific positron emission mammography (PEM) camera [28] is used to detect the two gamma-rays in coincidence (two events that are detected within ~ 12 ns). PEM is increasingly used in North America not only in cancer diagnosis but also in staging, planning and monitoring anticancer therapy. This information can be helpful not only in eliminating unnecessary axillary dissection [29] and biopsies but also in determining the appropriate treatment. The diagnosis of viable tumour tissue following chemotherapy is another application of PET [30, 31]. Imaging with 18F-FDG has shown considerable promise in breast cancer imaging, but the exact role is still in evolution. Wahl [32] recommended that it is best applied to solve difficult clinical cases in specific patients rather than routinely. There are a number of reasons that limit the wide use of PEM for routine cancer diagnosis: (1) the high cost (over $2 million) of PET coincidence imaging equipment, i.e. cyclotron, scanner and radiochemistry facility [27]; (2) the difficulty of producing and labelling the short half-life PET radionuclides [28]; (3) the lack of centres with the required experience to develop more advanced methodology appropriate for breast oncology—in particular, more data are needed about the metabolism of different PET radio-pharmaceuticals in breast tumours—and (4) the lack of oncologists with a high knowledge of PET methodology [32].

Scintimammography (SM) is a promising non-invasive functional imaging technique. It has been proposed to complement X-ray mammography and to improve patient selection for biopsy. This single-photon imaging of the breast involves injecting the patient in the arm vein with a small amount (555–740 MBq [33]) of radiopharmaceutical. The most commonly used radiopharmaceutical for SM is ^{99m}Tc labelled Sestamibi. After a period of time, the tracer distributes in the breast tissue as well as in the body organs. It accumulates more in the target object (lesion) with uptake ratio nearly 9:1 tumour-to-background ratio (TBR) [43]. A standard full-size clinical gamma camera is then used to scan the patient and thus measure the 3D distribution of the radioactivity. SM imaging using full-size clinical camera includes a range of different imaging approaches such as planar (2D) imaging or SPECT technique. The latter technique gives a 3D representation image but is not widely used because it is difficult with this technique to accurately localize the lesion [40]. In contrast, planar SM is the technique that is more widely used in clinical practice because it provides better lesion localization particularly the prone images with lateral views [34]. In this case the gamma camera is usually equipped with a LEHR parallel-hole collimator, and two views (prone and supine) are taken to the diagnosed breast. Since the energy imaged is 140 keV representing the photo peak, 20% energy window (symmetric ~10%) is often used and thus centred over the photo peak.

In brief, SM with a general-purpose camera has been introduced to evaluate patients with dense breast prior and in a least case after breast biopsy [35]. The technique may also be considered valuable for many clinical applications such as evaluating the axillary lymph nodes, investigating patients with microcalcifications [36], assessing multifocal and multi-centric breast cancer diseases [37]. It is also useful for imaging patients following surgery, chemotherapy, hormonal replacement therapy and radiotherapy as well as for patients with breast implants [34]. The technique may also assist in the differentiation of benign and malignant breast abnormalities by measuring radio-tracer uptake in the lesions as compared with surrounding breast tissues. Studies such as [38, 39] suggested that SM may be used as a second-line diagnostic test in cases where the sensitivity of mammography is decreased or there is doubt about the presence of lesion. In summary, SM using conventional camera may be considered as a useful complementary imaging modality to aid the diagnosis and the detection of breast cancer [40]. It may also help to assess in patient selection for biopsies, and this may reduce the number of unnecessary or negative breast biopsies. However, the major drawback of the current standard clinical gamma camera SM imaging systems is the use of mechanical collimator. This causes the camera imaging system to utilize a very small fraction, ~0.01%, of the total number of the emitted photons. This limits the statistics and hence the quality and diagnostic value of the observed images. The collimator sensitivity and resolution are a trade-off, and the camera is also limited by its intrinsic spatial resolution. As a result, these factors make it difficult to practically image cases of smaller, non-palpable, lesions (<1 cm) that may be deep seated or those close to the chest wall. These have stimulated the development of new dedicated (breast specific) instrumentations that are used for breast tumour imaging applications.

Recent years have seen considerable interest by scientists in developing new compact medical imaging detectors. These instruments were proposed for different clinical applications with the aim to improve image quality by building cameras of suitable size and shape for the part of the body under investigation. Among these designed detectors is the small dedicated gamma camera for functional breast tumour imaging. The justification for this development is that a standard full-size clinical gamma camera is designed for whole-body imaging and, thus, has not been optimized for breast tumour imaging. In other words, there are a number of shortcomings with such general-purpose gamma camera such as the limiting sensitivity (on average 50% [41]) for lesions <1 cm such as DCIS particularly the medially located tumours. In addition, several studies have pointed out that due to the large FoV of the camera and the bulky collimators, it is difficult to position the camera close to the breast, and thus, imaging breast tissue adjacent to the chest wall may not be possible. This may, ultimately, decrease the spatial resolution of the camera imaging system and thus affect the diagnostic value of the test in detecting such a small lesion size.

To overcome some of the limitations offered by conventional gamma camera on breast imaging, Gupta and colleagues [42] reported the first preliminary clinical data that are performed with breast-specific detectors and then compare it with the data obtained from standard full-size camera. A limited number of patients were investigated in this study but interestingly reported a higher sensitivity for the dedicated camera. Following this and due to the large research activities, new generation of detectors has been designed and developed for breast tumour imaging, for instance, the position-sensitive photo-multiplier tubes (PSPMT), semiconductor arrays and scintillation crystals coupled to an array of solid-state photo detectors.

The commercially available dedicated breast camera has two detectors and is designed and optimized to image only the breasts. It possesses a high intrinsic spatial resolution, and the camera is also equipped with ultra-high-resolution parallel-hole collimator and thus optimized for high-resolution SM. The main advantage of such cameras is the ability to separate the breast from the chest wall by positioning the camera close to the breast. Thus, the camera can be used in areas with limited space (e.g. medial view can be possible), where the use of a full-sized camera is impractical or impossible. The use of moderate breast compression capabilities may improve both the signal-to-nose ratio (SNR) and the spatial resolution [43] and thus increase the sensitivity for detecting smaller lesions. The proposed clinical indications for such dedicated cameras are similar to the full-size clinical gamma camera SM. There are some recent clinical studies associated with using these dedicated gamma cameras. For instance, a clinical preliminary study by Brem et al. [44, 45] using dedicated breast camera demonstrated a slight improvement in resolution and tumour sensitivity particularly for lesions~ 1 cm. Rhodes and colleagues reported [46] on SM performed on 40 women with small mammographic abnormalities (<2 cm) scheduled to undergo biopsy. The SM examination identified (33/36) malignant lesions confirmed at biopsy. The authors concluded that this preliminary study suggested an important role for the dedicated SM camera in women with dense breasts. In another study Brem and colleagues [47] evaluated 94 women (median age 55 years) presented with normal mammographic and physical examination results but all considered at high risk of developing breast cancer. Of these women 35 had a history of previous breast carcinoma or atypical ductal hyperplasia. The authors concluded that with this camera, they can depict small (8–9 mm) non-palpable lesions in women at high risk of breast cancer.

In summary, whilst these studies using breast-specific cameras are promising, all are considered preliminary in nature because they based on very few cases. Additional studies with a larger sample size are needed to accurately assess and reach scientific conclusions concerning these proposed cameras. They also need to be cost competitive with the general-purpose gamma cameras in order to be widely used in breast tumour imaging applications. In addition, the smallest lesion sizes that can be detected with these cameras claimed to be 3–3.3 mm [48] compared to 4–5 mm [49] with conventional camera. However, the evidence published to date did not demonstrate a statistically significant difference in lesion detection. The spatial resolution of these proposed cameras may further improve by increasing the pixel size, but there are however practical limitations in the development of cameras with small pixel sizes, including cost and detector design. More importantly due to the use of collimator, these dedicated cameras suffer from low detection efficiency. Nowadays, the latest revolution in the mammography field was announced by Dr. Jeffrey Shuren, director of the FDA's Center for Devices and Radiological Health, said on Friday, February 11, 2011 "Physicians can now access this unique and innovative 3-D technology that could significantly enhance existing diagnosis and treatment approaches". In addition, the US Food and Drug Administration approved on Friday the first X-ray mammography device that provides three-dimensional images of the breast for cancer screening and diagnosis.

3.1. Image reconstruction techniques

Screening and diagnostic mammography suffers from the limitation that the complex 3D breast structure is projected into a plane. Thus, lesions can be obscured by overlaying and underlying tissue structures which could cause a false negative, or dense overlapping tissue can mimic lesions, leading to an unnecessary recall of a patient. The proposed solution is 3D breast tumour image reconstruction techniques such as digital breast tomosynthesis (DBT) which is an emerging modality that produces 3D breast images. In DBT, lesion conspicuity is improved, which could potentially lead to earlier cancer detection and a more accurate diagnosis. In tomosynthesis, a volume image is created from a sequence of projection views acquired over a limited arc. Reconstruction from this data is challenging because the data is inherently incomplete. One-shot algorithms such as filtered back projection (FBP) have been developed for DBT image reconstruction. Though efficient, they tend to yield conspicuous artefacts. Iterative algorithms such as expectation maximization (EM) have also been employed with DBT. Such algorithms sacrifice efficiency but yield images with fewer artefacts. An additional drawback for EM, however, is that in general some form of regularization is needed which tends to reduce resolving power necessary for calcification detection.

3.2. Design details and preliminary results

3.2.1. Design details

The experimental system consists of a general radiography tube pointing at a given distance from the central axis of the breast. Four flat-panel digital detectors will be used to collect all the photon information (energy, flux, position) scattered by the phantom breast covering all possible area around it. The patient would lie on a table in the prone position with one breast drawn downwards through an opening to allow the X-ray tube and detector flat panels to be safely placed beneath the table (**Figure 1**).

During one irradiation of such phantom, we will investigate all the collected data to reconstruct the image in a 3D framework.

3.2.2. Preliminary results

As an illustrative example to indicate whether the proposed idea will work, we simulated a semi-spherical breast phantom including two air-filled cavities, irradiated with 10^8 photons. The photon energies imitate the standard spectrum of the commonly used X-ray source in mammography case studies. Monte Carlo sampling of the X-ray generator (30 kVp, Mo anode, filter 0.03 mm Mo and 1 mm Be) was carried out using the inverse cumulative method

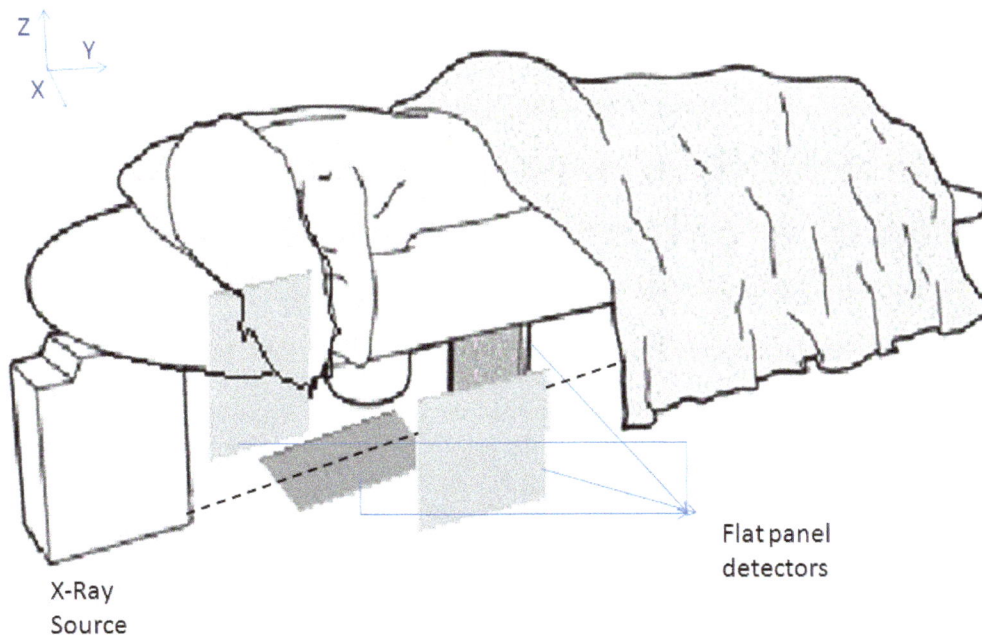

Figure 1. Schematic view of proposed setup design. Patient lies prone with one breast drawn downwards through opening in scanning device.

starting from experimental data sets. **Figure 2** shows the phantom (magenta colour) including two cavities (yellow) and surrounded with four flat-panel detectors (white). The two other faces contain the chest and the source beam zone.

The important data given by the scorers (flat-panel detector) numbers 2, 3 and 4 will contribute significantly on the final 3D image reconstruction process. **Figure 3** demonstrates how important the scattered photon statistics are for the given simulated setup.

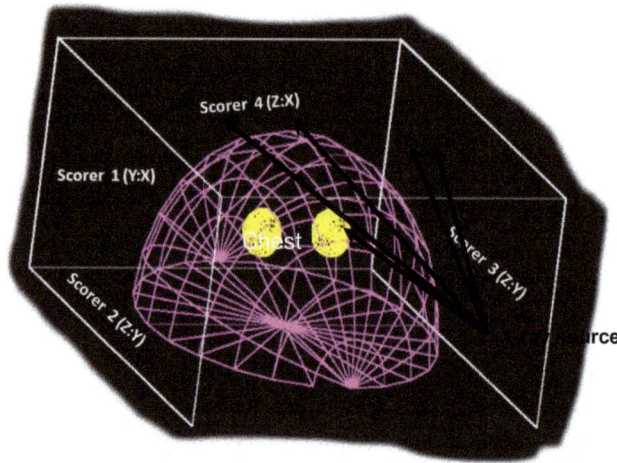

Figure 2. Simulated setup including the breast phantom (magenta), air cavities (yellow), X-ray photon (red) and the four scorers.

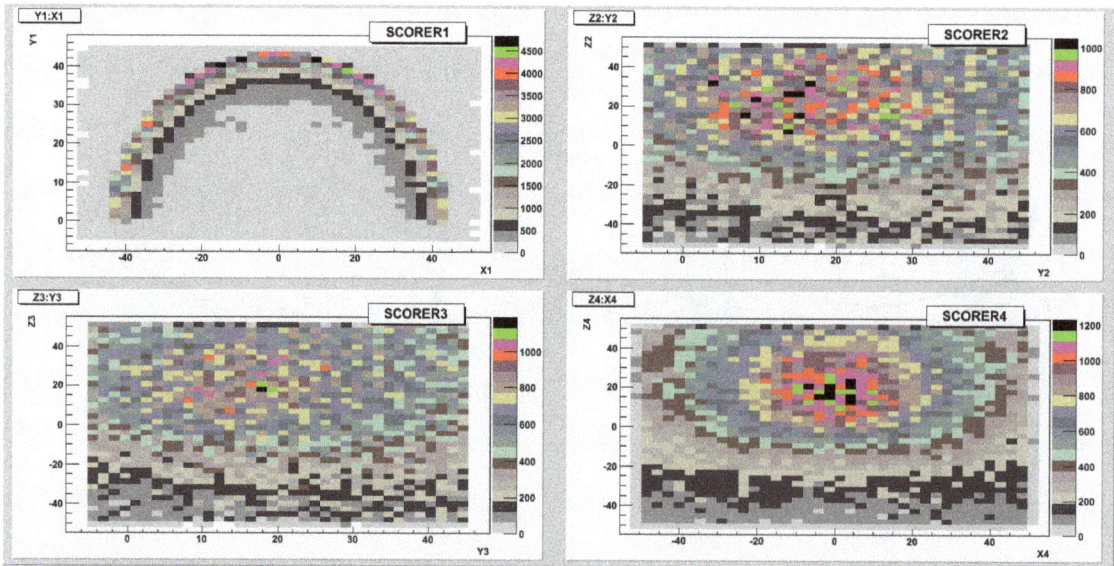

Figure 3. Simulated deposited energy using Geant4 Monte Carlo simulation toolkit for the four scorers. Bar scale indicates the specific magnitude of deposition.

Therefore, the goal of this project is to overcome all of the above limitations by providing a proof of concept for painless 3D mammography to be used as a screening and as diagnostic methods after commercialization. The proposed prototype includes (1) the detection system, which will be a set of semi-conductor arrays spatially distributed around each breast; (2) the X-Ray source; and (3) the convenient patients' test bed for painless exposition to X-rays. For that purpose, the first phase of the proposed project will focus on a versatile and widely used Monte Carlo simulation tool, Geant4, to optimize the detector arrays' chemical composition (CdZnTe, GaAs, etc.), spatial positioning around patient, source characterization (energy, spatial localization) and also the test-bed geometry to mainly fulfil the two conditions of radiation protection and painless positioning.

Secondly, we will use an iterative reconstruction algorithm to reconstruct the images of a mathematically breast phantom using the cluster network technique. Then, the experimental construction of the overall design will be carried out. Finally, the use of anthropomorphic breast phantoms to check the effectiveness prediction of the simulation will resume the project phases. Since most imaging modalities required a wide spectrum of capabilities which span biomedical sciences and physical sciences and clinical medicine, thus this project will be a collaborative cross-disciplinary research engaging together with scientist in universities and clinician in hospitals. Consequently, this proposal has the potential to score some successes in clinical imaging science. The project outputs will include the creation of a numerical platform able to more understand the breast disease problems and the development of an innovative prototype for painless breast imaging within a 3D framework. These allow the large communities of researchers and doctors to improve the breast imaging process and to build and to share some knowledge and experiences within that context. As a result, some international and national publications will be submitted to well-recognized journals.

Based on the assessment of current prevalence and projected incidence of diseases, cancer has been selected as medical and health-priority area for strategic intervention by the National Medical and Health Research Strategic Priorities (NMHRS) for the Kingdom. It is classified as a non-communicable disease [1]. Within that context, breast cancer is the second leading cause of cancer deaths in women today. About 1.3 million women are diagnosed annually worldwide, and about 465,000 will die from the disease. Incidence and mortality have reached a plateau and appear to be dropping in both United States and parts of Europe [1]. This decline has been attributed to several factors, such as the early detection. Despite the relatively low incidence in Saudi Arabia compared to other countries, breast cancer has been the most common cancer among Saudi females for the past decade (Saudi Cancer Registry, 1994–2005). The most concerned patients were aged between 40 and 50 years old. For that, a breast cancer screening programme will help all the female population, including the young one (having dense breast), for early detection and prevention advices.

So, the potential positive impacts on the economy and society of the current project are well defined in terms of decreasing the enormous burden to the healthcare-utilization costs.

Furthermore, the expertise to be developed through this project will be applied to the review of new digital radiographic imaging systems, the development of amendments to the diagnostic X-ray performance standard, the development of an advisory pertaining to national public breast cancer screening programmes and the joint planning of a consensus development conference on the 3D X-ray imaging modality with the King Saud University.

Also, investigating the computer-assisted diagnosis devices will provide the Kingdom with the scientific basis to effectively regulate this fast-growing field. In addition, this project may provide powerful tools of a commercial value for X-ray imaging application, especially with the development of such prototype, including the detectors, the source and the patient bed, that will meet to a 3D painless mammography.

Another benefit of such project concerns the supervision of two master's students and to create a locally competent talent capable of conducting novel medical and health sciences research. The creation of an infrastructure that supports and enables further research, in such medical field, will be an extra added benefit to the College of Applied Medical Sciences and to the King Saud University. The development and the setup of cooperative agreement by establishing collaborative research with advanced institutions such as the CERN and the University of Surrey will contribute to the technological opportunities transferred from over the world. Finally, the proposed project should participate in increasing national scientific discovery and productivity through promotion by publishing in peer-reviewed and reputable journals.

4. Valuable to the Kingdom

Based on the assessment of current prevalence and projected incidence of diseases, cancer has been selected as medical and health-priority area for strategic intervention by the National Medical and Health Research Strategic Priorities (NMHRS) for the Kingdom. It is classified as a non-communicable disease [1]. Within that context, breast cancer is the second leading cause of cancer deaths in women today. About 1.3 million women are diagnosed annually worldwide, and about 465,000 will die from the disease. Incidence and mortality have reached a plateau and appear to be dropping in both United States and parts of Europe [1]. This decline has been attributed to several factors, such as the early detection. Despite the relatively low incidence in Saudi Arabia compared to other countries, breast cancer has been the most common cancer among Saudi females for the past decade (Saudi Cancer Registry, 1994–2005). The most concerned patients were aged between 40 and 50 years old. For that, a breast cancer screening programme will help all the female population, including the young one (having dense breast), for early detection and prevention advices. So, the potential positive impacts on the economy and society of the current project are well defined in terms of decreasing the enormous burden to the healthcare-utilization costs.

Furthermore, the expertise to be developed through this project will be applied to the review of new digital radiographic imaging systems, the development of amendments to the diagnostic X-ray performance standard, the development of an advisory pertaining to national public breast cancer screening programmes and the joint planning of a consensus development conference on the 3D X-ray imaging modality with the King Saud University. Also, investigating the computer-assisted diagnosis devices will provide the Kingdom with the scientific basis to effectively regulate this fast-growing field.

In addition, this project may provide powerful tools of a commercial value for X-ray imaging application, especially with the development of such prototype, including the detectors, the source and the patient bed, that will meet to a 3D painless mammography.

Another benefit of such project concerns the supervision of two master's students and to create a locally competent talent capable of conducting novel medical and health sciences research. The creation of an infrastructure that supports and enables further research, in such medical field, will be an extra added benefit to the College of Applied Medical Sciences and to the King Saud University. The development and the setup of cooperative agreement by establishing collaborative research with advanced institutions such as the CERN and the University of Surrey will contribute to the technological opportunities transfer from over the world. Finally, the proposed project should participate in increasing national scientific discovery and productivity through promotion by publishing in peer-reviewed and reputable journals.

Author details

Mohammed Ali Alnafea

Address all correspondence to: alnafea@ksu.edu.sa

Department of Radiological Sciences, College of Applied Medical Sciences, King Saud University, Riyadh, Saudi Arabia

References

[1] King Abdulaziz City for Science and Technology. Strategic Priorities for Advanced Medical and Health Research, Doc. No. 39P0001-PLN-0001-ER01

[2] Apostolakis J, et al. GEANT – Detector Description and Simulation Tool, CERN Program Library Long Writeup W5013. Geneva, Switzerland: CERN; 1993

[3] Nelson WR, Rogers DW. Structure and operation of the EGS4 code system. In: Jenkins TM, Nelson WR, Rindi A, editors, Monte Carlo Transport of Electrons and Photons. New York: Plenum Press; 1988, pp. 287-305

[4] Briesmeister J. MCNP—A general Monte Carlo N-Particles Transport Code, LA 1265-M, Version 4B. Los Alamos, New Mexico, USA: Los Alamos National Laboratory; 1997

[5] Agostinelli S, et al. GEANT4—a simulation toolkit. Nuclear Instruments and Methods A. 2003;506:250-303

[6] Harris JR, Lippman ME, Verone U, Willett W. Breast cancer. New England Journal of Medicine. 1992;327:319-328

[7] The American Cancer Society. Cancer Facts and Figures 2006. Available from: http://www.cancer.org, retrieved on September; 2006

[8]   Cavalli F, Hansen HH, Kaye SB. Textbook of Medical Oncology. Martin Dunits Ltd; 1998. ISBN: 1853172901

[9]   Kelsey JL, Gammon MD. The epidemiology of breast cancer. Cancer. 1991;41:146-165

[10] Department of Health and Social Security, D. o. H. a. S., Ed., Breast Cancer Screening: Report of a Working group chaired by Professor Sir Patrick Forrest. London, UK: H. M. S. O; 1986

[11] Dufy SW, Tabr L, Chen HH, Holmqvist M, Yen MF, Abdsalah S, Epstein B, Frodis E, Ljungberg E, Hedborg-Melander C, Sundbom A, Tholin M, Wiege M, Kerlund A, Wu HM, Tung TS, Chiu YH, Chiu CP, Huang CC, Smith RA, Rosn M, Stenbeck M, Holmberg L. The impact of organized mammography service screening on breast carcinoma mortality in seven Swedish counties. Cancer. 2002;95:458-496

[12] Gøtzsche PC, Nielsen M. Screening for breast cancer with mammography. Cochrane Database of Systematic Reviews. 2009(4). Art. No.: CD001877. DOI: 10.1002/14651858. CD001877.pub3

[13] Kacl GM, Liu PF, Debatin JF, Garzoli E, Cadu RF, Krestin GP. Detection of breast cancer with conventional mammography and contrast-enhanced MR imaging. European Radiology. 1998;8(2):194-200

[14] Kopans DB. The positive predictive value of mammography. American Journal of Roentgen. 1992;158:521-526

[15] Hendee WR. History and status of X-ray mammography. Health Physics. 1995; 69(5)636-648

[16] Sankararaman S, Karellas A, Vedanthan S. Physical characteristics of a full-field digital mammography system. Nuclear Instruments and Methods in Physics Research A. 2004;533(14):560-570

[17] James JJ. The current status of digital mammography (Review). Clinical Radiology. 2004;59:1-10

[18] Adler DD, Wahl RL. New methods for imaging the breast: Techniques, findings, and potential. American Journal of Roentgenology. 1995;164:19-30

[19] Stefanoyiannis AP, Costaridou L, Skiadopoulos S, Panayiotakis G. A digital equalisation technique improving visualisation of dense mammary gland and breast periphery in mammography. European Journal of Radiology. 2003;45:139-149

[20] Pani R, Scopinaro F, Pellegrini R, Soluri A, Weinberg IN, De Vincentis G. The role of Compton background and breast compression on cancer detection in scintimammography. Anticancer Research. 1997;17(3B):1645-1649

[21] Alnafea MA, Wells K, Spyrou NM, Saripan MI, Guy M, Hinton P. Preliminary results from a Monte Carlo study of breast tumour imaging with low energy high-resolution collimator and a modified uniformly-redundant array-coded aperture. Nuclear Instrument and Method A. 2006;563:146-149

[22] Alnafea MA, Wells K, Spyrou NM, Guy M. Preliminary Monte Carlo study of coded aperture imaging with a CZT gamma camera system for scintimammography. Nuclear Instrument and Method A. 2007;573:122-125

[23] Kopans DB. The positive predictive value of mammography. American Journal of Roentgen. 1992;158:521-526

[24] Stavrous AT, Thickman D, Rapp CL, Dennis MA, Parker SH, Sisney GA. Solid breast nodule: Use of sonography to distinguish between benign and malignant lesions. Radiology. 1995;196:123-134

[25] Weinreb JC, Newstead G. MR imaging of the breast. Radiology. 1995;196:593-610

[26] Rankin SC. MRI of the breast. British Journal of Radiology. 2000;73(872):806-818

[27] Sharp PF, Gemmell HG, Smith FW. Practical Nuclear Medicine. USA: Oxford University Press. ISBN: 0-19-26284-0, 1-12; 1998

[28] Wahl RL. Current status of PET in breast cancer imaging, staging, and therapy. Seminars in Roentgenology. 2001;36(3)250-260

[29] Adler LP, Crowe JP, Alkaisi NK, Sunshine JL. Evaluation of breast masses and axillary lymph nodes with [F-18] 2-deoxy-2-uoro-D-glucose PET. Radiology. 1993;187(3):743-752

[30] Strauss LG, Conti PS. The application of PET in clinical oncology. Journal of Nuclear Medicine. 1991;32(4)632-648

[31] Strauss LG. PET in clinical oncology: Current role for diagnosis and therapy monitoring in oncology. The Oncologist. 1997;2:381-388

[32] Price P. Is there a future for PET in oncology? European Journal of Nuclear Medicine. 1997;24(6):587-589

[33] Bombardieri E, Aktolun C, Baum RP, Bishof-Delaloye A, Buscombe J, Chatal JF, Maoli L, Moncayo R, Mortelmans L, Reske SN. Breast scintigraphy: Procedure guidelines for tumour imaging. European Journal of Nuclear Medicine and Molecular Imaging. 2003;30(12):B107-B114

[34] Schillaci O, and Buscombe JR. Breast scintigraphy today: Indications and limitations. European Journal of Nuclear Medicine and Molecular Imaging. 2004;31:S35-S45

[35] Wiesenberger AG, Barbosa F, Green TD, Hoefer R, Keppel C, Kross B, Ma-jewski S, Popor V, Wojcik R, Wymer DC. A combined scintimammography/stereotactic core biopsy X-ray. Nuclear Science Symposium Conferece Record. 2000;3

[36] Fondrinier E, Muratet JP, Anglade E, Fauvet R, Breger V, Lorimier G, Jallet P. Clinical experience with 99mTc-MIBI scintimammography in patients with breast microcalci cations. Breast. 2004;13(4):316-320

[37] Schillaci O, Scopinaro F, Spanu A, Donnetti M, Danieli R, Di Luzio E, Madeddu G, David V. Detection of axillary lymph node metastases in breast cancer with 99mTc tetrofosmin scintigraphy. International Journal of Oncology. 2002;20(3):483-487

[38] Imbriaco M, Del Vecchio S, Riccardi A, Pace L, Di Salle F, Di Gennaro F, Salvatore M, Sodano A. Scintimammography with 99mTc-MIBI versus dynamic MRI for non-invasive characterization of breast masses. European Journal of Nuclear Medicine and Molecular Imaging. 2001;28(1)

[39] Buscome JR, Cwikla JB, Holloway B, Hilson AJW. Prediction of the usefulness of combined mammography and scintimammography in suspected primary breast cancer using ROC curves. Journal of Nuclear Medicine. 2001;42;3-8

[40] Fahey FH, Grow KL, Webber RL, Harkness BA, Harkness BA, Bayram E, Hemler PF. Emission tuned-aperture computed tomography: A novel approach to scintimammography. Journal of Nuclear Medicine. 2001;42(7):1121-1127

[41] Scopinaro F, Ierardi M, Porri LM, Tiberio NS, De Vincentis G, Mezi S, Cannas P, Gigliotti T, Marzetti L. 99mTc-MIBI prone scintimammography in patients with high and intermediate risk mammography. Anticancer Research. 1997;17:1635-1638

[42] Gupta P, Waxman A, Nguyen K, Phillips E, Yadagar J, Silberman A, Memsic L. Correlation of 99mTc-sestamibi uptake with histopathologic characteristics in patients with benign breast diseases [Abstract]. Journal of Nuclear Medicine. 1996;37(5):1122-1122

[43] Coover LR, Caravaglia G, Kunh P. Scintimammography with dedicated breast camera detects and localizes occult carcinoma. Journal of Nuclear Medicine. 2004;45(4):553-558

[44] Brem RF, Schoonjans JM, Kieper DA, Majewski S, Goodman S, Civelek C. High-resolution scintimammography: A pilot study. Journal of Nuclear Medicine. 2002;43:909-915

[45] Brem RF, Kieper DA, Rapelysea JA, Majewski S. Evaluation of a high-resolution, breast-specific, small-field-of-view gamma camera for the detection of breast cancer. Nuclear Instruments and Methods in Physics Research Section A. 2003;497(1):39-45

[46] Rhodes DJ, O'Connor MK, Phillips SW, Smith RL, Collins DA. Molecular breast imaging: A new technique using 99mTc-scintimammography to detect small tumours of the breast. Mayo Clinic Proceedings. 2005;80:24-30

[47] Brem RF, Rapelyea JA, Zisman G, Mohtashemi K, Raub J, Teal CB, Majewski S, Welch BL. Occult breast cancer: Scintimammography with high-resolution breast-specific gamma camera in women at high risk for breast cancer. Radiology. 2005;237(1):274-280

[48] Scopinaro F, Pani R, De Vincentis G, Soluri A, Pellegrini R, Porfri LM. High-resolution scintimammography improves the accuracy of technetium-99m methoxy-isobutylisonitrile scintimammography: Use of a new dedicated gamma camera. European Journal of Nuclear Medicine and Molecular Imaging. 1999;40:1279-1288

[49] Taillefer R. The role of 99mTc-sestamibi and other conventional radiopharmaceuticals in breast cancer diagnosis. Seminars in Nuclear Medicine. 1999;XXIX(1):16-40

12

Advances in Breast Thermography

Siva Teja Kakileti, Geetha Manjunath,
Himanshu Madhu and
Hadonahalli Venkataramanappa Ramprakash

Abstract

Thermography-based breast cancer screening has several advantages as it is non-contact, non-invasive and safe. Many clinical trials have shown its effectiveness to detect cancer earlier than any other modality. Historically, thermography has only been used as an adjunct modality due to the high expertise required for manual interpretation of the thermal images and high false-positive rates otherwise found in general use. Recent developments in thermal sensors, image capture protocols and computer-aided software diagnostics are showing great promise in making this modality a mainstream cancer screening method. This chapter describes some of these advances in breast thermography and computer-aided diagnostics that are poised to improve the quality of cancer care.

Keywords: breast cancer, thermography, analytics, machine learning, artificial intelligence, medical imaging, breast thermography, computer-aided diagnostics

1. Introduction

Breast cancer is the leading cause of cancer deaths in women today. According to WHO, 1 in every 12 women have the risk of a breast abnormality in her lifetime. It is well established that early diagnosis is very critical to increase survival rates. For example, a study sponsored by Australian Government found that the breast cancer survival is strongly associated with tumor size at detection. In Australia in 1997, five-year relative survival was 98, 95, 93, 88 and 73% for women with tumors of size 0–10, 11–15, 16–19, 20–29 and 30 mm or greater, respectively [1]. Unfortunately, 70% of the breast cancer cases are detected when the tumor size is over 30 mm [2]. Therefore, there is a critical need for a method that can detect early-stage breast cancer.

Thermography is a method of cancer screening that has been known to detect early-stage cancer [3]. However, there is a lot of variation in the results of clinical studies based on thermography and many show low specificity. A medical scientist and deep expert in thermography, Dr. Gautherie, observed that the lack of technical skill and expertise to interpret thermal images leads to this low diagnostic accuracy [3]. Recent developments on high-resolution thermal cameras and computer algorithms for thermal analysis are making the interpretation process more factual. With increased computation power, automated diagnostics is also able to decrease the false-positive rates. Hence, thermal imaging along with computer-aided diagnostics is showing a promise of upgrading breast thermography to main stream usage. In this chapter, we study these recent trends in advanced thermal imaging as well as the advances in imaging algorithms.

2. Introduction to thermography

Infrared thermography is the recording of temperature distribution of a body using the infrared radiation emitted by the surface of that body at wavelengths between 7 and 14 μm. With this information, it is possible to create a visual map or thermogram of the distribution of temperatures on the surface of the object imaged. The sensitivity of modern infrared cameras is such that temperature differences to 0.025°C can be detected.

Thermography can be used for breast cancer screening based on the fact that the temperature of the tumor is about 2°C higher than the neighboring tissues and blood vessel activity surrounding a developing cancer is almost always higher than in normal breast tissue. Since breast tissue is part of the skin, vascular alterations due to cancer result in temperature changes on the surface of the breast which can be captured with infrared thermography. Thermal abnormalities identified with thermal imaging are among the earliest signs of a precancerous or cancerous lesion of the breast.

Thermal imaging is a noncontact, noninvasive and extremely privacy aware. Since thermal cameras are small, they are very portable and can be used for screening in rural camps.

There are many certified thermographers and thermologists who continue to practice using thermal analysis for breast cancer diagnosis [4].

3. Comparison with mammography

Most common methods used for cancer screening today is clinical examination, mammography and ultrasound. Among them, mammography is considered as a gold standard for breast cancer screening. It uses X-rays to screen the breast region and digitizes the density difference in image format. Typically, cancerous tumor has high density compared to surrounding region and can be easily distinguished from other regions. Studies [5–7] show that it gives a sensitivity of 68% to 88% (or as low as 48% for extremely dense breasts) and specificities ranging from 82% to 98%. In addition, it has the following disadvantages:

1. *Low sensitivity toward younger women:* In order to clearly detect tumors using X-rays, the density of the lump should be higher than the surrounding tissue density. Breast tissue density in younger women is high and decreases with age and exposure to hormonal changes [8]. This makes mammography mainly applicable for women with age greater than 45 years.

2. *Risk of radiation:* X-rays can cause genetic change in the tissues, and these mutations increase with increased dosage of radiation and duration of exposure. A study presented at an annual meeting of Radiology Society of North America (RSNA) observed that high-risk women exposed before age 20 or with five or more exposures were 2.5 times more likely to develop breast cancer than high-risk women not exposed to low-dose radiation [9]. This limits the mammography as a frequent screening modality.

3. *Fear and pain:* To get proper mammograms, breast region should be compressed. An approximate of 15–20 pounds of pressure is applied on the breast region to image. Due to high compression involved, sometimes it might also lead to rupture of tumor. Many surveys described this as painful screening method that subjects would like to avoid [10].

4. *Privacy:* Apart from pain and fear of radiation, it is reported in Ref. [11] that nearly 38% among women from different ethnic groups and with more than 60% among South Asian countries like India and Pakistan do not go for screening due to embarrassment of disrobing.

Thermography overcomes the above issues and enables more people to go for screening. It can work on women of all age groups. It is a non-contact, non-invasive modality with passive infrared measurement, which does not involve any radiation, hence a safe screening method. Since the thermal images can essentially be captured from a laptop connected to the thermal camera, it is also extremely privacy aware.

Among other modalities, clinical breast exam can detect tumors only once they are large enough to be palpable and result in many false positives. Effective use of sono-mammography (ultrasound) for cancer detection requires location of the lump. Hence, ultrasound is best used as a correlation modality. Once a lump is detected either through mammography or thermography or clinical breast examination, ultrasound will be very useful to reconfirm malignancy or not.

4. Biological explanation

Cancer cells release nitric oxide [12, 13] into the blood and lead to alteration in microcirculation. This nitric oxide coupled with aggressiveness of cancer to grow increases the blood circulation by dilating the vessels and leads to creation of new blood vessels (neo-angiogenesis) and dormant vessel recruiting. Experimentally, Folkman [14, 15] observed this dependency of tumor growth with angiogenesis by implanting tumour cells in mice. Large volume of blood flow in these vessels connected to tumor makes them hotter when compared to normal blood vessels. This large flow distorts the vessel structure, and vessels become dilated as well as elongated, causing the increase in the dimension of vessel caliber and length [16, 17]. This elongation combined with the large flow deviates the vessel structure from normal vessels by making them more tortuous due to formation of bends [18–20]. In fact, it is experimentally evident that this high tortuosity is observed much before angiogenesis [18].

In addition, it has been empirically observed that tumor temperature is higher than the neighboring temperatures with the help of contact temperature measurements. In Ref. [21], Gautherie claimed that this high heat is due to high metabolic activity at tumor location. Hence, this region appears brighter and hotter in thermographic images when compared to surroundings. It is also observed that tumor temperature is warmer compared to the blood vessels feeding the tumor region [21]. Aggressiveness of cancer cells makes the boundary of tumor irregular as they break the boundary formed by basal laminas to invade the neighboring tissues [19, 20]. This is not seen in case of benign tumors whose cells behave similar to normal cells. This makes the benign tumor boundaries regular.

The size of tumor indicates the stage of cancer and largely affects the survival rate. A survey conducted by Narod [2] observed drastic decrease in survival rate with increase in tumor size. Early detection of cancer increases the chances of survival. Thermography outperforms other modalities when it comes to early detection. Changes such as vasodilation, neo-angiogenesis and high tortuosity of blood vessels which are found in initial stages of cancer result in thermal impressions and hence can be detected in thermography [15–19]. These might not be observed in other modalities which depend upon detecting architectural distortions that appear only when tumor is sufficiently grown. A study by Gautherie and Gros [3] over 58,000 patients for 12 years showed that thermography detected breast cancer five years earlier in around 400 patients than mammography and ultrasonography.

Abnormality in thermogram is not the sole criterion for malignancy. Increase in heat pattern might even be observed due to hormonal response, lactation and presence of benign tumors such as fibrocystic and fibroadenoma. However, these non-malignant conditions have different projections in the thermographic image when compared to malignant tumors. Unlike in malignant breasts where there is asymmetrical heat map, heat response is mostly symmetrical across the two breasts with high hormonal response. Estrogen released during hormonal activity produces nitric oxide that causes increase in heat and vessel dilation [12]. Similar activity happens in the case of lactating mothers except that a little asymmetry in heat map is seen due to uneven lactation in both breasts. There is an increase in heat signature even in benign cases such as fibrocystic and fibroadenoma [21, 22]. In contrast to malignant tumors, these cells are not aggressive and behave similar to normal cells [19, 23]. Other than these cases, abnormal heat pattern leading to vasodilation and angiogenesis can also occur during inflammation caused by infection or wound healing [12, 14]. Though these abnormalities are formed, they have distinct features compared to malignancy that can be distinguished.

Some recent explorations have shown that thermography can even help in prognosis. Since the increase of temperature in malignant tumors is primarily due to the release of nitric oxide, which is caused due to hormonal activity, the temperature distribution on the breasts also provides signals on the hormonal receptor status of malignant tumors. Zore et al. [9] have studied the effect of hormone receptor status of malignant tumors on thermograph through a quantitative analysis of average or maximum temperatures of the tumor, the mirror tumor site and the breasts. While no statistically significant difference was found in the overall temperature distribution in breasts with hormone receptors being positive or negative, they report a significant difference in average and maximum tumor temperature measurements. Another computer-aided study [24] reported an accuracy of more than 80% for automated estimation of hormonal receptor status of malignant tumors. This shows the potential of a non-invasive way of predicting the hormone receptor status of malignancies through thermal imaging, before going through Immuno-Histo-Chemistry (IHC) analysis on the tumor samples after surgery.

5. Protocols for capturing thermal images

A standard imaging protocol has to be followed for any modality to make it a repeatable and operator agnostic procedure that can reduce subjectivity and errors in image capture. Likewise, a set of instructions has to be followed in thermography as well [25, 26].

Most importantly, before capturing the images, patient must be cooled for minimum period of 10–15 min in a room maintained at a temperature of 16-22 °C. This helps in attaining thermal equilibrium with the surrounding environment [25]. Cooling is mandatory as it helps in removal of extraneous heat caused due to external reasons such as tight clothing, apparel and friction from a hand bag or outside temperature. Cooling also helps in enhancing the temperature pattern of tumorous regions compared to non-tumourous regions [27–30]. It is observed that normal tissue reacts quickly to external cooling, whereas malignant reacts slowly, making it appear hotter compared to rest of the breast region. For quick cooling of images, cold challenge can be used where patient hands are immersed in cold water causing the regulation of body temperature with sympathetic stimulus [30].

When it comes to capturing the actual thermal images, imaging protocols can be categorized into discrete and continuous imaging protocols.

Discrete imaging protocols: These protocols are interested in specific set of static fixed views. The basic views which are observed in most discrete protocols include frontal view (0°), oblique views (±30°) and lateral views (±90°). Some variations of different protocols in the way of the mentioned views are captured, such as (a) seated position, (b) supine position, (c) standing position and (d) combinations of {a,b,c}. Subset of mentioned views/changing the angle of views/ adding more view angles are also being used in some studies.

A tumor has less effect with cooling compared to normal tissues whose heat signatures decrease drastically [28, 30]. To study the nature of cancer cells further, some protocols include the above combinations of different views after cooling the breasts. Some protocols consider only fully cooled breasts, while some capture the breast image before and after cooling and analyze the thermal patterns of the cooled breast and uncooled breasts [31].

Continuous imaging protocols: Continuous imaging protocols capture videos of the breast as they are cooled, instead of static images. These protocols are not as popular as discrete due to the large processing time needed to analyze. However, much larger information can be captured in a video. For example, tumorous regions do not cool as fast as rest of the tissues.

6. Advances in thermal cameras

Medical thermography is also benefiting from the rapid advancement in the quality of thermal imaging too. Temperature capture has evolved from a complicated probe-based method to a camera-based registration.

Over the years, improvements in silicon technology have made a huge impact on the technology used in IR detectors. Many use cases of thermal imaging are evolving in biomedical, transport, energy and environmental applications, and they have been the key business driver for this growth, as well. **Figure 1** depicts the history of development of infrared sensors, which is very well described in Ref. [32]. The real breakthroughs were focal plane arrays and bi-dimensional arrays improving spatial resolution and thermal sensitivity.

Broadly, infrared cameras can be divided into cooled and uncooled detectors. Cooled thermal cameras have infrared detectors integrated with cryocoolers and enable measurement of very low temperatures as well as very high resolution and improved sensitivity as thermally-induced noise is reduced. However, cooled cameras are expensive and may be needed only for applications that require very high resolution and high sensitivity.

Microbolometer focal plane arrays (FPAs) have tremendously modified the way of image capture by allowing an array of sensors at the focal plane of lens to detect the LWIR wavelengths [32, 33]. This integration has led to the development of uncooled infrared detectors that are typically small, handheld and also restricted the need for expensive cooling techniques. The current uncooled cameras work on the principle of change in resistance or voltage or current due to the emitted infrared radiation. The resolution is direct function of number of pixels in the microbolometer array per unit area. With the advances in silicon technology, these digital infrared uncooled cameras have massively transformed from a low resolution to high resolution of 640 × 480 pixels to 1024 × 768 pixels or more. The current cameras also have improved the sensors to obtain a thermal sensitivity and accuracy error of at most 20 mK and 1°C respectively. To detect the infrared radiation, vanadium oxide (VOx) and amorphous silicon are common materials in microbolometer [32].

The lens is costly compared to lens found in normal video-shoot cameras, since normal glass cannot be used to make the lens due to its property of blocking LWIR radiation and reflecting the LWIR incident on the lens. Hence, Germanium (Ge), Chalcogenide glass, Zinc Selenide (ZnSe) and Zinc Sulfide (ZnS) that are LWIR-transmissive are used for the lens preparation.

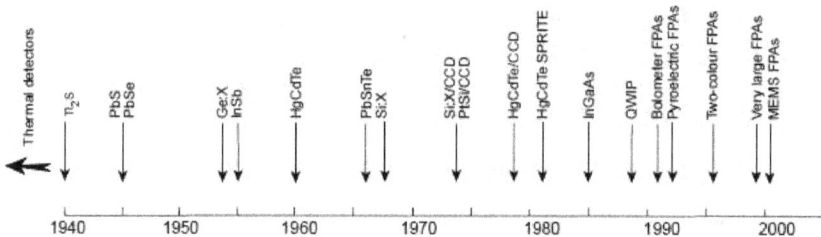

Figure 1. Advances in thermal sensor technology (reproduced from Ref. [32]).

These uncooled cameras have also reduced the cost and heavy maintenance that would be needed for the cooled detectors. Some popular camera models used for medical purposes are shown in **Figure 2**. Today, FLIR, Fluke and Meditherm are thermal camera vendors preferred by thermographers for medical thermography as many of these camera models are already FDA-certified for tele-thermology.

6.1. Visual interpretation of thermal images

There are different protocols followed by thermographers for analyzing and interpreting thermal images, especially for breast cancer screening. Most of this work in creating the protocols have taken place in the 1970s and 1980s, such as the Marseille protocol [13–15], Hobbins protocol [30], Gautherie protocol [21], Hoekstra protocol [34] and, more recently, with newer thermal cameras, the Villa Marie protocol [12]. An attempt to obtain an agreement of different experienced thermographers was also made in 1975 to provide a consistent set of observations to be noted [17].

All of these protocols give different thermographic category ratings of four to five levels, starting from normal to highly suspicious of malignancy. Multiple criteria are noted, using both vascular and non-vascular observations. These criteria are generally qualitative rather than quantitative. The visual interpretation necessitates heuristic rules to combine these observations to determine a thermographic category. Some protocols assign numbers to each observation and combine them using a mathematical function for categorization. This also shows the need for experience and proper training for thermographic interpretation.

Regardless of the variations across protocols, these criteria can be broadly classified into vascular and non-vascular criteria, with some generality in these criteria, as follows:

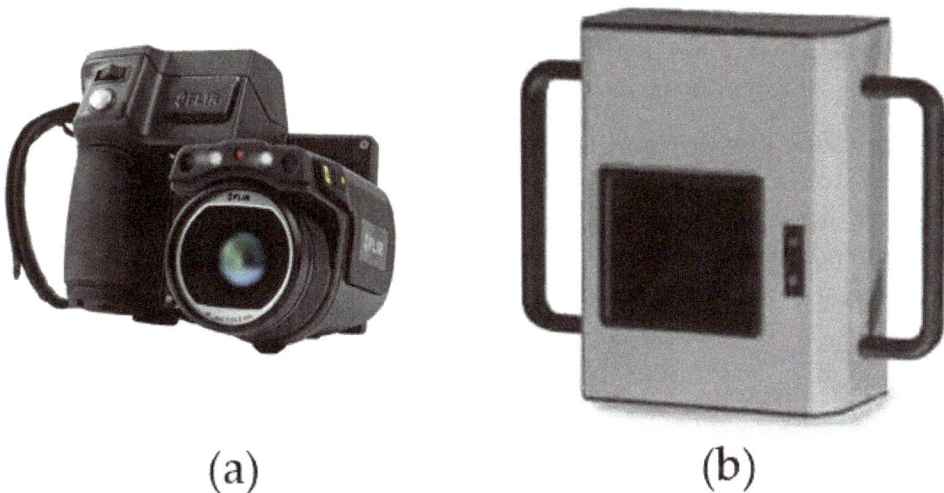

(a)   (b)

Figure 2. Two thermal camera models from different vendors (a) FLIR T650SC (b) Meditherm IRIS 2000.

Non-vascular criteria:

1. Focal increase in temperature by a fixed interval, e.g., 1, 2, 3°C

2. Global increase in temperature compared to the contralateral breast by, say, 1.5°C

3. Regional increase in temperature, including specific quadrants

4. Differences in temperature between contralateral regions or between different quadrants/regions in the same side

5. Abnormal location of focal increase including areolar regions or along edges/bulges

6. Abnormal physical observations: bulging/size variation, retraction

Vascular criteria:

1. Vascular asymmetry

2. Vascular anarchy, including tortuous or serpentine or loops or clusters or bifurcations

3. Increased vascular density

4. Abnormal directions of clusters of vessels, such as vertical, horizontal

5. Number of vessels

6. Caliber of vessels

7. Abnormal location of vascularity and avascularity

The general interpretation from these protocols is that with few and mild abnormal findings, the categorization is toward normal and likely benign. With increased abnormality, the observations tend toward increased suspicion of malignancy. Another important point to note is that benign diseases also exhibit some abnormal thermal vascular/non-vascular criteria [30]. The diagnosis for benign conditions is made by follow-up of thermography over a few months, by which time the abnormal thermal findings change or reduce or disappear.

Due to these multiple diverse metrics used by practitioners and no standardized way of interpretation across different expert thermographers, the thermological interpretation becomes very subjective and many times results in high false positives. Many efforts are therefore underway to remove subjectivity using computer-aided diagnostic methods—some of which are described later in this chapter.

7. Clinical validations

Thermography is not a new technique for breast cancer screening. Its presence has been there since 1960 [26]. There have been many longitudinal and clinical trials performed to show its efficacy. In 1982, FDA approved thermography as an adjunct modality for breast cancer screening. **Table 1** lists out the studies that has been done to show the potential of thermography. This technique is undervalued due to the difficulty in interpreting the thermograms with naked eye. The interpretation varies from observer to observer and needs high expertise to correctly validate the diagnosis result, limiting to few thermographers. With advent of technology, in both hardware and software, automated analysis of thermograms is emerging to obtain high sensitivity and specificity.

Studies	Subjects	Follow-up	Results	Comments
Gershon–Cohen [41], 1967	1924	No follow-up	Sensitivity—91.6% Specificity—92.4%	
Stark and Way [42], 1974	4621	No follow-up	Sensitivity—98.3% Specificity—93.5%	–
Spitalier [43, 44], 1982	61,000	10-Year period	Sensitivity—89% Specificity—89%	They reported that thermography was the first alarm in 60% cancer cases and stated that abnormal thermogram represents
Haberman [45], 1980	39,802	3-Year period	Sensitivity—85% Specificity—70%	30% of cancers showed their initial signs in thermography compared with traditional screening
Gros and Gautherie [3, 21, 46, 47], 1980	85,000	5-Year period for 58,000 patients	Sensitivity—90% Specificity—88%	Out of 1245 women that showed –ve signs with traditional screening in their first visit, more than 33% have got cancer in this 5-year period
Jones [48], 1983	70,000	No follow-up	Sensitivity—87% Specificity—85%	
Parisky [37], 2003	769	No follow-up	Sensitivity—97%	
Rassiwala [49], 2014	1008	No follow-up	Sensitivity—97.6% Specificity—99.2%	

Table 1. List of large-scale studies.

8. Advances in software technology

As seen in the clinical validation, the sensitivity observed with visual analysis is acceptable, but specificity is lower than desired with visual interpretation. Further, visual observations and heuristic categorization are subject to human error and variation through subjective interpretation. To solve these problems, there are automated and semiautomated approaches for diagnostics [35]. We review some of the software tools available from companies who are intending to provide a replicable method of interpreting thermal images.

We review the technology used in three such software tools from Niramai health, Total vision and Mammo vision. All these approaches use static images obtained after cooling the subject with discrete imaging protocols.

8.1. Visualization tools for thermal interpretation

Given that a thermologist has to look at five colored images, where the temperature differences between neighboring regions need to be identified by minute color variations, interpretation of thermal breast images is a huge cognitive overload and very error prone. So, software tools that aid in visualization and capturing of the observations about thermal patterns are becoming available.

Total vision software from Med-hot.com gives an excellent visualization of the thermal images and additional support for a thermographer to systematically look for specific abnormal thermal pattern alongside a rule-based decision-making support to simplify the interpretation process. However, it does not have any automation of the diagnosis.

Mammo vision [31] is a semi-automated tool that tries to identify the non-vascular abnormal thermal patterns during dynamic thermography with cold challenge. It considers 10 images in total, 5 images before cooling and 5 images after cooling, for the analysis. An elliptical grid is used to approximate breast region, and it automatically extracts the lateral symmetry, isothermia in each quadrant, areolar temperature, nipple temperature, temperature decrease with cooling and hotspot parameter. Additionally, the clinician can manually identify the vascularity in the breast by looking at grayscale thermal image, which is then used by the tool to categorize the subjects into five groups. The tool defines assessment criteria called Breast Infrared Assessment System (BIRAS) with which they categorize the images into five groups with BIRAS 1 being low risk and BIRAS 5 being high risk.

8.2. Use of sophisticated computer-aided diagnostics

Use of sophisticated artificial intelligence algorithms for enabling automatic diagnosis or clinical interpretation guidance is most needed to reduce subjectivity in interpretation [37]. Niramai Thermalytix software is one such advanced software tool with a technology that enables end-to-end fully automated approach for the diagnosis [38–40]. The Niramai tool uses complex computer algorithms for the following five key aspects of automated diagnostics.

1. Autotagging

Since one single view may not be sufficient to capture tumor region in different parts of the breast region, multiple views are taken. Typically, there are five thermal images in multiple views that are captured; one of the common mistakes done by clinicians is to name the image wrongly. It is observed that many a times humans are confused with classification of right and left sides of breast in the image correctly and resulting in improper tagging of lateral and oblique views. Hence, Niramai software provides an automated tagging support. This reduces the error in naming or false tagging, which in turn would have resulted in other errors such as segmentation error and misclassification of subjects. Their software automatically tags the views based on the body border curvature and body area.

2. Detecting the region of interest

The thermal image is captured with the patient sitting about three feet from the camera. This captures the thermal signature of the top part of body of the subject starting from neck region. A tool like Niramai that does automatic analysis of breast cancer has to accurately crop the region of interest (ROI), namely the breast tissue region. For this, Niramai tool removes inframammary fold, axilla, sternum and thyroid regions that are usually warm regions and might unnecessarily cause false positives. Additional heuristic based on the shape of body gives accurate segmentation of the ROI as shown in **Figure 3**. There is considerable research in the detection of ROI for single view [35], and tools that provide manual support through freehand segmentation and adjustable and draggable ellipse that the clinician can use mark the region of interest. Niramai software automatically detects the breast region using a polygon approximation of region that makes it easier for a clinician to edit, if needed.

3. Tumor localization

Once the region of interest for analysis is determined, next technical challenge is to accurately identify the exact location of an abnormality or a lesion. This usually means detecting regions having warm and hot temperature pixels in the image and analyzing the heat pattern around the same. The heat patterns found in the thermal images are then analyzed for specific tumor properties. Tumor-specific patterns include multiple important thermal patterns or features that typically help in discriminating malignancy versus benign conditions [38].

Symmetry plays a significant role in detecting whether a hot patch is abnormal. So, a subset of the ROI showing a significant increase in temperature as compared to the neighboring areas and contralateral sides is identified. In NIRAMAI, two varieties of abnormal regions

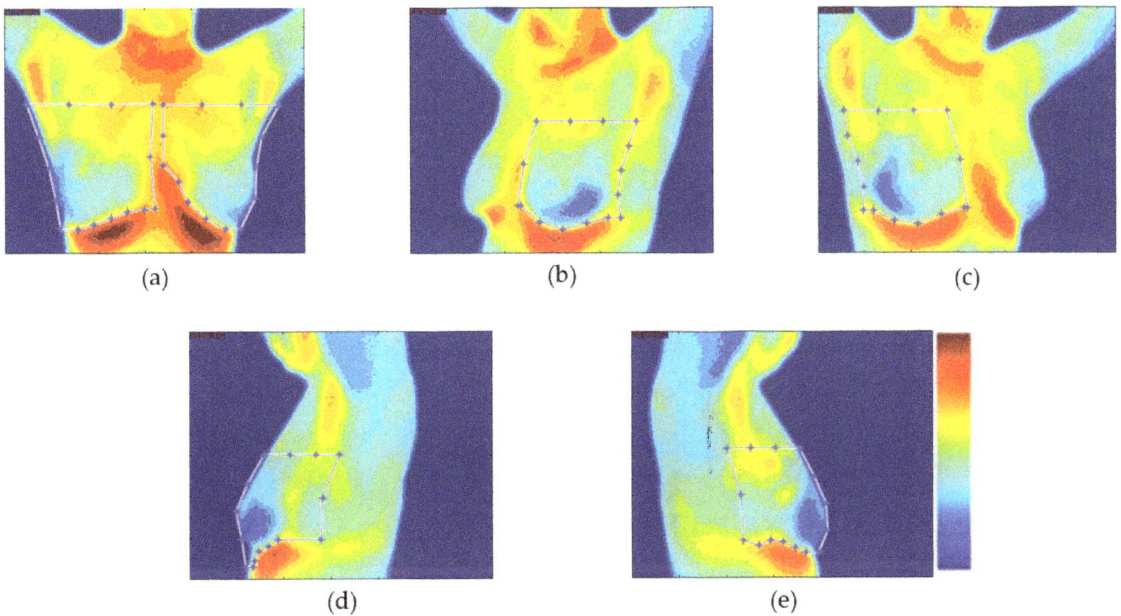

Figure 3. Results of automated segmentation in different views. (a) Frontal (b) Left Oblique (c) Right Oblique (d) Left Lateral (e) Right Lateral.

are extracted, hot-spots and warm-spots, based on the degree of their thermal response. This categorization helps to increase sensitivity with low thermal response tumors without increasing the false positives. Hot-spots correspond to high-temperature regions segmented using a combination of temperature-based thresholds. Warm-spots correspond to slightly lower temperature regions as compared to hot-spots with a change in parameters. One way of categorizing the same is using the modes and maximum temperature values, as shown in Eqs. (1) and (2).

$$T_a = T_{overallmax} - T \tag{1}$$

$$T_b = \Gamma + P(T_{overallmax} - \Gamma) \tag{2}$$

In above equations, Γ refers to the mean of the modes of the ROI temperature histograms in all views, and $T_{overallmax}$ represents the overall maximum temperature in all views. (P, T) are parameters chosen depending on the dataset.

Niramai tool detects hot-spots and warm-spots in each view of the subject. The best views of hot-spots and warm-spots are defined as the view in which the normalized size of the detected abnormal regions with respect to the ROI is maximum. **Figure 4** shows some sample subject images with their corresponding hotspots identified by NIRAMAI tool. From the detected hot-spots in multiple views, the hot-spots and warm spots corresponding to the best view are usually used to extract core features. Since symmetry places an important role, features are also extracted using the best view and its contralateral side view.

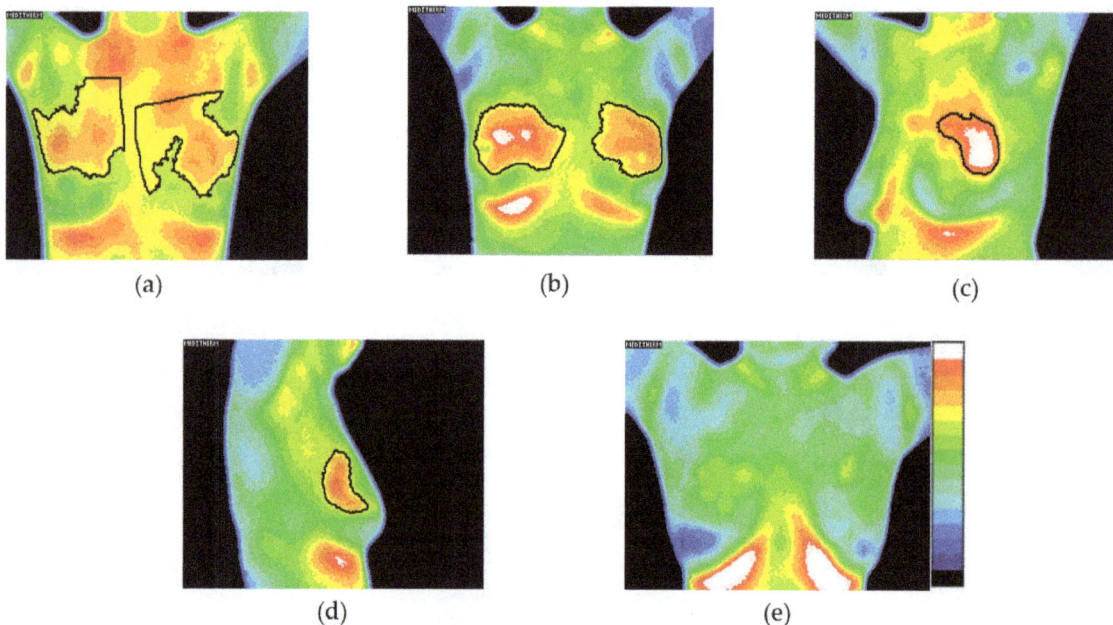

Figure 4. Sample subject images for (a) hormone-sensitive tissues showing warm-spots, (b) lactating case showing warm-spots, (c) malignant case showing hot-spots, (d) benign case showing warm-spots and (e) normal case.

4. Feature extraction

Once the hot- and warm-spots showing potential lesion is detected, three high-level properties of the lesion are extracted. These are boundary features, thermal symmetry and temperature distribution.

Malignant tumor cells are aggressive in nature, which makes them to invade surrounding tissues by rupturing through the boundary formed by basal laminas [19]. This makes the boundary irregular for malignant cases compared to non-malignant and benign cases which behave similar to normal cells.

In the case of malignant tumors, benign tumors, inflammation or wound-healing cases, an increase in temperature in the abnormal regions is observed. This leads to a difference in thermal heat patterns compared to the contralateral breasts. However, similarity in thermal heat patterns is seen for normal, hormonal, lactating conditions [12, 22, 36] due to the presence of similar hormone-sensitive tissues in both the breasts. This property is captured by including symmetrical features.

Finally, the mean temperature difference between the detected abnormal region and the remaining region of interest is calculated to get the relative increase in temperature compared to the neighboring region. In addition, many other temperature parameters of the abnormal region can be used for analysis.

5. Automated classification

Computer algorithms based on artificial intelligence and machine learning are making huge inroads in automated diagnostics [38]. Many methods of supervised classification are being developed where a small group of patient data is used to train a probabilistic model that represents the decision criteria based on the extracted features. A simple such classifier is a random forest that is able to identify the significant discriminatory features and learns a combination of the features and feature groups that helps decide on malignancy subjects. Other classifiers include support vector machines, Kmeans classifiers and deep learning.

9. Conclusions

In the recent years, use of Information Technology in healthcare diagnostics is proving to be very effective in improving efficiency and quality of care. Thermography is highly suited for breast cancer screening owing to its ability to detect cancer much earlier than any other modality, patient safety and privacy. The complexity and subjectivity in interpretation of thermal imaging has been a major deterrent in wide acceptance of the usage of thermography. Use of computer-aided diagnostics for automated thermography interpretation is just round the corner. With software support, thermal analysis and interpretation can be more efficient, effective and non-subjective. This chapter described some of the recent developments in both the hardware and the software of a thermographic solution that shows great promise that breast thermography will be a mainstream cancer screening modality very soon.

Author details

Siva Teja Kakileti[1], Geetha Manjunath[1]*, Himanshu Madhu[1] and Hadonahalli Venkataramanappa
Ramprakash[2]

*Address all correspondence to: geetha@niramai.com

1 NIRAMAI Health Analytix Pvt Ltd, Bangalore, India

2 Central Diagnostics Research Foundation, Bangalore, India

References

[1] Nickson C, Kavanagh AM. Tumor size at detection according to different measures of mammographic breast density. Journal of Medical Screening. 2009;**16**(3):140-146. DOI: 10.1258/jms.2009.009054

[2] Narod SA. Tumor size predicts long-term survival among women with lymph node-positive breast cancer. Current Oncology. 2012;**19**(5):249-253

[3] Gautherie M, Gros CM. Breast thermography and cancer risk prediction. Cancer. 1980;**45**(1):51-56. DOI: 10.1002/cncr.2820450110

[4] American College of Clinical Thermology. ACCT Approved Thermography Clinics [Internet]. Available from: http://www.thermologyonline.org/Breast/breast_thermography_clinics.htm [Accessed: March 25, 2017]

[5] Kolb TM, Lichy J, Newhouse JH. Comparison of the performance of screening mammography, physical examination, and breast US and evaluation of factors that influence them: An analysis of 27 825 patient evaluations. Radiology. 2002;**25**(1). DOI: 10.1148/radiol.2251011667

[6] Skaane P. Studies comparing screen-film mammography and full-field digital mammography in breast cancer screening: Updated review. Acta Radiology. 2009;**50**(1):3-14. DOI: 10.1080/02841850802563269

[7] Svahn TM, Chakraborty DP, Ikeda D, Zackrisson S, Do Y, Mattsson S, Andersson I. Breast tomosynthesis and digital mammography: A comparison of diagnostic accuracy. The British Journal of Radiology. 2017;**85**(1019):e1074–e1082. DOI: 10.1259/bjr/53282892

[8] Ginsburg OM, Martin LJ, Boyd NF. Mammographic density, lobular involution, and risk of breast cancer. British Journal of Cancer. 2008;**99**(9):1369-1374. DOI: 10.1038/sj.bjc.6604635

[9] Zore Z, Boras I, Stanec M, Orešić T, Zore IF. Influence of hormonal status on thermography findings in breast cancer. Acta Clinica Croatica. 2013;**52**(1):35-42

[10] Collins K, Winslow M, Reed MW, Walters SJ, Robinson T, Madan J, Green T, Cocker H, Wyld L. The views of older women towards mammographic screening: A qualitative and quantitative study. British Journal of Cancer. 2010;**102**(10):1461-1467

[11] Forbes LJL, Atkins L, Thurnham A, Layburn J, Haste F, Ramirez AJ. Breast cancer awareness and barriers to symptomatic presentation among women from different ethnic groups in East London. British Journal of Cancer. 2011;**105**(10):1474-1479. DOI: 10.1038/bjc.2011.406

[12] Kennedy DA, Lee T, Seely D. A comparative review of thermography as a breast cancer screening technique. Integrative Cancer Therapies. 2009;**8**(1):9-16. DOI: 10.1177/1534735408326171

[13] Thomsen LL, Miles DW, Happerfield L, Bobrow LG, Knowles RG, Moncada S. Nitric oxide synthase activity in human breast cancer. British Journal of Cancer. 1995;**72**(1):41

[14] Folkman J. What is the evidence that tumors are angiogenesis dependent? Cancer Spectrum Knowledge Environment. 1990;**82**(1):4-6

[15] Folkman J. Tumor angiogenesis: Therapeutic implications. New England Journal of Medicine. 1971;**285**(21):1182-1186

[16] Konerding MA, Malkusch W, Klapthor B, van Ackern C, Fait E, Hill SA, Parkins C, Chaplin DJ, Presta M, Denekamp J. Evidence for characteristic vascular patterns in solid tumors: Quantitative studies using corrosion casts. British Journal of Cancer. 1999;**80**(5-6):724

[17] Goel S, Duda DG, Xu L, Munn LL, Boucher Y, Fukumura D, Jain RK. Normalization of the vasculature for treatment of cancer and other diseases. Physiological Reviews. 2011;**91**(3):1071-1121

[18] Li C-Y, Shan S, Huang Q, Braun RD, Lanzen J, Hu K, Lin P, Dewhirst MW. Initial stages of tumor cell-induced angiogenesis: Evaluation via skin window chambers in rodent models. Journal of the National Cancer Institute. 2000;**92**(2):143-147

[19] Baish JW, Jain RK. Fractals and cancer. Cancer Research. 2000;**60**(14):3683-3688

[20] Bullitt E, Zeng D, Gerig G, Aylward S, Joshi S, Smith JK, Lin W, Ewend MG. Vessel tortuosity and brain tumor malignancy: A blinded study. Academic Radiology. 2005;**12**(10):1232-1240

[21] Gautherie M. Thermobiological assessment of benign and malignant breast diseases. American Journal of Obstetrics and Gynecology. 1983;**147**(8):861-869

[22] Keyserlingk JR, Ahlgren PD, Yu E, Belliveau N, Yassa M. Functional infrared imaging of the breast. IEEE Engineering in Medicine and Biology Magazine. 2000;**19**(3):30-41

[23] Harvey L, et al. Cancer. In: Harvey L, editor. Molecular Cell Biology. 7th ed. New York: W.H. Freeman and Co.; 2013. pp. 1113-1148

[24] Kakileti S, Venkataramani K, Madhu H. Automatic determination of hormone receptor status in breast cancer using thermography. In: 19th International Conference on Medical Image Computing and Computer-Assisted Intervention—MICCAI. Vol. 9900. Springer; 2016. DOI: 10.1007/978-3-319-46720-7_74

[25] Ring EFJ, Ammer K. The technique of infrared imaging in medicine. Thermology International. 2000;**10**(1):7-14

[26] Amalu WC, Hobbins WB, Head JF, Elliot RL. Infrared imaging of the breast. In: Diakides M, Bronzino JD, Peterson DR, editors. Medical Infrared Imaging: Principles and Practices. CRC Press; Taylor & Francis Group, Boca Raton, Florida. 2012. pp. 10.1-10.22. DOI: 10.1201/b12938-11

[27] Gautherie M. Thermopathology of breast cancer: Measurement and analysis of in vivo temperature and blood flow. Annals of the New York Academy of Sciences. 1980; **335**(1):383-415

[28] Laaperi E, Laaperi AL, Strakowska M, Wiecek B, Przymusiala P. Cold provocation improves breast cancer detection with IR thermography: A pilot study. Thermology International. 2012;**22**(4):152-156

[29] Ohashi Y, Uchida I. Applying dynamic thermography in the diagnosis of breast cancer. IEEE Engineering in Medicine and Biology Magazine. 2000;**19**(3):42-51

[30] Hobbins WB. Thermography of the breast—A skin organ. In: Thermal Assessment of Breast Health. proceedings of an international conference held in Washington, DC, USA, July 20-24, 1983. pp. 40-48

[31] Berz R, Schulte-Uebbing C. MammoVision (infrared breast thermography) compared to X-ray mammography and ultrasonography. In: Diakides M, Bronzino JD, Peterson DR, editors. Medical Infrared Imaging: Principles and Practices. CRC Press; 2012. pp. 12.1-12.12. DOI: 10.1201/b12938-13

[32] Rogalski A. Infrared detectors: Status and trends. Progress in Quantum Electronics. 2003;**27**(2):59-210

[33] Corsi C. Infrared: A key technology for security systems. Advances in Optical Technologies. 2012;**2012**. DOI: 10.1155/2012/838752

[34] Carmeliet P, Jain RK. Angiogenesis in cancer and other diseases. Nature. 2000;**407** (6801):249-257

[35] Borchartt TB, Conci A, Lima RCF, Resmini R, Sanchez A. Breast thermography from an image processing viewpoint: A survey. Signal Processing. 2010;**93**(10):2785-2803

[36] Gautherie M. Improved system for the objective evaluation of breast thermograms. Progress in Clinical and Biological Research. 1982;**107**:897

[37] Parisky YR, Sardi A, Hamm R, Hughes K, Esserman L, Rust S, Callahan K. Efficacy of computerized infrared imaging analysis to evaluate mammographically suspicious lesions. American Journal of Roentgenology. 2003;**180**(1):263-269. DOI: 10.2214/ ajr.180.1.1800263

[38] Madhu H, Kakileti ST, Venkataramani K, Jabbireddy S. Extraction of medically interpretable features for classification of malignancy in breast thermography. In: 2016 IEEE 38th Annual International Conference of the Engineering in Medicine and Biology

Society (EMBC); August; Orlando, Florida. IEEE; 2016. pp. 1062-1065. DOI: 10.1109/EMBC.2016.7590886

[39] Kakileti ST, Venkataramani K. Automated blood vessel extraction in two-dimensional breast thermography. In: 2016 IEEE International Conference on Image Processing (ICIP); September; Phoenix, Arizona. IEEE; 2016. pp. 380-384. DOI: 10.1109/ICIP.2016.7532383

[40] Venkataramani K, Mestha LK, Ramachandra L, Prasad SS, Kumar V, Raja PJ. Semi-automated breast cancer tumor detection with thermographic video imaging. In: 37th Annual International Conference of the IEEE Engineering in Medicine and Biology Society (EMBC). IEEE; 2015. pp. 2022-2025

[41] Gershon-Cohen J, Haberman-Brueschke JA, Brueschke EE. Medical thermography: A summary of current status. Radiologic clinics of North America. 1965;3(3):403

[42] Stark, Agnes M, Way S. The screening of well women for the early detection of breast cancer using clinical examination with thermography and mammography. Cancer. 1974;33(6):1671-1679. DOI: 10.1002/1097-0142(197406)33:6<1671::AID-CNCR2820330630>3.0.CO;2-4

[43] Spitalier H, Giraud D, et al. Does infrared thermography truly have a role in present day breast cancer management?. In: Liss AR, editor. Biomedical Thermology. New York: 1982. pp. 269-278.

[44] Amalric R, Giraud D, Altschuler C, Amalric F, Spitalier JM, Brandone H, Ayme Y, Gardiol AA. Does infrared thermography truly have a role in present-day breast cancer management?. Progress in Clinical and Biological Research. 1981;107:269-278

[45] Haberman, JoAnn D, Love, Francis TJ, John E. Screening a rural population for breast cancer using thermography and physical examination techniques: Methods and results-A preliminary report. Annals of the New York Academy of Sciences. 1980;335(1):492-500. DOI: 10.1111/j.1749-6632.1980.tb50774.x

[46] Sciarra J. Breast cancer: Strategies for early detection. In: Thermal Assessment of Breast Health (Proceedings of the International Conference on Thermal Assessment of Breast Health); MTP Press LTD; 1983. pp. 117-129

[47] Louis K, Walter J, Gautherie M. Long-term assessment of breast cancer risk by thermal imaging. In: Liss AR, editor. Biomedical Thermology; New York: 1982. pp. 279-301

[48] Jones CH. Thermography of the female breast. Diagnosis of Breast Disease. Baltimore: University Park Press; 1983. pp. 214-234

[49] Rassiwala M, Mathur P, Mathur R, Farid K, Shukla S, Gupta PK, Jain B. Evaluation of digital infra-red thermal imaging as an adjunctive screening method for breast carcinoma: A pilot study. International Journal of Surgery. 2014;12(12):1439-1443. DOI: http://dx.doi.org/10.1016/j.ijsu.2014.10.010

Permissions

All chapters in this book were first published in BI, by InTech Open; hereby published with permission under the Creative Commons Attribution License or equivalent. Every chapter published in this book has been scrutinized by our experts. Their significance has been extensively debated. The topics covered herein carry significant findings which will fuel the growth of the discipline. They may even be implemented as practical applications or may be referred to as a beginning point for another development.

The contributors of this book come from diverse backgrounds, making this book a truly international effort. This book will bring forth new frontiers with its revolutionizing research information and detailed analysis of the nascent developments around the world.

We would like to thank all the contributing authors for lending their expertise to make the book truly unique. They have played a crucial role in the development of this book. Without their invaluable contributions this book wouldn't have been possible. They have made vital efforts to compile up to date information on the varied aspects of this subject to make this book a valuable addition to the collection of many professionals and students.

This book was conceptualized with the vision of imparting up-to-date information and advanced data in this field. To ensure the same, a matchless editorial board was set up. Every individual on the board went through rigorous rounds of assessment to prove their worth. After which they invested a large part of their time researching and compiling the most relevant data for our readers.

The editorial board has been involved in producing this book since its inception. They have spent rigorous hours researching and exploring the diverse topics which have resulted in the successful publishing of this book. They have passed on their knowledge of decades through this book. To expedite this challenging task, the publisher supported the team at every step. A small team of assistant editors was also appointed to further simplify the editing procedure and attain best results for the readers.

Apart from the editorial board, the designing team has also invested a significant amount of their time in understanding the subject and creating the most relevant covers. They scrutinized every image to scout for the most suitable representation of the subject and create an appropriate cover for the book.

The publishing team has been an ardent support to the editorial, designing and production team. Their endless efforts to recruit the best for this project, has resulted in the accomplishment of this book. They are a veteran in the field of academics and their pool of knowledge is as vast as their experience in printing. Their expertise and guidance has proved useful at every step. Their uncompromising quality standards have made this book an exceptional effort. Their encouragement from time to time has been an inspiration for everyone.

The publisher and the editorial board hope that this book will prove to be a valuable piece of knowledge for researchers, students, practitioners and scholars across the globe.

List of Contributors

Lulu Wang and Hu Peng
School of Instrument Science and Opto-electronics Engineering, Hefei University of Technology, Hefei, China

Jianhua Ma
School of Biomedical Technology, Southern Medical University, Guangzhou, China

Mohammed Ali Alnafea
Department of Radiological Sciences, College of Applied Medical Sciences, King Saud University, Riyadh, Saudi Arabia

Alexander Karpov, Andrey Kolobanov and Marina Korotkova
Clinical Hospital, Yaroslavl, Russia

Nebojsa Duric
Karmanos Cancer Institute, Wayne State University, Detroit, MI, USA

Peter Littrup
Crittenton Hospital, Troy, MI, USA

José María Celaya Padilla and Cesar Humberto Guzmán Valdivia
Autonomous University of Zacatecas/ CONACyT – Universidad Autónoma de Zacatecas (CONACyT – UAZ), Jardín Juarez, Centro, Zacatecas, Zacatecas, Mexico

Jorge Issac Galván Tejada, Carlos Eric Galván Tejada and Hamurabi Gamboa Rosales
Electric Engineering Department, Autonomous University of Zacatecas (UAZ), Jardín Juarez, Centro, Zacatecas, Zacatecas, Mexico

Juan Rubén Delgado Contreras
Superior Technical Institute of Zacatecas South (ITSZaS), Las lomitas, Tlaltenango, Zacatecas, Mexico

Antonio Martinez-Torteya
Engineering Department, Monterrey University (UdeM), Morones Prieto Pte, Jesús M. Garza, San Pedro Garza García, Nuevo Leon, Mexico

Jorge Roberto Manjarrez Sánchez
Computer Engineering Systems Department, Superior Technical Institute of Jerez (ITSJ) Libramiento Fresnillo-Tepetongo, Fracc. Los Cardos, Jerez de García Salinas, Zacatecas, Mexico

Idalia Garza-Veloz and Margarita L. Martinez-Fierro
Health Sciences Department ,Human Medical School, Autonomous University of Zacatecas (UAZ), Jardín Juarez, Centro, Zacatecas, Zacatecas, Mexico

Victor Treviño and Jose Gerardo Tamez-Peña
Bioinformatic group, Medical School, Monterrey Institute of Technology (ITESM), Eugenio Garza Sada, Monterrey, Nuevo Leon, Mexico

Michael Friedrich and Stefan Kraemer
Department of Obstetrics and Gynecology, HELIOS Medical Center, Krefeld, Germany

Stefan Kraemer
Breast Unit, HELIOS Hospital, Lutherplatz, Krefeld, Germany

Shinya Tajima, Ichiro Maeda, Akira Endo, Motohiro Chosokabe and Masayuki Takagi
Department of Pathology and Radiology, St. Marianna University School of Medicine, Kawasaki City, Kanagawa, Japan

Shinya Tajima, Keiko Kishimoto, Yoshihide Kanemaki and Takafumi Ono
Department of Radiology, St. Marianna University School of Medicine, Kawasaki City, Kanagawa, Japan

Koichiro Tsugawa
Department of Breast and Endocrine Surgery,
St. Marianna University School of Medicine,
Kawasaki City, Kanagawa, Japan

Azlena Ali Beegan and Gozie Offiah
Royal College of Surgeons in Ireland,
Education and Research Centre, Beaumont
Hospital, Dublin, Ireland

**Ryusuke Murakami, Hitomi Tani and
Shinichiro Kumita**
Department of Radiology, Nippon Medical
School, Tokyo, Japan

Nachiko Uchiyama
Department of Radiology, National Cancer
Center, Tokyo, Japan

Jocelyn A. Rapelyea
Breast Imaging & Intervention, George
Washington University Medical Faculty
Associates, Washington, DC, USA

Department of Radiology, George Washington
University School of Medicine & Health
Sciences, Washington, DC, USA

Christina G. Marks
University of Mississippi Medical Center,
Jackson, MS, USA

Mohammed Ali Alnafea
Department of Radiological Sciences, College
of Applied Medical Sciences, King Saud
University, Riyadh, Saudi Arabia

**Siva Teja Kakileti, Geetha Manjunath
and Himanshu Madhu**
NIRAMAI Health Analytix Pvt Ltd, Bangalore,
India

Hadonahalli Venkataramanappa Ramprakash
Central Diagnostics Research Foundation,
Bangalore, India

Index